Dedication

To my husband Jerry, for his continual support in all of my professional pursuits, and whose devotion and enduring patience has meant the world to me.

To my grandchildren, who have enriched my life and have been the inspiration for this text: Alex, Tate, Eleanor, Theodore, Samuel, Sophia, and Sydney.

Pediatric Physical

Examination

Health

Assessment

N, CPNP
te Professor
Professions
egis College
Weston, Massachusetts

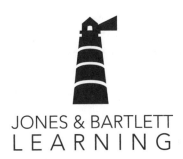

JONES & BARTLETT
LEARNING

World Headquarters
Jones & Bartlett Learning
40 Tall Pine Drive
Sudbury, MA 01776
978-443-5000
info@jblearning.com
www.jblearning.com

Jones & Bartlett Learning
Canada
6339 Ormindale Way
Mississauga, Ontario L5V 1J2
Canada

Jones & Bartlett Learning
International
Barb House, Barb Mews
London W6 7PA
United Kingdom

Jones & Bartlett Learning books and products are available through most bookstores and online booksellers. To contact Jones & Bartlett Learning directly, call 800-832-0034, fax 978-443-8000, or visit our website, www.jblearning.com.

Substantial discounts on bulk quantities of Jones & Bartlett Learning publications are available to corporations, professional associations, and other qualified organizations. For details and specific discount information, contact the special sales department at Jones & Bartlett Learning via the above contact information or send an email to specialsales@jblearning.com.

The author, editor, and publisher have made every effort to provide accurate information. However, they are not responsible for errors, omissions, or for any outcomes related to the use of the contents of this book and take no responsibility for the use of the products and procedures described. Treatments and side effects described in this book may not be applicable to all people; likewise, some people may require a dose or experience a side effect that is not described herein. Drugs and medical devices are discussed that may have limited availability controlled by the Food and Drug Administration (FDA) for use only in a research study or clinical trial. Research, clinical practice, and government regulations often change the accepted standard in this field. When consideration is being given to use of any drug in the clinical setting, the health care provider or reader is responsible for determining FDA status of the drug, reading the package insert, and reviewing prescribing information for the most up-to-date recommendations on dose, precautions, and contraindications, and determining the appropriate usage for the product. This is especially important in the case of drugs that are new or seldom used.

Production Credits
Publisher: Kevin Sullivan
Acquisitions Editor: Amy Sibley
Editorial Assistant: Rachel Shuster
Production Editor: Amanda Clerkin
Rights and Permissions Supervisor: Christine Myaskovsky
Associate Marketing Manager: Katie Hennessy
V.P., Manufacturing and Inventory Control: Therese Connell
Composition: Arlene Apone and Paw Print Media
Cover Design: Kate Ternullo
Cover Image: © experimental/ShutterStock, Inc.
Printing and Binding: Malloy, Inc.
Cover Printing: Malloy, Inc.

Library of Congress Cataloging-in-Publication Data
Sawyer, Susan, 1945-
 Pediatric physical examination and health assessment / Susan Sawyer.
   p. ; cm.
 Includes bibliographical references and index.
 ISBN 978-0-7637-7438-7 (pbk.)
 1. Children—Medical examinations. 2. Children—Diseases—Diagnosis. I. Title.
 [DNLM: 1. Physical Examination—methods. 2. Child. 3. Infant. WS 141 S271p 2011]
 RJ50.S29 2011
 618.92'0075—dc22
                                2010025283
6048

Printed in the United States of America
15 14 13 12 11   10 9 8 7 6 5 4 3 2 1

Contents

Dianna M. Jones

Rosemarie A. Fuller

Acknowledgments

Many thanks to all of my students for their thoughtful questions, valuable feedback, and for providing me with continual intellectual growth and development.

I am particularly grateful for the thorough and enriching contributions of those professionals that reviewed each chapter. Your guidance and recommendations have been appreciated and greatly enhanced the professional overview of this text.

In addition many thanks to all of the children and adolescents who have enriched my pediatric career, broadened my perspective, and enlightened my view in understanding their needs, both physical and emotional.

Contributors

David B. Brown, MD
Senior Attending
Department of Orthopedic Surgery
Bridgeport Hospital
Bridgeport, Connecticut

Elise Buckley, MSN, CPNP-AC/PC
Orthopedics
Children's Hospital
Boston, Massachusetts

Rosemarie A. Fuller, RNC, MSN, NNP-BC, PNP-BC
Clinical Educator
Neonatal Intensive Care Unit
Caritas St. Elizabeth's Medical Center
Boston, Massachusetts

Gregory L. Holmes, MD
Chief, Section of Neurology
Dartmouth Medical School
Lebanon, New Hampshire

Dianna M. Jones, MSN, CFNP-BC
Director of Health Services
Nursing Faculty
Regis College
Weston, Massachusetts

Patricia R. Lawrence, RN, MS, CPNP-AC/PC
Cardiology
Children's Hospital,
Boston, Massachusetts

Daniel McCarthy, BS, CPT
Exercise Physiologist
Natick, Massachusetts

Deborah Summers, CPNP
Pediatric Health Care
Brockton, Massachusetts

Preface

This textbook was born out of the need for a guide designed to describe how to conduct a physical examination on a pediatric patient with emphasis on assessment techniques. This text, devoted solely to the assessment and examination of the pediatric patient, hopes to fill the void left by texts that focus on adult physical examination.

The text describes the many techniques used in examining the infant and child, and explains how physical findings are altered in the pediatric patient. The text is designed as a beginning guide for those learning to perform physical examination on patients from birth through adolescence. The reader will find an in-depth review of anatomy, physical assessment, and examination techniques, including differentiation of normal and abnormal findings. The text assumes that the examiner has had basic courses in human anatomy, physiology, and general health assessment of the adult.

Taking a course in physical assessment and learning how to obtain a comprehensive history and physical exam for a child can be a daunting experience, whether you are interacting with a toddler or an adolescent. It is important to remember that the physical exam continues to be the backbone of education for healthcare providers. With the technical advances in health care, the art of clinical observation and physical diagnosis is often replaced by the reliance on radiographic and laboratory data. Although a variety of tests can be ordered, good clinical judgment and thoughtful attention to the art of physical diagnosis are still based on the findings of a thorough history and comprehensive physical examination. Developing the ability to auscultate lung sounds in a crying child, palpate an abdomen, or inspect the ears takes patience, fortitude, and much practice. Attainment of these assessment skills is crucial in examining a child, as is having a grasp of developmental milestones. Developing rapport and putting the child at ease through your comfort and expertise in physical assessment are critical to building the provider–patient relationship and ultimately earning the patient's trust and confidence.

Approaching a child with comfort and ease is essential to developing a relationship that affords you the opportunity to perform a skilled examination. Patient compliance, whether the patient is a toddler or an adolescent, is a critical component of the patient–provider relationship.

In focusing on the examination of the pediatric patient, this text addresses the differences in anatomic and physiologic growth and how these varying parameters affect different body systems. It is the process of growth and development and the anatomic and physiologic changes that make the pediatric patient so unique.

With this being said, the key concept underlying each chapter is to seize the opportunity. These are key words when performing a physical examination on a child, particularly an infant and/or toddler. *Seize the opportunity* means assessing that part of the body that is readily available without being intrusive or causing fear and discomfort to the child. Although this textbook is written with cephalocaudal progression, the examination need not proceed in that order. Remember, the child who is calm, comfortable, and trusting will allow you the opportunity to perform a comprehensive examination.

Case Studies

At the end of each chapter, a case history is presented that incorporates diagnostic reasoning and critical thinking, and is supported by evidence-based care. Using established clinical practice guidelines in conjunction with what is best for the child based on cultural views, the child's developmental needs, and the family's choices are all part of critical thinking in formulating your diagnostic reasoning.

Family Dynamics

Introduction

This chapter considers issues that arise from the relationships and interactions of the developing family. The intention is to provide an overview of the given topics, rather than an in-depth discussion.

SUBJECTS TO BE ADDRESSED:

- The vulnerable child and child abuse
- Discipline
- Developmental screening
- Mealtime/eating behavior

Family dynamics are based on family system theory, which examines the relational components that guide family interactions. For the purposes of this text, family dynamics refers to family health and the subsystems within this setting such as parent–child relationships. How a family interacts to ensure adequate growth and development for the child is a key component to understanding family dynamics. Important concerns of the family are first and foremost to provide the child with the necessities of food and shelter, followed by family health promotion of wellness and disease prevention.

In today's world, the interrelatedness and dynamics of the family can vary widely, from the traditional family to the single-parent family to the gay and lesbian family to the foster and adoptive family. As a health professional caring for diverse family units, we must be tolerant, understanding, and sensitive to this broad range of lifestyles and diversity of family relationships.

To understand the characteristics of these modern family units, the basic concept of social attachment comes into play, specifically during the newborn period. This concept was first described by Bowlby, who stated that "the earliest bonds formed by the child and their caregivers have a tremendous impact that continues throughout one's life . . . resulting in lasting psychological connectedness between human beings" (1969, p. 194). These early bonds strengthen continuity and stability by promoting connectedness in family relationships. Fostering meaningful relationships based on Bowlby's view further emphasizes that experiences in childhood influence one's development and behavior in life.

Initial attachment styles are established in early childhood, and the promotion of positive, secure relationships contribute to cognitive development and socialization. A key consideration in view of this is that parents want to do what is best for their children. Families make decisions based on life experience, their emotional well-being, their intelligence, and their communal and personal support systems. Whether they make good or bad decisions for their child, parents generally use the resources and information at hand to promote what they feel is the best outcome for their family.

Much research has demonstrated that the central theme of attachment theory is that when mothers are responsive to their infant's needs, a sense of security is established. The infant knows that the mother is dependable, which ultimately creates a secure base for the child to then explore the world. The question arises regarding what happens to the child in families where there is failure to form secure attachments early in life. Research has suggested that failure to form these early attachments can have a negative impact on behavior in later childhood and throughout life. According to Murray Bowen (1978), children diagnosed with oppositional-defiant disorder (ODD), conduct disorder (CD), or post-traumatic stress disorder (PTSD) often have attachment problems.

Encouraging good communication, appropriate coping mechanisms, problem solving, constructive limit setting, and motivation to achieve all contribute to the development of positive self-esteem and a sense of security. This interplay of family connectedness is evident as the child develops and seeks approval and support from not just family members, but society at large.

The many variations in family dynamics are based on cultural issues, genetic background, geographic determinants, and economic conditions. The child's level of adaptation to stressors of family dynamics, which include adherence to rules and expectations, management of anger and aggression, non-violent resolution of conflict, development of healthy sexuality, and respect for others, is due to the differences in the child's temperament as well as his or her emotional, biologic, and cognitive development. Poor parent–child relationships are frequently characterized by parents who may be rigid, controlling, secretive, and/or isolated. An important characteristic of the parent–child relationship that affects attachment is the concept of "fit." The goodness or "synchrony of fit" between a parent and child describes the degree to which the child's real temperament matches the parent's expectations of that child. There are four types of childhood temperament:

- *EASY*: These children are approachable, have positive moods, and are easy to console.
- *SLOW TO WARM UP*: These children may be shy, may be less active and adaptable, and have negative moods.
- *DIFFICULT*: These children may avoid interactions, may be less adaptable, and have negative moods.
- *INTERMEDIATE*: These children present with a combination of the "slow to warm up" and "difficult" temperament styles.

The Vulnerable Child: Abuse

Vulnerability or vulnerable child syndrome refers to the parent–child relationship and the parent's perception of the child's illness. This term was first defined by Green and Solnit (1964), who stated that "the psychological sequalae was the parent's reaction to the life-threatening episode and their altered perception of the child. The parental reaction was seen to represent pathologic after-effects of a persistent disguised mourning reaction." Since then, research has demonstrated that the risk factors for the vulnerablility of the child are based on the parent's perception, rather than the child's.

With that in mind, children's vulnerability is based on physical characteristics that make them prone to specific types of injury and that affect the severity of the injuries they experience. The following are examples of anatomic characteristics specific to the young child:

SKIN: The skin of the very young child is characterized by decreased elastin and collagen fibers, increased fluid content, increased permeability and fragility, and a higher pH level. These characteristics increase the risks of and damage from mechanical, chemical, and burn injuries.

GENITAL TISSUE: The genital tissue of children is highly distensible and heals rapidly so that physical assessment often does not reveal evidence of abuse. In addition, the *cervix* of young and adolescent girls contains a large amount of columnar epithelium, which is highly prone to infection from sexually transmitted diseases (STDs).

BONES: The bones of young children differ from those of adults in that they are not calcified until 20 years of age (Ball & Bindler, 2008). This means that children's bones are more flexible and can absorb more impact than can adult bones. It also means that the types of injuries seen in accidental injury will differ compared to those of intentional injury; adults are more likely to sustain compression fractures, whereas children experience buckle and torsion fractures. These types of fractures occur typically at the ends of the long bones as a result of twisting or impact on the bones. Children with chronic illnesses who may be confined to bed or a wheelchair exhibit demineralization of bones and are at risk for bone injury. These children may fracture bones quite easily even with routine care.

BRAIN AND SKULL: The brain and skull of the child are highly vulnerable to injury, particularly from shaking. Shaken baby syndrome (SBS) is a common type of abuse seen in children between the ages of 4 and 9 months. Characteristics of the child's brain that impact the severity of injury experienced during shaken baby syndrome include:

1. Unmyelinized, softer brain tissue
2. Higher water content
3. Smoother fossae
4. Shallow subarachnoid space
5. Larger mass and surface area compared with the body
6. Weaker neck muscles
7. Fragile cerebrovasculature and delicate bridging vessels
8. Pliable skull
9. Open cranial sutures (until the age of about 18 months)

There are protective mechanisms, however, that minimize harmful damage due to accidental falls and injuries. These mechanisms include elasticity of the skull, which increases the skull's tolerance of compression but distributes forceful injury over a wider area of the brain. A shorter standing height and the presence of the parachute and righting reflexes also provide some protection during accidental falls (Giardino & Giardino, 2002).

Developmental Considerations

The achievement of developmental milestones may be helpful to consider when differentiating accidental versus intentional injury.

Infants

Infants work to develop physiologic stability and trust in the caregiver. Some developmental milestones to watch for in infancy include:

- Visually following an object to midline: 2 months
- Lifting head when lying prone: 2 months
- Rolling from stomach to back: 4 months
- Babbling, reaching for objects, and grasping objects placed within reach: 6 months
- Pulling self to stand and creeping: 9 months
- Cruising (walking while supporting self): 12 months

An injury sustained when an infant rolls off of a surface such as a bed or couch is common to around 4–6 months of age but not typical before that time. Burn injuries of the hand may be seen at about 6 months when the infant develops reaching skills. Injuries from cruising or walking, milestones normally seen between 9 and 12 months, generally do not occur in children younger than that age.

Toddlers

Toddlers are intent on developing independence, but they still seek proximity with their parents. Temper tantrums are frequently seen at this age, and safety issues are a concern due to rapidly developing motor abilities. Walking and language development are also important developmental tasks at this age. Other important developmental milestones in this age group include:

- Developing a vocabulary of 2–3 words: 15 months
- Scribbling: 18 months
- Climbing stairs one at a time, obeying two-step commands, and standing from a squatting position: 2 years
- Kicking a ball: 3 years

Burns affecting children who have pulled a container of hot liquid onto themselves or who have turned on the hot water faucet in the bathtub are not generally seen after 2 years of age. Toddlers and preschool children may also present with injuries acquired as a result of their greater mobility and physical activity. A toddler's fracture is a common accidental spiral fracture of the distal end of the tibia, which results from falling off a slide or step.

Preschool-Age Children

Preschool-age children are refining their fine motor skills and beginning to develop the ability to socialize with peers. Due to immature cognitive and ethical skills, lying is a normal finding in this age group, as is magical thinking. Children in this age group are often able to provide some history around abuse events. Some important developmental milestones include:

- Becoming aware of gender of self and others
- Dressing self, brushing teeth, and performing other self-care activities: 4–5 years
- Climbing stairs using alternating feet: 4–5 years
- Riding tricycle

School-Age Children

School-age children are at a point of intellectual and social growth. Biking and skating injuries are common in school-age children, and injuries due to sports are seen in older children. In contrast to intentional injury, accidental injuries are less severe and are commonly found on the shins, forearms, knees, elbows, and forehead. Intentional injuries occur in places where the child would not normally be injured, such as the back of the hands and legs, and the buttocks.

Adolescents

Adolescents are in a second stage of independence, and peer pressure is a great influence on them. Concerned about body image, they should be assured of privacy during the history and examination. These children are often hesitant to report abuse but are usually able to provide clear history around the events (Bickley, Szilagyi, & Stackhaus, 2002; Giardino & Giardino, 2002).

Physical Abuse

Behavioral Findings

Often the earliest indicators of abuse in a child are behavioral changes. In the younger child, these changes may include sleep disturbances, toilet training difficulties, temper tantrums, or aggressive behaviors. In the older child, behaviors such as anorexia or bulimia, oppositional-defiant or conduct disorders, phobias, school problems, promiscuity, truancy or running away, and depression or suicidal ideation may indicate long-term abuse.

Adolescents who have experienced abuse often present with behavioral changes, most commonly depression or suicidal ideation. Depression is a pervasive condition, characterized by changes in mood, appetite, sleep, and behavior. Pediatric patients manifest depression differently than do adults; in adults it is marked by depressed mood or decreased pleasure in activities, whereas in pediatric patients it is marked by feelings of powerlessness and pessimism. Irritability and agitation may also be noted in children (Hamarman & Bennett, 2000; Horner, 2001a; Stevens-Simon & Barrett, 2001).

Physical Examination

Once the child's condition has been stabilized, if necessary, and a history has been obtained, a physical assessment should be performed, which includes comprehensive and systematic review of the child, looking for obvious and subtle injury patterns. Injuries common to physical abuse include soft tissue injuries, bruises, burns, bite marks, fractures, impact injuries to the mouth or abdomen, and brain injuries. Many injuries may be due to intended discipline, such as that administered around the time of toilet training, a peak time for abuse to occur.

Hallmark Findings in Intentional Abuse

BRUISES: Bruises form distinctive patterns from identifiable objects such as cords, switches, and finger marks from open-handed slaps. Common sites where these types of injuries may be found include the face (particularly bruises that occur on both sides of the face), chest, thighs, abdomen, and buttocks. Circumferential injuries to the wrists or ankles may be due to restraints. Intra-oral injuries in infants result from excessive force used in feeding or inserting a pacifier in the mouth of a crying infant. Although accidental bruises are typically found on the forehead, forearms, knees, and shins, extensive bruising in these areas should be evaluated carefully. Multiple bruises of different ages, or occurring on multiple body parts, or bruises that are inconsistent with the stated history should also be investigated.

Although the progression of bruise healing is not as exact as was once thought, in general a bruise that contains yellow coloration is about 18–20 hours old. The colors blue, black, and red may appear at any time during healing and do not predict the age of the bruise. Factors that may make it difficult to identify the age of a bruise include the age of the child, the force and depth of the impact, the degree of vascular involvement, the amount of bleeding, the body part involved, and the child's healing abilities. Bruising that occurs on different body parts of the same child may also heal at different rates so that the timing of these types of bruises may be difficult to identify (Giardino & Giardino, 2002).

BURNS: Burns classified as greater than second degree that present in a glove, stocking, or doughnut pattern are typical of intentional immersion in scalding water, as are burns found on the backs of the hands. Palm and finger burns are usually sustained accidentally, resulting from a child grabbing a hot object. Burns sustained by young children who pull a container of hot liquid onto themselves will develop in a pattern consistent with splashing liquid. Children rarely allow themselves to come into contact with scalding water or other hot objects for longer than a few seconds, so will not usually sustain a serious burn (Giardino & Giardino, 2002).

BITE MARKS: Bite marks that occur on the back, buttocks, or genitalia and that may be accompanied by sucking marks are indicative of physical or sexual abuse. Bites received from another child leave a smaller impression compared with those received from adults, and animal bites are usually found on the face or lower extremities. Animal bites also produce lacerations or deeper punctures, which are not seen in human bites (Giardino & Giardino, 2002).

ORAL INJURIES: Head, face, and neck injuries occur in over 50% of abuse cases. Oral injuries most commonly associated with abuse include abrasion, lacerations, and burn marks due to eating utensils and scalding liquids. Damage to teeth, the jaw, the frenulum, the palate, and the tongue are also noted. The mouth may be a focus of abuse due to the significance of speech and nutrition (American Academy of Pediatrics, 2005).

HAIR LOSS: Hair loss accompanied by breakage of the shaft of the hair and erythema or swelling of the underlying scalp indicates forceful pulling.

FRACTURES: After soft tissue injury, fractures are the second most common type of injury associated with abuse. Fractures indicative of abuse include those that occur in a "bucket handle" or chip pattern at the ends of long bones; spiral fractures of long bones in nonambulatory children; rib fractures, particularly posterior rib fractures in infants; and fractures of the spinous processes and the sternum. Also indicative are multiple fractures and fractures at different stages of healing. Shaking of a young child or infant will result in pulling of the ligaments and tendons on the ends of the long bones, resulting in chipping of the ends of these bones. In bucket handle fractures, the metaphysis (the upper end of the long bones) separates from the diaphysis (the shaft of the long bones), lifting up and creating a rounded gap, which may be seen on x-ray and gives the fracture its name. Spiral fractures of long bones occur during violent twisting of the extremity. The age of a fracture can be identified by the formation of calcium deposits at the site of the injury. These deposits are usually formed at about 7–10 days after the fracture occurs and can assist in identifying the age of the fracture. Skull fractures are common in both accidental and intentional injury, so a careful history is recommended (Giardino & Giardino, 2002; Jenny, 2006).

SPINAL CORD INJURIES: In suspected spinal cord injuries of children whose bones have not yet calcified, there may be no evidence of fracture or cord injury. This condition is given the mnemonic SCIWORA—spinal cord injury without radiological abnormality. These children should be treated as though they have a spinal cord injury until this diagnosis can be ruled out (Snider, 1997).

INTRA-ABDOMINAL INJURIES: Bruises or tears of the liver or spleen as a result of blunt trauma are indicative of intentional injury, such as punching, when the history is not consistent with an accidental injury (Reece & Ludwig, 2001).

EYE INJURIES: Periorbital bruising, orbital fractures, and visual loss may result from intentional abuse (Giardino & Giardino, 2002).

Shaken Baby Syndrome

Shaken baby syndrome (SBS) is a specific type of abuse that is seen in children younger than 2 years and commonly in children younger than 6 months. One-third of these children sustain few or no sequelae, one-third sustain permanent or significant injury, and one-third of these children die as a result of their injuries. Risk factors include parents—most often the father or male caregiver—who are young, uneducated, or have minimal parenting skills. The child may have a difficult temperament, be colicky, or not meet the parents' expectations.

The precipitating factor is often a crying child who is difficult to console. Unable to quiet the child and growing increasingly frustrated, the caregiver shakes the child, usually without intent to do harm. Interviews with perpetrators reveal that they believed shaking was less harmful to the child than spanking or hitting. In SBS the child is typically grasped by the upper arms or around the chest and shaken back and forth. The rotational acceleration–deceleration forces result in cerebral edema, shearing of the gray and white matter of the brain, and diffuse brain injury. The optic nerve is frequently affected, which results in the retinal hemorrhages characteristic of this condition. Other physical findings include posterior rib fractures, multiple skull fractures if impact occurred after the shaking episode, subdural or subarachnoid hemorrhages, visual disturbances, breathing difficulty, seizures, or behavioral changes. The child often presents with vomiting, dehydration, and altered level of consciousness. There may also be multiple bruises and fractures in various stages of healing along with other injuries.

Tin ear syndrome may also be seen with SBS when the shaking is followed by impact on one side, resulting in erythema and swelling of the ear, subdural hematoma, and cerebral swelling on the affected side as well as retinal damage. (Alexander & Smith, 1998; American Academy of Pediatrics, 2001b).

Neglect

The incidence of neglect is difficult to assess because it is frequently not reported. Parents who neglect their children frequently exhibit poor parenting and problem-solving skills, have poor support systems, or may be socially isolated. In addition, parents with developmental or psychosocial disabilities may be unable to care for themselves or their children, as are parents who abuse drugs or alcohol. Poverty, however, is more closely correlated with neglect than with any other type of abuse. Although many children living in poverty are not abused or neglected, poverty and lack of education are considered risk factors. Children who are quiet, are non-interactional, have chronic medical conditions, or have a poor temperament fit with their parents are likely to be neglected as well. The underlying psychosocial factor in neglect is attachment failure. Unlike bonding, which is unilateral from mother to newborn, attachment describes a reciprocal bond between mother and child. In neglect, the mother (or caregiver) does not bond with the child, so the child does not develop a reciprocal attachment to the mother. This lack of attachment is manifested by avoidant behaviors in the child as well as the mother. The clinician observing the mother may notice poor cue reading, poor eye contact, failure to engage with the child, and avoidance of physical contact or expression of disgust or displeasure with the child. It may require several visits before the diagnosis is identified.

Intervention in neglect is based on three criteria:

- The child's unmet needs of food, shelter, medical care, education, protection, and nurturing
- The repetitiveness or chronicity of the neglect
- The degree of potential or actual harm

In many families both parents work and, due to job and child-care pressures, may be unintentionally neglectful, resulting in harm to the child. Examples have been seen in the news of harried parents who leave their babies unattended in a car seat in their car or van for hours, forgetting that their child is in the vehicle. Although this type of neglect does not meet the criterion of chronicity, the degree of harm is significant enough to warrant intervention. In more severe cases of neglect, legal action is required (Cheung, 1999).

Hallmark Findings in Neglect

There are three types of neglect: *failure to thrive, medical neglect, and educational neglect.*

FAILURE TO THRIVE: Failure to thrive is defined as abnormal growth, identified by decrease in growth velocity that crosses two or more percentiles downward on standard growth charts. Failure to thrive may have inorganic causes (25% of cases), organic causes (50% of cases), or mixed causes (25% of cases). Organic causes such as metabolic illness (see also "Conditions That May Be Mistaken for Abuse" later in this chapter) include metabolic, genetic, or acquired conditions in which the child will demonstrate *symmetrical* growth lag—that is length, weight, and head circumference lags that are similar. Children who suffer from neglect, however, demonstrate first a drop in weight, then a decrease in length and head circumference. This *asymmetric* growth lag is a result of brain sparing and is the body's way of attempting to nourish the brain at the expense of body weight gain. Physical findings in failure to thrive may also include poor interactional skills such as poor eye contact or self-stimulatory behaviors, poor hygiene, diaper rash or other untreated skin conditions, wasted extremities, protruding ribs, or flat occiput due to supine positioning. Because the brain and immune system are affected by malnutrition, cognitive development and immune system impairments may also be noted. In the assessment of malnutrition, it is often helpful to observe a feeding and obtain a feeding diary to calculate the child's caloric intake.

MEDICAL NEGLECT: Medical neglect involves failure to obtain medical care when it is needed or noncompliance with prescribed care. Failure to maintain needed immunizations or comply with chronic care procedures is included in this category, as is failure to obtain needed dental care. However, care should be taken to identify and appropriately manage those families who may be noncompliant for religious reasons or those families who may not have the resources to be compliant. Religious objections to health care or specific aspects of care may be overridden when the refused treatment is superior to the alternative therapy, if any, when side effects of the recommended medical therapy are minimal, and when the failure to treat is expected to result in serious harm or death to the child. In these cases, custody of the child may be temporarily granted to a representative of the medical facility while vital care is provided to the child.

Healthcare providers must also guard against noncompliance due to lack of judgment or resources of the family. A careful assessment of parental resources as well as education regarding the need for and provision of therapies may go a long way in assuring compliance with medical therapies. In 1997 there were approximately 11 million children in the United States who were uninsured. These children were found to be the most vulnerable and at risk for preventable health problems including abuse and neglect. The Balanced Budget Act of 1997 initiated a plan, the Children's Health Insurance Program (CHIP), to facilitate enrollment of uninsured children into both Medicaid and state–federal (matching fund) programs. Criteria for inclusion into the CHIP program include noneligibility for Medicaid, children 19 years of age or younger, and family income below the federal poverty level (FPL). Healthcare providers should be proactive in identifying and enlisting families who are eligible for this type of support.

EDUCATIONAL NEGLECT: Educational neglect is diagnosed when the parent fails to provide required education or allows the child to be truant.

Consequences of Neglect

The consequences of neglect are profound. Inadequate nutrition leads to poor growth, impaired cognitive ability, impaired immunity, impaired socialization skills, and impaired cognitive development. Educational neglect results in impaired self-esteem, poor skill acquisition, and difficulty obtaining or maintaining job skills and income, thus continuing the cycle of poverty and neglect (Giardino & Giardino, 2002; Reece & Ludwig, 2001).

Emotional Abuse

Emotional abuse is the most common but most difficult type of abuse to identify and includes a wide range of behaviors. It is important to recognize that many parents may inflict emotional abuse unintentionally in isolated instances; however, sustained and repeated episodes of this type require intervention. Research indicates that intent and resulting harm are key factors to identify in emotional abuse. If there is no intent to cause harm and minimal or no harm is produced, then counseling may provide sufficient treatment; if there is intent to cause harm and severe harm is produced, then the abuse must be reported through the proper channels. Emotional abuse includes the following (Hamarman & Bennett, 2000; Nelms, 2001):

- *REJECTING AND IGNORING*: Failure to show affection or provide appropriate stimulation and attention to the child
- *ISOLATING*: Denying the child human contact, including not involving the child in peer or family activities and celebrations
- *TERRORIZING*: Threatening the child verbally or with the use of weapons such as guns or knives
- *CORRUPTING*: Promoting antisocial behaviors, such as sexually explicit or criminal behaviors, child pornography, and prostitution
- *VERBALLY ASSAULTING*: Exposing the child to demeaning, sarcastic, or humiliating comments that diminish the child's self-esteem and sense of worth

Hallmark Findings in Emotional Abuse

Hallmark findings in emotional abuse are similar to those found in other types of abuse and include sudden change in school achievement and eating, sleeping, and behavioral changes. In general, the younger the child when the emotional abuse begins, the more severe the symptoms. Social isolation and interactional difficulties (or, conversely, emotional dependence), eating disorders, and self-respect problems are common. In severe emotional abuse, the child may develop failure to thrive, antisocial or violent behaviors, psychiatric disorders such as borderline personality, and self-destructive behaviors (Stevens-Simon & Barrett, 2001; Wilson & Knight, 2002).

Sexual Abuse

Sexual abuse is frequently perpetrated by an individual known to the child and can include rubbing or fondling, exposure or visualization of genitalia, or incomplete penetration. Young children may experience multiple abuses, whereas adolescent victims tend to present after a single event. Shame or fear often prevents children from reporting this type of abuse. Because penetration may not be complete and the genital tissues of young children heal so rapidly, there may be no or minimal physical evidence of sexual abuse, particularly if an examination is delayed beyond 24 hours after the assault. Often these children are identified through reported behavioral changes or disclosure by the child or a caregiver. Behavioral changes include unexplained anxiety, depression, worsening school performance, and physical complaints, particularly involving the genital area. In older children, suicidal ideation, drug and alcohol abuse, and risky sexual behaviors may be seen.

The increase of child pornography sites on the Internet has had an impact on sexual abuse. The availability of explicit images and the ease with which they may be accessed desensitize offenders as well as children to the violence of these images. Children may be lured into "chat rooms" by sexual offenders, where it then becomes easier to attempt a real-life contact. Many images are accessed involuntarily and are upsetting to youngsters. Strategies to decrease the availability of pornographic images to children may be managed through filtering and blocking programs and parental controls, although such measures do not prevent children from accessing these sites from a computer outside the home (Horner, 2001a; Horner, 2001b; Hymel & Jenny, 1996).

Hallmark Findings in Sexual Abuse

Three hallmark physical findings in sexual abuse include vaginal or anal distention along with decreased sphincter tone, fissures or scarring, and the presence of sexually transmitted diseases (STDs) in a child older than 1 year. Prior to that age, the possibility of perinatally acquired STDs should be considered. The perinatal transmission of human papillomavirus (HPV) may result in the typical warty, flesh-colored genital lesions up to 2 years of age; gonorrhea may present as neonatal conjunctivitis in the first week of life with copious purulent drainage; and chlamydia presents with mild conjunctivitis and pneumonia up to 3 years of age. Severe perinatally acquired illness usually presents as systemic disease, chorioretinitis, pneumonia, and skin lesions. The finding of lesions or discharge in the genital region or lesions consistent with STDs found in the mouth or hands in a child older than 1 year is diagnostic of sexual abuse. Typical findings in STDs include painful, grouped oral or genital vesicles herpevirus.

Conditions That May be Mistaken for Abuse

In identifying abuse, other diagnoses should be excluded. The following is a partial list of differential diagnoses for which abuse may be mistaken.

Bruising

BLEEDING PROBLEMS: Examples include hemophilia, von Willebrand disease, or vitamin K deficiency. These illnesses may involve joint pain, warmth, and swelling, and are identified by history and appropriate lab studies. Idiopathic thrombocytopenia and leukemia also result in bruising.

BIRTH MARKS: Examples include Mongolian spots or nevi. These marks are usually localized and do not blanch with applied pressure. Bruises typically blanch when pressure is applied over the area, and there is usually underlying tenderness.

CULTURAL BEHAVIORS: Examples include cupping or coining. These behaviors are practiced in many cultures and are believed to relieve signs and symptoms of illness. Coining involves the rubbing of a coin over the affected area. The resulting abrasion is linear and may be mistaken for intentional bruising unless the examiner specifically asks the family about cultural treatments in a nonjudgmental manner. Cupping involves heating of a small cup that is then placed over the affected area. The resulting imprint may resemble an intentional burn. These types of findings occur frequently on the upper back or chest in pulmonary disease.

DRUG REACTIONS: Examples include Stevens-Johnson syndrome or Henoch-Schönlein purpura, which may be identified by history of illness treated with antibiotics. Other symptoms of illness may be seen, such as fever, lethargy, upper respiratory symptoms, nausea, and vomiting.

ORAL LESIONS: Examples include stomatitis, which may resemble inflicted injury or STDs (Giardino & Giardino, 2002).

Fractures

TODDLER'S FRACTURE: This is a spiral fracture at the distal end of the tibia due to a fall. The history and lack of other findings help identify this condition.

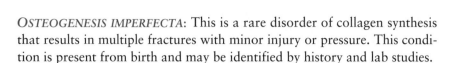

OSTEOGENESIS IMPERFECTA: This is a rare disorder of collagen synthesis that results in multiple fractures with minor injury or pressure. This condition is present from birth and may be identified by history and lab studies.

CHRONIC ILLNESS: Some chronic illnesses may result in immobility, demineralization of bone, and fractures.

BIRTH TRAUMA: Fractures of the clavicles, humerus, femur, and skull may occur during a difficult birth, particularly in larger babies (Jenny, 2006; Snider, 1997).

Burns

IMPETIGO OR NUMMULAR ECZEMA: Lesions seen in these conditions are circular and may be accompanied by weeping or crusting. These conditions may be identified by history.

PHOTODERMATITIS: A type of dermatitis that occurs in people when exposed to light; they require certain medications. This diagnosis is excluded by history.

CONTACT OR IRRITANT DERMATITIS: This condition may appear as a burn (Giardino & Giardino, 2002).

Bite Marks

Bite marks less than 3 cm in diameter are typical of those sustained by children. Animal bites usually involve the lower extremities and may be accompanied by lacerations (Giardino & Giardino, 2002).

Hair Loss

TRICHOTILLOMANIA: A child may twist or twirl a portion of his or her hair. This condition does not have the accompanying signs of forceful pulling such as erythema and swelling of the underlying scalp.

TINEA CAPITUS: Ringworm of the scalp may be differentiated by the presence of circular silvery plaques at the site of hair loss.

ALOPECIA AREATA: This is a clinical condition in which hair loss involves a larger area of the scalp without the accompanying signs of trauma.

TIGHT BRAIDS: Tight braids may cause some breaking of the hair shaft without the accompanying erythema or swelling.

POSITIONAL HAIR LOSS: Babies kept on their backs may have posterior hair loss. As an isolated finding, this is indicative of positional hair loss; however, when other signs such as chronic skin conditions and failure to thrive are present, neglect should be considered (Giardino & Giardino, 2002).

Failure to Thrive

The most common cause of inorganic failure to thrive is insufficient intake caused by inexperienced parents who may be mixing powdered or concentrated formulas incorrectly or underfeeding a quiet baby. Intake may also be insufficient to meet increased caloric needs in conditions such as sepsis or hyperthyroidism, gastroesophageal reflux, hepatitis, lactose intolerance, or other genetic and metabolic illnesses. Organic causes of failure to thrive may be identified by history and lab studies and may also be ruled out if the child gains weight with identified adequate intake (Giardino & Giardino, 2002).

Sudden Infant Death Syndrome

Sudden infant death syndrome (SIDS) is defined as the sudden death of a previously healthy child who is less than 1 year of age. It is the most common cause of death in babies between 1 and 6 months of age. The cause is believed to be physiologic instability in cardiorespiratory coordination. The baby is usually found after a nap or bedtime. There is usually watery or serosanguinous discharge from the mouth or nose, and skin mottling of independent portions of the child's body. Death from abuse may be difficult to distinguish from SIDS, and a history is invaluable in identifying inconsistent information and a past history of deaths or near-death episodes while children were under the care of the same person. In contrast to the watery discharge seen in SIDS, bloody discharge may be noted from the child's mouth or nose (American Academy of Pediatrics, 2001a).

Other Causes of Neglect

UNINTENTIONAL NEGLECT may occur when parents are anxious, inexperienced, or cognitively challenged. These families may be identified by observing parent–child interaction and diet logs. These families respond well to counseling and appropriate education.

ACCIDENTAL INJURY may result in the intracranial hemorrhages and retinal damage seen in SBS (Giardino & Giardino, 2002).

Sexual Abuse

PRENATALLY ACQUIRED STDS: It is particularly important to educate young pregnant women about STDs as transmission of STDs during pregnancy can occur before, during or after birth.

BICYCLE OR HORSE RIDING may produce genital abrasions or injury.

EXPLORATION and placing of objects into the vagina by the child or other young children may be seen in the early preschool years as a part of normal development.

PERIANAL STREPTOCOCCAL ERYTHEMA is seen during group A beta-hemolytic streptococcal (GABHS) pharyngitis or strep throat infection. In this illness, the streptococcal bacteria are swallowed, resulting in abdominal pain, and they are later released during defecation. The perianal area becomes reddened as a result of contact with the bacteria, and the condition may appear as anal trauma.

NORMAL VARIATIONS OF THE HYMENAL ORIFICE may appear as sexual trauma. Such variations include crescent, annular, or fimbriated appearance; hymenal tags; and labial adhesions due to low estrogenization of the tissue (Emans, Laufer, & Goldstein, 1998; Hymel & Jenny, 1996).

In the appendix there is a copy of the "Department of Children & Families" (DCF) form used in the state of Massachusetts when filing a report on child abuse.

Discipline

The American Academy of Pediatrics (AAP) Committee on Psychosocial Aspects of Child and Family Health (1998) describes discipline as an approach to help the child learn rules, regulations, and goals of living in a world with others—not just setting limits and punishing. The AAP goes on to state that discipline should include three components:

1. Positive, supportive, nurturing caregiver–child relationship
2. Positive reinforcement techniques to increase desirable behaviors
3. Removal of reinforcement or use of punishment to reduce or eliminate undesirable behaviors

Parenting style and discipline are intertwined: The manner of parenting affects the approach to discipline. The personality characteristics, birth order, gender, and temperament of children affect how a parent disciplines. The following is a brief review of differing parenting styles.

AUTHORITARIAN: These parents put much emphasis on obedience and punitive measure for disobedience. They expect deference and respect to be exhibited toward authority figures. They are less expressive emotionally and demonstrate harsh disapproval and withdrawal of love when the child disobeys. Children of this parenting style tend to be dependent and passive, lack social competence, and demonstrate less intellectual curiosity.

DEMOCRATIC: These parents focus on providing a sense of autonomy and decision making for their children. They are consistent in limit setting and clear on expectations. They discuss their rationale for decisions and household rules. They foster a sense of independence but are receptive to a child's needs. Children of this parenting style are self-reliant, have high self-esteem, and are socially competent.

INDULGENT: These parents place few demands on their children, have limited restraints, and allow the child much freedom. They encourage the child to develop personal standards of behavior, providing little input or direction. Children of this parenting style often do not develop internal controls and lack a sense of direction. They tend to be disrespectful, defiant of authority, and irresponsible.

INDIFFERENT: These parents are self-absorbed and are focused primarily on their own life and needs with little investment in their children. They devote minimal time and energy toward their children, often avoiding or rejecting the child's needs. These children receive limited discipline and guidance and often demonstrate impulsive behavior leading to delinquent acts. They demonstrate disregard and an insensitivity to others (Maccoby & Martin, 1983).

Encouraging acceptable behavior in children is based on setting realistic expectations that are defined by the age of the child and by the child's developmental level. All too often discipline and punishment are related to the educational level of the parent, the age of the parent, family income and culture, as well as the sex of the child. There are common strategies to use when disciplining, but most importantly they need to be age appropriate. *Reasoning or explaining* to a child why a behavior is inappropriate is necessary so the child can understand why he or she is being punished. Explaining and reasoning with the child at the appropriate cognitive level reinforces what is expected in the child's behavior. For example, if the child wants to wear flip-flops to school, the parent may say, "You have to wear shoes, but you can choose between the brown ones or the black ones."

Behavior modification, another means of disciplining, means ignoring certain negative behaviors or complimenting and reinforcing the positive behavior. This approach ultimately encourages the child to behave in an acceptable way. Using time-out allows the child to learn important lessons by experiencing consequences when misbehaving. Time-out is a means of punishment. The general rule is the child must be placed away from toys and other distractions for a specific length of time. The length of time recommended is 1 minute per year of age. Taking a toy away or limiting certain privileges makes this method of behavior very concrete for the child. *Scolding* (i.e., using harsh language) and *spanking* (i.e., inflicting pain) are not recommended means of discipline. They send a negative message that violence is acceptable. *Disapproval of behavior*, either verbal or nonverbal, can be effective. Tone of voice, facial expression, and body language can send the message of unacceptable behavior. Raising your voice and frequently reprimanding for minor issues loses its significance over time and eventually reinforces the undesirable behavior by drawing attention to the child.

Effective disciplinary practices mean not just setting limits and saying *no*, but praising good behavior, being constructive, guiding desired behavior, and, overall, showing the child how to cooperate. Although discipline is generally viewed in a negative light, when viewed constructively it offers structure, safety barriers, limitations, and a sense of security that the child wants and needs. *When disciplining, set clear and developmentally appropriate expectations, ones that the child understands and can follow; doing so can avoid frustration, distrust, and further problems.* Always explain the consequences when the behavior occurs again so that the child knows what to expect. Institute the consequences soon after the situation has occurred. Do not delay the discipline action until later; the child may forget exactly what occurred, and the importance of the situation may not have the same significance. When reprimanding and instituting a punishment, do not become angry or raise your voice. Remaining calm will be more effective. Based on research, the goal of discipline is to teach children, not to punish them. Always remember to praise children when they behave in an acceptable manner and demonstrate appropriate behavior. Encourage problem solving in children by allowing them to make choices and decisions, whether it is what clothes to wear or relinquishing one toy for another. Review the steps of problem solving from defining the problem, expressing the needs, discussing the alternatives, agreeing on a solution, and following through with an agreed-upon plan. Working through this process builds confidence in the child.

When establishing discipline practices, be consistent, ensuring that the punishment is equal to the behavior. Do not punish today for the same incident that was not punished for yesterday. Be consistent!

Developmental Screening

The basic principles of growth and development address a cephalocaudal and proximodistal progression in conjunction with maturation of the central nervous system. Child development is a very complex process with much variability from child to child, and child theorists have addressed these many facets, each focusing on different observations and stages. (Theoretical understanding of child development goes beyond the scope of this textbook.) Understanding of *maturation*, *growth*, and *human development* provides a pathway for interpreting the various physiologic, psychological, and cognitive changes that occur as a child develops.

Maturation refers to the process of cell division, from the unfolding of biologic events in an organism to the maturation from a simple to a more complex organism. Maturation is based on the cellular changes that occur due to genetic inheritance. As providers, one monitors the maturation of the central nervous system as the child matures. **Growth** refers to actual change in physical growth measured in height, weight, and head circumference. **Development** refers to the changes that occur in a child, from physiologic, psychosocial development such as the ability to walk and kick a ball to the development of language skills to the development of reasoning and intellectual processing. During the process of assessment of the child, developmental surveillance is a key component that includes monitoring of the child's overall development as described by Dworkin (1989):

- Obtaining a relevant developmental history
- Making accurate and informative observations of children
- Eliciting and attending to parental concerns
- Sharing opinions and concerns with other relevant professionals

Areas of development that are monitored through developmental screening include perceptual/fine motor skills, gross motor skills, cognitive and language skills, and social/emotional skills. Screening provides a snapshot of the child's progress and helps to identify strengths, as well as areas of weakness that need to be addressed. It is important to keep in mind that how children learn and their developmental progression are affected by those around them, such as parents, grandparents, and siblings. Although children generally follow an upward progression of development, most often they face many peaks and valleys in their attainment of developmental milestones.

A list of screening tools follows that can be used in the office during a well-child visit for children from birth to 21 years of age:

- *AGES AND STAGES QUESTIONNAIRE: SOCIAL-EMOTIONAL (ASQSE):* Administered by the parent for children ages 3–60 months (http://www.brookespublishing.com/tools/asqse/index.htm)
- *BRIEF INFANT AND TODDLER SOCIAL AND EMOTIONAL ASSESSMENT (BITSEA):* Administered by the parent for children ages 12–36 months (http://harcourtassessment.com/HAIWEB/cultures/en-us/productdetail.htm)
- *CHILD BEHAVIOR CHECKLIST (CBCL):* Advocated by the Achenbach System of Empirically Based Assessment; administered by the parent or youth for children ages 1.5 through 20 years (http://www.ASEBA.org)

- *DENVER DEVLOPMENT SCREENING TOOL (DDST)*: Administered by the healthcare provider for children 1 month through 6 years.
- *CAR, RELAX, ALONE, FORGET, FRIENDS, TROUBLE (CRAFFT)*: Administered by the youth for children ages 14–18 years (http://www.ceasar-boston.org/clinicians/crafft.php)
- *PARENTS' EVALUATION OF DEVELOPMENTAL STATUS (PEDS)*: Administered by the parent for children ages birth to 8 years (http://pedstest.com/content.php?content=peds-intro.html)
- *MODIFIED CHECKLIST FOR AUTISM IN TODDLERS (M-CHAT)*: Administered by the parent for children ages 16–30 months (http://www.dbpeds.org/articles/detail.dfm?TextID=377)
- *PATIENT HEALTH QUESTIONNAIRE-9 (PHQ-9)*: Administered by self for children ages 18–20 years (http://www.pfizer.com/pfizer/download/do/phq-9.pdf)
- *PEDIATRIC SYMPTOM CHECKLIST (PSC)*: Administered by the parent or youth for children ages 4–16 years (http://psc.partners.org/)

In the appendix there is a copy of the pediatric symptom checklist (PSC), the youth self-report pediatric symptom checklist (Y-PSC), and the Denver Developmental Screening Tool (DDST).

Mealtime/Eating Behaviors

Mealtime is an opportunity for parents to establish good eating habits through the variety of foods offered, the tone that is set, and the table etiquette that is expected. In today's hurried world, dinnertime with everyone gathered around the table is unfortunately not always possible for a variety of reasons. Hectic schedules, families where both parents work, and after-school commitments all impinge on the traditional dinnertime.

To provide healthy, nutrient-rich meals, parents should set guidelines and dietary expectations for their children. In conjunction with providing an environment that makes mealtime pleasant and welcoming, parents are responsible for choosing the types and amounts of foods they make available. Children learn their eating habits by observation and patterning what their parents do. If nutrient-rich foods such as fruits and vegetables are presented and caregivers indicate interest and pleasure in eating them, children will adopt these values. Basic eating patterns are established early in life, generally during the toddler period when the child is off baby food and eating primarily table food. If empty calories and fast food are routinely offered to the child, the child will develop a taste for and comfort with these foods.

Dietary requirements for the preschooler and early school-age child differ considerably from those of the infant. The baby's birth weight doubles by 6 months and triples by 12 months. Also, the infant's length increases by approximately 50% during the first year. Body weight is not doubled again until around 4 years of age. The average weight increase during childhood is 2–3 kg/year until 9 to 10 years of age. During this same period, height increases 6–8 cm/year until the child reaches puberty. During this period of preschool and school-age years, the child experiences spurts in height and weight accompanied by changes in appetite. During quiescent periods when there is decreased growth, there is decreased appetite as well. *These variations in growth and dietary intake cause much concern for parents, creating a prime opportunity for teaching regarding nutrient needs in conjunction with growth spurts.* During these periods, children continue to grow and develop bones, muscles, teeth, and blood; they therefore have an increased need for nutrient-rich foods.

In conjunction with growth spurts, there are gradual changes in body proportions: The arms and legs lengthen considerably, the trunk growth slows, and there is minimal head growth. As the legs lengthen, they straighten and the abdominal and back muscles strengthen and tighten in order to support the taller child.

Because children are continually growing, periodic height, weight, and body mass index are plotted on the National Center for Health Statistics (NCHS) growth charts. This provides an ongoing basis by which to assess the child's growth and identify developmental trends early. Intervention can then be instituted to ensure that adequate growth is not compromised.

During the preschool and school-age period, body composition remains fairly constant, with fat gradually decreasing until age 6 years. During the early school years, body fat gradually increases in preparation for the pubertal growth spurt. Females have a higher percentage of fat in the early years, and males have more lean body mass per centimeter of height. These differences do not become significant until puberty is achieved during adolescence.

Toddlers and Preschoolers

Toddlers' and preschoolers' diets are influenced by the family, environment, media (such as television), and societal trends. For the toddler, the family is the primary influence. A toddler or early school-age child is not stopping at the neighborhood store to purchase snack foods. Children this age eat only what is presented to them or is available in the home. What the parent buys is what the child eats. Parents and older siblings are role models for young children, who imitate what they see and learn in their environment.

Through exposure to healthy foods, the child has the opportunity to try various tastes and textures and eventually to make better choices.

It is important, as mentioned previously, for the parent to remember that the child's appetite has fluctuations associated with growth spurts, and at times the child may overindulge in certain foods, neglecting others. Forcing children to eat certain foods and requiring them to remain at the table until they are finished establishes negative feelings around mealtime. High expectations regarding mealtime manners, arguments, and emotional stress associated with occasional spills also lead to much disruption and anger for both the child and the parent. Remember that senses such as odor, color, texture, and temperature all contribute to which foods are accepted by the toddler. Many children during this age do not want different foods touching each other on the plate or will reject food if it is cut differently than they usually see it. Young children fill up quickly and should not be given a snack or drink within 1.5 hours of a meal (Mahan & Stump, 2001) because it will decrease their appetite for more nutrient-rich foods.

Today, due to working parents, many toddlers spend the majority of the day in child-care centers, Head Start programs, or preschool programs. During group feeding in these settings, children who tend to be poor eaters at home generally eat what is presented to them, either from peer pressure or imitation. They also may experience new foods in these settings.

School-Age Children

School-age children generally have a slow but steady growth rate. Their likes and dislikes are established during this period, so offering a wide variety of foods is important to expose them to various tastes, colors, and textures. These children spend the majority of their day in school and therefore carry their lunch or participate in the school lunch program. Studies have shown that lunches made at home have fewer nutrients but less fat than the school lunches and that less variety is seen in lunches made at home.

Television has a big influence on determining what foods a child will like, such as the sugared cereals often presented during children's viewing hours. To avoid distractions during mealtime, turn off the television and serve meals at the table rather than in front of the television. For a picky eater, encourage the child to help plan the meals, offering the child several options to choose from. Because this is a period when eating habits are more solidly established, promotion of fruits and vegetables, whole-grain products, low-fat dairy products, legumes and lean meat, fish, and poultry should be emphasized.

To support recommended food intake and reduce the incidence of chronic disease late in life, the Food Guide Pyramid is part of many educational curriculums. In addition, the Centers for Disease Control and Prevention (CDC) has developed guidelines for schools to promote adequate nutritional intake.

Nutritional concerns are heightened by the epidemic public health problem of obesity in children. In 2006 the Third National Health and Nutrition Examination Survey found that 11–15% of children, including adolescent groups, were overweight or fell at or above the 95th percentile for body mass index (U.S. Department of Health and Human Services, 2006). There are many contributing factors, including increased fast food consumption, sedentary behavior of young people, increased television viewing, and media influence such as advertisements for less healthy foods, to name a few. As healthcare providers, it is our role to *first* identify those children who are overweight or at risk for becoming overweight based on family genetics. *Secondly*, we must establish accurate height, weight, and body mass index to confirm an accurate diagnosis. Suggestions established by the American Association of Pediatric Nurse Practitioners (Small, Anderson, Gance-Cleveland, 2009) include the following:

- Plan the desired weight goal with your healthcare provider.
- Make changes slowly and one or two at a time.
- Always eat breakfast.
- Include vegetables with each meal.
- Have plenty of fresh fruits, vegetables, and whole grains in the home.
- Limit chips, cookies, carbonated beverages, and other sweetened and fatty snacks.
- Plan meals ahead and eat together as a family.
- Integrate physical activity into daily life.
- Consult with a healthcare provider regularly.

Adolescents

During adolescence, it is particularly important to develop healthy eating habits because of the increased rate of growth. As adolescents go through the pubertal process, the composition of the body changes. Due to the variation in achieving pubertal growth, Tanner stages are used to evaluate growth and developmental age during this period. In addition, participation in sports, pregnancy, use of alcohol and drugs, dieting, and obsession with body image may all place increased nutritional demands on the body. Teens often have many dietary concerns and are preoccupied with their body size and shape based on the media portrayal of the ideal body as thin. Easy access to fast foods, soda, and sweets contribute to poor eating habits.

Teens frequently skip breakfast, stating that they do not have time in the morning or that they feel sick after eating breakfast. They skip lunch at school, as well, often ending up drinking a soda late in the morning and having one large meal at the end of the day.

Studies have demonstrated that adolescents with a normal-appearing physique may in fact have a very different body image (Emmons, 1994). *As clinicians, we need to be sensitive to this disparity and try to assess the extent of inappropriate eating and exercise behaviors, as it is during these years when issues of independence and control occur, leading to eating disorders such anorexia nervosa and bulimia.* Teens may need help realistically assessing their body weight. Because teens are at increased risk for developing eating disorders, they are also at risk for subsequent complications caused by inadequate nutrition. These complications can affect brain development and bone growth and can ultimately lead to malnutrition. See the Appendix 1-6 for a questionnaire for screening eating disorders.

Dietary Guidelines

New dietary guidelines established by the U.S. government are easily accessible through the Web site MyPyramid.gov, which provides meal plans based on age. It offers recommendations regarding caloric intake and consumption of fruits, vegetables, grains, meat/beans, and milk. Meal plans are specifically designed with foods that the toddler and school-age child will enjoy, but that also are nutrient rich.

Some examples for breakfast "on the run," recommended by the Children's Hospital, Boston, include the following:

- Fruit
- Milk
- Bagel
- Cheese toast
- Cereal
- Peanut butter sandwich
- Yogurt

Some examples for after-school snacks include the following:

- Fruit
- Vegetables and dip
- Yogurt
- Sandwich
- Cheese and crackers
- Milk and cereal

References

Alexander, R., & Smith, W. (1998). Shaken baby syndrome. *Infant and Young Child, 1,* 1–9.

American Academy of Pediatrics, Committee on Child Abuse and Neglect. (2001a). Distinguishing sudden infant death syndrome from child abuse fatalities. *Pediatrics, 107,* 437–441.

American Academy of Pediatrics, Committee on Child Abuse and Neglect. (2001b). Shaken baby syndrome: Rotational cranial injury. *Pediatrics, 8,* 206–210.

American Academy of Pediatrics, Committee on Child Abuse and Neglect. (2005). Oral and dental aspects of child abuse and neglect. *Pediatrics, 116.*

American Academy of Pediatrics, Committee on Psychosocial Aspects of Child & Family Health. (1998). *Pediatrics, 101*(4), 231–241.

Ball, J.W., Bindler, R. (2008). *Pediatric nursing,* (4th ed.). Upper Saddle River, NJ: Prentice Hall.

Bickley, L., Szilagyi, P., & Stackhaus, J. (2002). *Bates' guide to physical examination and history taking* (8th ed.). Philadelphia: Lippincott Williams & Wilkins.

Bowen, M. (1978). *Family therapy in clinical practice.* Northvale, NJ: Jason Aronson.

Bowlby, J. (1969). *Attachment* (Vol. 1). New York: Basic Books.

Cheung, K. (1999). Identifying and documenting findings of child abuse and neglect. *Journal of Pediatric Health Care, 13,* 142–143.

Children's Hospital Boston. (n.d.). Nutrition for school-aged children. Retrieved from http://www.childrenshospital.org/az/Site1563/mainpageS1563P0.html

Dworkin, P. H. (1989). British and American recommendations for developmental monitoring: The role of surveillance. *Pediatrics, 83,* 619–622.

Emans, S. J., Laufer, M. R., & Goldstein, D. (1998). *Pediatric and adolescent gynecology* (4th ed.). Philadelphia: Lippincott Williams & Wilkins.

Emmons, L. (1994). Predisposing factors differentiating adolescent dieters and non dieters. *Journal of American Dietetic Association,* (7), 725–728.

Giardino, A. P., & Giardino, E. R. (2002). *Recognition of child abuse for the mandated reporter* (3rd ed.). St. Louis, MO: GW Medical Publishing.

Hamarman, S., & Bennett, W. (2000). Evaluation and reporting of emotional abuse in children. *Journal of the American Academy of Child and Adolescent Psychiatry, 39,* 928–930.

Horner, G. (2001a). Child sexual abuse: Psychological risk factors. *Journal of Pediatric Health Care, 16,* 187.

Horner, G. (2001b). Repeated sexual abuse allegations: A problem for primary health care providers. *Journal of Pediatric Health Care, 15,* 71–76.

Hymel, K. P., & Jenny, C. (1996). Child sexual abuse. *Pediatric Review,* 17, 236–249.

Jenny, C. (2006). Evaluating infants and young children with multiple fractures. *Pediatrics, 118*(3).

Maccoby, E. E., & Martin, J. A. (1983). Socialization in the context of the family: Parent–child interaction. In P. H. Mussen (Ed.) & E. M. Hetherington (Vol. Ed.), *Handbook of child psychology: Vol. 4. Socialization, personality, and social development* (4th ed., pp. 1–101). New York: Wiley.

Mahan, L. K, & Stump, S. E. (2000). *Krause's food, nutrition, & diet therapy* (10th ed.). Philadelphia: W.B. Saunders.

Nelms, B. (2001). Emotional abuse: Helping prevent the problem. *Primary Health Care, 15*, 103–104.

Reece, R. M., & Ludwig, S. (Eds.). (2001). *Child abuse: Medical diagnosis and management* (2nd ed.). Philadelphia: Lippincott Williams & Wilkins.

Small, L., Anderson, D. Gance-Cleveland, B. (2009). Pediatric nurse practitioners assessment and management of childhood overweight/obesity: Results from 1999 and 2005 cohort surveys. *Journal of Pediatric Health Care, 23*(4), 231–241.

Snider, R. (Ed.). (1997). *Essentials of musculoskeletal care*. Rosemont, IL: American Academy of Orthopaedic Surgery.

Stevens-Simon, C., & Barrett, J. (2001). Comparison of psychological resources of adolescents at low and high risk of mistreating their children. *Journal of Pediatric Health Care, 15*(6), 299–303.

U.S. Department of Health Services (2006). Centers for Disease Control and Prevention. National Health and Nutrition Examination Survey 2003–2006. Retrieved from http://www.cdc.gov/nchs/nhanes.htm

Wilson, C., & Knight, J. (2002). Early child abuse linked to behavioral problems in adolescence. *Archives of Pediatrics and Adolescent Medicine, 156*, 824–830.

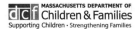
MASSACHUSETTS DEPARTMENT OF
Children & Families
Supporting Children · Strengthening Families

Report of Child(ren) Alleged to be Suffering from Serious Physical or Emotional Injury by Abuse or Neglect

Massachusetts law requires an individual who is a mandated reporter to immediately report any allegation of serious physical or emotional injury resulting from abuse or neglect to the Department of Children and Families by:

1. Immediately reporting by oral communication; and
2. Completing and sending this written report to the appropriate Department of Children and Families office within 48 hours of making the oral report.

Please complete all sections of this form. If some data is unknown, please signify. If some data is uncertain, place a question mark after the entry.

▼ **DATA ON CHILDREN REPORTED**

Name	Current Location/Address	Sex	Age or Date of Birth
		❑ Male ❑ Female	
		❑ Male ❑ Female	
		❑ Male ❑ Female	
		❑ Male ❑ Female	
		❑ Male ❑ Female	

▼ **DATA ON MALE GUARDIAN OR PARENT**

Name: _____
        First   Last   Middle

Address: _____
        Street & Number   City/Town   State   Zip Code

Phone #: _____   Age: _____

▼ **DATA ON FEMALE GUARDIAN OR PARENT**

Name: _____
        First   Last   Middle

Address: _____
        Street & Number   City/Town   State   Zip Code

Phone #: _____   Age: _____

▼ **DATA ON REPORTER/REPORT**

Report Date: _____   ❑ Mandatory Report   ❑ Voluntary Report

Reporter's Name: _____
        First   Last   Middle
(If the reporter represents an institution, school or facility, please indicate)

Reporter's Address: _____
        Street & Number   City/Town   State   Zip Code

Phone #: _____

Has reporter informed caretaker of report   ❑ Yes   ❑ No

▼ What is the nature and extent of injury, abuse, maltreatment, or neglect, including prior evidence of same? (Please cite the source of this information if not observed firsthand.)

_____

_____

_____

_____

_____

_____

▼ What are the circumstances under which the reporter became aware of the injuries, abuse or maltreatment, or neglect?

_____

_____

_____

_____

_____

_____

▼ What action has been taken thus far to treat, shelter, or otherwise assist the child(ren) to deal with the situation?

_____

_____

_____

_____

_____

_____

▼ Please give other information that you think might be helpful in establishing the cause of the injury and/or the person(s) responsible for it. If known, please provide the name(s) of the alleged perpetrator(s)?

_____

_____

_____

_____

_____

_____

_____

Signature of Reporter:

Source: Massachusetts Department of Children and Families

Pediatric Symptom Checklist (PSC)

Emotional and physical health go together in children. Because parents are often the first to notice a problem with their child's behavior, emotions, or learning, you may help your child get the best care possible by answering these questions. Please indicate which statement best describes your child.

Please mark under the heading that best describes your child:

		Never	Sometimes	Often
1. Complains of aches and pains	1	____	____	____
2. Spends more time alone	2	____	____	____
3. Tires easily, has little energy	3	____	____	____
4. Fidgety, unable to sit still	4	____	____	____
5. Has trouble with teacher	5	____	____	____
6. Less interested in school	6	____	____	____
7. Acts as if driven by a motor	7	____	____	____
8. Daydreams too much	8	____	____	____
9. Distracted easily	9	____	____	____
10. Is afraid of new situations	10	____	____	____
11. Feels sad, unhappy	11	____	____	____
12. Is irritable, angry	12	____	____	____
13. Feels hopeless	13	____	____	____
14. Has trouble concentrating	14	____	____	____
15. Less interested in friends	15	____	____	____
16. Fights with other children	16	____	____	____
17. Absent from school	17	____	____	____
18. School grades dropping	18	____	____	____
19. Is down on him or herself	19	____	____	____
20. Visits the doctor with doctor finding nothing wrong	20	____	____	____
21. Has trouble sleeping	21	____	____	____
22. Worries a lot	22	____	____	____
23. Wants to be with you more than before	23	____	____	____
24. Feels he or she is bad	24	____	____	____
25. Takes unnecessary risks	25	____	____	____
26. Gets hurt frequently	26	____	____	____
27. Seems to be having less fun	27	____	____	____
28. Acts younger than children his or her age	28	____	____	____
29. Does not listen to rules	29	____	____	____
30. Does not show feelings	30	____	____	____
31. Does not understand other people's feelings	31	____	____	____
32. Teases others	32	____	____	____
33. Blames others for his or her troubles	33	____	____	____
34. Takes things that do not belong to him or her	34	____	____	____
35. Refuses to share	35	____	____	____

Total score _____

Does your child have any emotional or behavioral problems for which she or he needs help?   ( ) N   ( ) Y

Are there any services that you would like your child to receive for these problems?   ( ) N   ( ) Y

If yes, what services? _____

Source: http://www.brightfutures.org

Pediatric Symptom Checklist—Youth Report (Y-PSC)

Please mark under the heading that best fits you:

			Never	Sometimes	Often
1.	Complain of aches or pains	1			
2.	Spend more time alone	2			
3.	Tire easily, little energy	3			
4.	Fidgety, unable to sit still	4			
5.	Have trouble with teacher	5			
6.	Less interested in school	6			
7.	Act as if driven by motor	7			
8.	Daydream too much	8			
9.	Distract easily	9			
10.	Are afraid of new situations	10			
11.	Feel sad, unhappy	11			
12.	Are irritable, angry	12			
13.	Feel hopeless	13			
14.	Have trouble concentrating	14			
15.	Less interested in friends	15			
16.	Fight with other children	16			
17.	Absent from school	17			
18.	School grades dropping	18			
19.	Down on yourself	19			
20.	Visit doctor with doctor finding nothing wrong	20			
21.	Have trouble sleeping	21			
22.	Worry a lot	22			
23.	Want to be with parent more than before	23			
24.	Feel that you are bad	24			
25.	Take unnecessary risks	25			
26.	Get hurt frequently	26			
27.	Seem to be having less fun	27			
28.	Act younger than children your age	28			
29.	Do not listen to rules	29			
30.	Do not show feelings	30			
31.	Do not understand other people's feelings	31			
32.	Tease others	32			
33.	Blame others for your troubles	33			
34.	Take things that do not belong to you	34			
35.	Refuse to share	35			

M-CHAT

Please fill out the following about how your child **usually** is. Please try to answer every question. If the behavior is rare (e.g., you've seen it once or twice), please answer as if the child does not do it.

1. Does your child enjoy being swung, bounced on your knee, etc.?   Yes   No

2. Does your child take an interest in other children?   Yes   No

3. Does your child like climbing on things, such as up stairs?   Yes   No

4. Does your child enjoy playing peek-a-boo/hide-and-seek?   Yes   No

5. Does your child ever pretend, for example, to talk on the phone or take care   Yes   No
   of dolls, or pretend other things?

6. Does your child ever use his/her index finger to point, to ask for something?   Yes   No

7. Does your child ever use his/her index finger to point, to indicate interest in something?   Yes   No

8. Can your child play properly with small toys (e.g. cars or bricks) without   Yes   No
   just mouthing, fiddling, or dropping them?

9. Does your child ever bring objects over to you (parent) to show you something?   Yes   No

10. Does your child look you in the eye for more than a second or two?   Yes   No

11. Does your child ever seem oversensitive to noise? (e.g., plugging ears)   Yes   No

12. Does your child smile in response to your face or your smile?   Yes   No

13. Does your child imitate you? (e.g., you make a face—will your child imitate it?)   Yes   No

14. Does your child respond to his/her name when you call?   Yes   No

15. If you point at a toy across the room, does your child look at it?   Yes   No

16. Does your child walk?   Yes   No

17. Does your child look at things you are looking at?   Yes   No

18. Does your child make unusual finger movements near his/her face?   Yes   No

19. Does your child try to attract your attention to his/her own activity?   Yes   No

20. Have you ever wondered if your child is deaf?   Yes   No

21. Does your child understand what people say?   Yes   No

22. Does your child sometimes stare at nothing or wander with no purpose?   Yes   No

23. Does your child look at your face to check your reaction when   Yes   No
    faced with something unfamiliar?

© 1999 Diana Robins, Deborah Fein, & Marianne Barton

Please refer to: Robins, D., Fein, D., Barton, M., & Green, J. (2001). The Modified Checklist for Autism in Toddlers: An initial study investigating the early detection of autism and pervasive developmental disorders. <u>Journal of Autism and Developmental Disorders, 31</u> (2), 131–144.

I.D. # _____

National Eating Disorders Screening Program
Screening Questionnaire©

Section A

1. Age: _____   Sex: ❏ male   ❏ female

2. Ethnic/Racial Group I most closely identify with:
   ❏ African American   ❏ Asian/Pacific Islander   ❏ Caucasian
   ❏ Latino/Latina/Hispanic ❏ Native American/Alaskan Native ❏ Other _____

3. If enrolled at a college or university, are you a:
   ❏ Freshman   ❏ Sophomore   ❏ Junior   ❏ Senior   ❏ Graduate student

   If not enrolled at a college or university, level of education completed:
   ❏ Elementary School   ❏ High School   ❏ Technical/some college   ❏ College   ❏ Graduate School

4. Have you ever been diagnosed with or treated for an eating disorder?
   ❏ No   ❏ Yes

Section B

5. Height: _____/feet _____/inches

6. Weight: _____ lbs

7. Highest past weight within the last 6 months: _____ lbs

8. Lowest past weight at current height: _____ lbs
   Was this within the last 6 months?   ❏ No   ❏ Yes

9. **Women Only:**
   Have you missed two or more menstrual periods within the last six months?   ❏ No   ❏ Yes

Section C

10. Do you worry about gaining weight?
    ❏ never/rarely   ❏ some of the time   ❏ much of the time   ❏ all of the time

11. Do you avoid foods because of the fat, carbohydrate, or sugar content in them?
    ❏ never/rarely   ❏ some of the time   ❏ much of the time   ❏ all of the time

12. How often do you think about wanting to be thinner?
    ❏ never/rarely   ❏ some of the time   ❏ much of the time   ❏ all of the time

13. Are you bothered by the thought of having fat on your body?
    ❏ never/rarely   ❏ some of the time   ❏ much of the time   ❏ all of the time

14. Do you feel guilty after eating?
    ❏ never/rarely   ❏ some of the time   ❏ much of the time   ❏ all of the time

15. Do you feel that food controls your life?
    ❏ never/rarely   ❏ some of the time   ❏ much of the time   ❏ all of the time

Section   D

16. During the past six months, have you had episodes when <u>both</u> of the following applied:

   a) you have eaten an *unusually* large amount of food within a two hour period, and
   b) you have felt unable to control how much you were eating within these periods?
   ❑ never   ❑ less than once a month   ❑ about once a month   ❑ about once a week   ❑ two or more times a week

   If <u>never</u>, please skip to question #18

17. If you have had binge-eating episodes (as defined in question #16), were they associated with:

Eating much more rapidly than usual?	❑ No	❑ Yes
Eating until feeling uncomfortably full?	❑ No	❑ Yes
Eating large amounts of food when not feeling physically hungry?	❑ No	❑ Yes
Eating alone because of being embarrassed by how much you were eating?	❑ No	❑ Yes
Feeling disgusted with yourself, depressed, or very guilty after over-eating?	❑ No	❑ Yes

18. During the past six months, have you ever done any of the following?

   Self-induced vomiting in an attempt to control your weight?
   ❑ never   ❑ less than once a month   ❑ about once a month   ❑ about once a week   ❑ two or more times a week

   Taken laxatives in an attempt to control your weight?
   ❑ never   ❑ less than once a month   ❑ about once a month   ❑ about once a week   ❑ two or more times a week

   Restricted your eating in an attempt to control you weight?
   Restrictive eating = eating less than 500 calories a day <u>or</u> skipping 2 or more meals a day
   ❑ never   ❑ less than once a month   ❑ about once a month   ❑ about once a week   ❑ two or more times a week

   Taken diuretics (water pills) *in an attempt to control your weight?*
   ❑ never   ❑ less than once a month   ❑ about once a month   ❑ about once a week   ❑ two or more times a week

   Exercised in an attempt to control your weight?
   ❑ never   ❑ about 1 hour a day   ❑ about 2 hours a day   ❑ about 3 hours a day   ❑ more than 3 hours a day

19. During the past six months, have you exercised to control your weight even when injured, sick, or against a doctor's orders?
   ❑ never   ❑ some of the time   ❑ much of the time   ❑ all of the time

   During the past six months, has exercising to control your weight significantly interfered with other activities?
   ❑ never   ❑ some of the time   ❑ much of the time   ❑ all of the time

---

Section   E

20. Do your concerns or behaviors about eating or weight interfere with your:

   Relationships (e.g., Avoiding family members and/or friends to have time and privacy for binging, purging, or exercising)?
   ❑ never   ❑ some of the time   ❑ much of the time   ❑ all of the time

   Academic/Work performance?
   ❑ never   ❑ some of the time   ❑ much of the time   ❑ all of the time

21. Do your concerns or behaviors about eating or weight cause you a great deal of distress?
   ❑ never   ❑ some of the time   ❑ much of the time   ❑ all of the time

ARE YOU DYING TO BE THIN?

Due to an increase in public awareness, ANOREXIA NERVOSA (key symptoms: refusal to maintain a minimally healthy body weight, intense fear of gaining weight, and a significant disturbance in the perception of the shape or size of owns body) and BULIMIA NERVOSA (key symptoms: binge eating—eating what the individual considers to be too much food in a way that feels out of control, followed by inappropriate compensatory behaviors (e.g., self-induced vomiting, excessive exercise) are becoming more and more openly acknowledged.

The following questionnaire will tell you whether or not you think or behave in a way that indicates that you have tendencies toward anorexia nervosa or bulimia nervosa.

DIRECTIONS: Answer the questions below honestly. Respond as you are now, not the way you used to be or the way you would like to be. Write the number of your answer in the space at the left. Do not leave any questions blank unless instructed to do so.

_____ 1. I have eating habits that are different from those of my family and friends.

   1) Often 2) Sometimes 3) Rarely 4) Never

_____ 2. I find myself panicking if I cannot exercise as I planned, because I am afraid that I will gain weight if I don't.

   1) Often 2) Sometimes 3) Rarely 4) Never

_____ 3. My friends tell me that I am thin, but I don't believe them because I feel fat.

   1) Often 2) Sometimes 3) Rarely 4) Never

_____ 4. (Females only) My menstrual period has stopped or become irregular due to no known medical reasons.

   1) True 2) False

_____ 5. I have become obsessed with food to the point that I cannot go through a day without worrying about what I will or will not eat.

   1) Almost always 2) Sometimes 3) Rarely 4) Never

_____ 6. I have lost more than 15% of what is considered to be a healthy weight for my height (e.g., female, 5'4" tall loses 20 pounds when a healthy weight for her is approximately 122 pounds.)

   1) True 2) False

_____ 7. I would panic if I got on the scale tomorrow and found that I had gained two pounds.

   1) Almost always 2) Sometimes 3) Rarely 4) Never

_____ 8. I find that I prefer to eat alone or when I am sure that no one will see me, and thus make excuses so that I can eat less and less often with friends or family.

   1) Often 2) Sometimes 3) Rarely 4) Never

_____ 9. I find myself going on uncontrollable eating binges during which I consume large amounts of food to the point that I feel sick and make myself vomit.

   1) Never 2) Less than 1 time per week 3) 1–6 times per week 4) 1 or more times per day

_____ 10. I find myself compulsively eating more than I want to while feeling out of control and/or what I am doing.

    1) Never 2) Less than 1 time per week 3) 1–6 times per week 4) 1 or more times pei

_____ 11. I use laxatives or diuretics as a means of weight control.

    1) Never 2) Rarely 3) Sometimes 4) On a regular basis.

_____ 12. I find myself playing games with food (e.g. cutting it up in tiny pieces, hiding food so pe think I ate it, chewing it and spitting it out without swallowing it, keeping hidden stashes have determined that there are "safe" foods that are okay for me to eat and "bad" foods

    1) Often 2) Sometimes 3) Rarely 4) Never

_____ 13. People around me have become very interested in what I eat and I find myself getting ¿ them for pushing me to eat more.

    1) Often 2) Sometimes 3) Rarely 4) Never

_____ 14. I have felt more depressed and irritable recently than is typical for me and/or have beei an increasing amount of time alone.

    1) True 2) False

_____ 15. I keep a lot of my fears about food and eating to myself because I am afraid no one wo understand.

    1) Often 2) Sometimes 3) Rarely 4) Never

_____ 16. I enjoy making gourmet and/or high calorie foods for others as long as I don't have to ε myself.

    1) Often 2) Sometimes 3) Rarely 4) Never

_____ 17. The most powerful fear in my life is the fear of gaining weight or becoming fat.

    1) True 2) False

_____ 18. I exercise a lot (more than 4 times per week and/or more than 4 hours per week as a n weight control).

    1) True 2) False

_____ 19. I find myself totally absorbed when reading books or magazines about dieting, exercisi or calorie counting to the point that I can spend hours studying them.

    1) Often 2) Sometimes 3) Rarely 4) Never

_____ 20. I tend to be a perfectionist and am not satisfied with myself unless I do things perfectly.

    1) Often 2) Sometimes 3) Rarely 4) Never

_____ 21. I go through long periods of time without eating (fasting) or eating very little as a mean; control.

    1) Often 2) Sometimes 3) Rarely 4) Never

_____ 22. It is important for me to try to be thinner than all of my friends.

    1) Almost always 2) Sometimes 3) Rarely 4) Never

Source: © 1982: K. Kim Lampson, Reprinted with permission

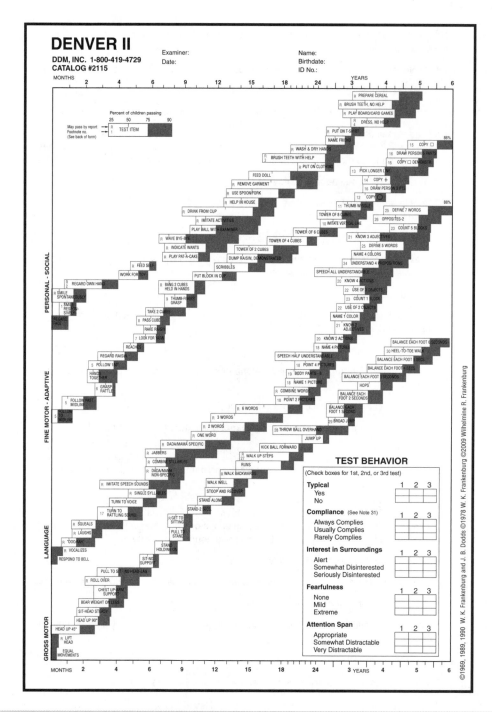

DIRECTIONS FOR ADMINISTRATION

1. Try to get child to smile by smiling, talking or waving. Do not touch him/her.
2. Child must stare at hand several seconds.
3. Parent may help guide toothbrush and put toothpaste on brush.
4. Child does not have to be able to tie shoes or button/zip in the back.
5. Move yarn slowly in an arc from one side to the other, about 8" above child's face.
6. Pass if child grasps rattle when it is touched to the backs or tips of fingers.
7. Pass if child tries to see where yarn went. Yarn should be dropped quickly from sight from tester's hand without arm movement.
8. Child must transfer cube from hand to hand without help of body, mouth, or table.
9. Pass if child picks up raisin with any part of thumb and finger.
10. Line can vary only 30 degrees or less from tester's line. |/
11. Make a fist with thumb pointing upward and wiggle only the thumb. Pass if child imitates and does not move any fingers other than the thumb.

| 12. Pass any enclosed form. Fail continuous round motions. | 13. Which line is longer? (Not bigger.) Turn paper upside down and repeat. (pass 3 of 3 or 5 of 6) | 14. Pass any lines crossing near midpoint. | 15. Have child copy first. If failed, demonstrate. |

When giving items 12, 14, and 15, do not name the forms. Do not demonstrate 12 and 14.

16. When scoring, each pair (2 arms, 2 legs, etc.) counts as one part.
17. Place one cube in cup and shake gently near child's ear, but out of sight. Repeat for other ear.
18. Point to picture and have child name it. (No credit is given for sounds only.)
    If less than 4 pictures are named correctly, have child point to picture as each is named by tester.

 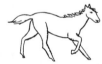

19. Using doll, tell child: Show me the nose, eyes, ears, mouth, hands, feet, tummy, hair. Pass 6 of 8.
20. Using pictures, ask child: Which one flies?...says meow?...talks?...barks?...gallops? Pass 2 of 5, 4 of 5.
21. Ask child: What do you do when you are cold?...tired?...hungry? Pass 2 of 3, 3 of 3.
22. Ask child: What do you do with a cup? What is a chair used for? What is a pencil used for?
    Action words must be included in answers.
23. Pass if child correctly places _and_ says how many blocks are on paper. (1,5).
24. Tell child: Put block **on** table; **under** table; **in front of** me, **behind** me. Pass 4 of 4.
    (Do not help child by pointing, moving head or eyes.)
25. Ask child: What is a ball?...lake?...desk?...house?...banana?...curtain?...fence?...ceiling? Pass if defined in terms of use, shape, what it is made of, or general category (such as banana is fruit, not just yellow). Pass 5 of 8, 7 of 8.
26. Ask child: If a horse is big, a mouse is ___? If fire is hot, ice is ___? If the sun shines during the day, the moon shines during the ___? Pass 2 of 3.
27. Child may use wall or rail only, not person. May not crawl.
28. Child must throw ball overhand 3 feet to within arm's reach of tester.
29. Child must perform standing broad jump over width of test sheet (8 1/2 inches).
30. Tell child to walk forward, ⚮⚮⚮➞ heel within 1 inch of toe. Tester may demonstrate.
    Child must walk 4 consecutive steps.
31. In the second year, half of normal children are non-compliant.

OBSERVATIONS:

Source: Reprinted with permission from William K. Frankenburg, M.D., Denver Developmental Materials, Inc. Denver, CO.

Interview Process and Health History

Setting the Tone: The Interview Process

To obtain a medical history and perform an examination on a child, understanding the child's physical, social, and cognitive development is key. Awareness of the parent's concerns and interaction with the child is equally important. Your approach as you walk into the room can set the tone for the visit. A professional demeanor is always important. A lab coat, while worn in an adult setting, is not necessary when interviewing children. A more casual, but professional attire is often appropriate and less intimidating to the child.

Before entering the room, review the chart to familiarize yourself with the patient's history and the reason for his or her visit. While talking to the parent or asking questions of a child, nonverbal communication plays an important role. Sit on a stool or chair so that you are eye level with the child. Be attentive to what the parent is telling you; close the chart and have a conversation by asking open-ended questions of the parent and/or the child if the child is old enough to respond to your questions.

Remember that the order of the exam should conform to the age and temperament of the child. Often, infants less then 6 months of age can be managed easily on the exam table without much fuss, whereas a child 2 or 3 years of age is better managed performing the exam on the parent's lap. In a young child, save the ears and throat for last and start by listening to the lungs and heart while the child is quiet. Try to examine the abdomen before crying starts. It is always helpful to make a game out of the exam, whether you are looking for monkeys in the child's ears or listening for birdies in the child's chest. You can whistle or play peekaboo games—anything that will distract your patient so that you can obtain necessary information. A slow, easy approach is always beneficial in helping to facilitate the exam.

Infants

When examining an infant, use a soothing voice. Do not unwrap the child immediately; do it gradually and allow the child to accommodate to the room air. While the infant is lying quietly, start with nonintrusive parts of the exam such as auscultation. Have a pacifier available or use a gloved finger. Turn on a musical toy if necessary. Wash your hands with warm water before you begin. There is nothing more unsettling to the child than being touched by icy cold fingers. Encourage the parent to stand beside the exam table. It is reassuring to the child to see and make eye contact with the parent, as well as to hear the parent's voice.

Toddlers

It is not unusual for the toddler to start screaming as you enter the room. Remain calm and make a joke such as, "Do you want me to leave already? I just walked in." Talk to the parent in a calm, assured manner, asking questions about the child. Encourage the child to touch and explore your stethoscope, particularly if you have a small toy attached to the tubing, or allow the child to play with your reflex hammer. Do not separate the child from the parent, and reassure the parent that he or she may hold the child on his or her lap during the exam. If the parent feels comfortable during the visit, this feeling is conveyed to the child as well.

Preschoolers

When examining a preschooler, encourage the child to be an active participant by using a hand-over-hand technique while listening with the stethoscope (i.e., allow the child to hold the diaphragm of the stethoscope and put your hand over the child's). Allow the child to play with the equipment. Explain in simple terms what you are doing and make a game out of it. The child is curious about you but also worried about what you are going to do. Allow the child some choices, such as, "Can I feel your tummy now or should I feel your legs first?" always using a slow, deliberate approach.

A preschooler may be interested in putting your stethoscope in his or her ears or imitating use of the reflex hammer as part of imitation play.

School-Age Children

In the examination of a school-age child, ask the child direct questions and explain what you are going to do using simple terms. Ask the child about school, their favorite subject, what sports they like to play, whether they have a best friend, or what they like to do when not in school, encouraging them to be part of the conversation. Tell the child what you are going to do next and when something is going to hurt or be uncomfortable. Reassure the child that the exam will not hurt; this allows the child to relax and allows you to perform a more comprehensive exam.

Remember, the rapport you develop with the parent helps set the tone during the visit as well as establish a level of comfort and reassurance for the child. When assessing a pediatric patient, you are establishing a relationship with both the parent and the child.

Adolescents

Adolescents like to be treated more as an adult than a child. Address them directly and indicate early in the visit that you will review some general questions with the parent and child. Then gently, but firmly suggest that the parent wait in the waiting room while you perform the physical exam. While interviewing the adolescent, ask open-ended questions to encourage conversation. Always start with nonthreatening topics such as school, sports, and friends, and gradually move to more delicate topics such as drugs, dating, sexual behavior, use of contraception, and STDs. Be respectful of the teen's modesty and maintain privacy during the exam. If a teen is uncomfortable talking about sexual issues, consider asking questions while performing the exam, such as while looking in the ears, then review the topics when you are finished. Often, not making direct eye contact and asking questions in a casual nonthreatening manner sets a more comfortable tone for adolescents, and they will be more likely to answer you truthfully. Remember to use terminology they understand and are familiar with.

The most important part of the exam is confirming to the adolescent that the interview will be confidential unless there is a problem that needs to be addressed for his or her health.

Your comfort level and professionalism convey a sense of confidence that goes a long way in building trust with your families. Once trust is established, you can begin your medical history. If this is a new patient, introducing yourself and telling the patient a little about yourself helps break the ice and is the first step in establishing a relationship with your new family. **Figure 2-1** shows the different stages of development for infants through adolescence.

Stages of Cognitive Development. Piaget identified four Stages in Cognitive Development:

Stage	Characteristics
Infant	**Sensorimotor stage:** In this period (which has 6 stages), intelligence is demonstrated through motor activity without the use of symbols. Knowledge of the world is limited (but developing) because its based on physical interactions/experiences. Children acquire object permanence at about 7 months of age (memory). Physical development (mobility) allows the child to begin developing new intellectual abilities. Some symbolic (language) abilities are developed at the end of this stage.
Toddler and early childhood	**Pre-operational stage:** In this period (which has two substages), intelligence is demonstrated through the use of symbols, language use matures, and memory and imagination are developed, but thinking is done in a nonlogical, nonreversable manner. Egocentric thinking predominates.
Elementary and early adolescence	**Concrete operational stage:** In this stage (characterized by 7 types of conservation: number, length, liquid, mass, weight, area, volume), intelligence is demonstrated through logical and systematic manipulation of symbols related to concrete objects. Operational thinking develops (mental actions that are reversible). Egocentric thought diminishes.
Adolescence and adulthood	**Formal operational stage:** In this stage, intelligence is demonstrated through the logical use of symbols related to abstract concepts. Early in the period there is a return to egocentric thought. Only 35% of high school graduates in industrialized countries obtain formal operations; many people do not think formally during adulthood.

Stages of Sullivan's Interpersonal Theory of Development		
Stage	**Age**	**Characteristics**
Infant	Birth to 18 months	Learns to rely on others, especially mother; "good me/bad me" emerges
Early childhood	18 months to 6 years	Learns to clarify communication; recognizes approval or disapproval; delays gratification
Late childhood	6 to 9 years	Increasing intellectual abilities: learns to control behavior and own place in the world
Preadolescence	9 to 12 years	Vulnerable to teasing; "chum" important
Early adolescence	12 to 15 years	Mastering independence; develops relationships with persons of opposite gender
Late adolescence	15 to 19 years	Masters expression of sexual impulses; forms responsible and satisfying relationships with others

Figure 2-1(a) Stages of Sullivan's Interpersonal Theory of Development

Source: Adapted from Evans III, B.F. Harry Stack Sullivan: Interpersonal Theory and Psychother. Routledge, 1996.

Figure 2-1(c) Stages of Sullivan's Interpersonal Theory of Development

Source: Adapted from Evans III, B.F. Harry Stack Sullivan: Interpersonal Theory and Psychother. Routledge, 1996.

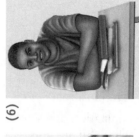

(4)

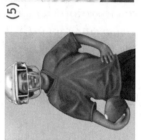

(5)

(6)

(1)

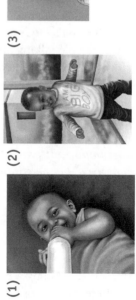

(2)

(3)

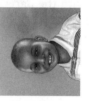

Figure 2-1(b) Stages of Sullivan's Interpersonal Theory of Development

Medical Interview Process

When examining a new patient, the history can take quite a bit of time, whereas a follow-up or return visit for a known patient requires less time to update the history. Components of a routine health history follow. The questions and specific information are dependent upon the age of the child. For example, a toddler's history may include questions focused on play and environmental safety, whereas an adolescent's history will focus more on sexual development, STDs, social/emotional issues, and school concerns.

Reason for the visit
Maternal concerns
Interval history
History of present illness (HPI) (there may not be one if this is a well-child visit)
Review of systems (ROS)
Past medical history:
    Immunizations
    Allergies
    Accidents/injuries
    Hospitalizations
    Illnesses (chronic)
    Prenatal history
    Labor and delivery history
    Family history
    Social history
Activities of daily living (ADLs)
    Nutrition
    Sleep
    Elimination
    Development
Screenings
    Height and weight
    Head circumference
    Vision
    Hearing
    Lead
    Hematocrit
    Tuberculosis (TB)
Physical exam
Assessment
Plan

Development

A basic understanding of developmental milestones is necessary. Monitoring developmental milestones of cognitive, social/emotional, fine and gross motor, and language skills is a fundamental part of each well-child visit.

The following are overviews of developmental theorists including: Piaget, Erikson, Freud, Sullivan, and Kohlberg. See **Figure 2-2** for further details.

Development is a reciprocal and ongoing process that occurs between the child and his or her environment. The following developmental principles (Cech & Martin, 2002) help us understand that one's development is dependent upon genetic background, intrauterine and extrauterine factors, as well as psychosocial factors. After discussing these principles, an overview of age-related developmental accomplishments is presented.

Developmental Theory			
Age	**Kohlberg**	**Freud**	**Erikson**
Birth–18 months	**"Amoral"** Moral reasoning cannot begin until the child reaches a certain level of cognitive development.	**Oral** Primary body zone: mouth Activities: sucking and eating Major conflict: weaning Interpersonal focus: self; minimal differentiation from others	**Trust vs. Mistrust** Trust develops when needs are met consistently by a loving, caring person. Mistrust develops when needs are not met or are met inconsistently. With trust, infant develops sense of hope and optimism.
18 months–3 years	**Preconventional: Obedience and Punishment Orient.** Behavioral decisions made based on fear of punishment; good and bad defined in terms of physical consequences.	**Anal** Primary body zone: anal area Activities: elimination (expulsion vs. retention) Major conflict: toilet training Interpersonal focus: rebellion vs. compliance with parental demands	**Autonomy vs. Shame and Doubt** Autonomy is developed as child gains increasing control of body and wants to use their power to control their environment. Shame and doubt appear when child is forced to be dependent in areas in which he/she has capability of control. Positive outcome is seen in sense of self-control and will-power.
3–6 years	**Preconventional: Instrumental Relativist Orientation** Behavioral decisions made based on concern or self and egocentric satisfaction, although may occasionally do something to please another if there are advantages for self.	**Phallic** Primary body zone: genital area Activities: genital exploration, fantasy Major conflict: Oedipal complex Interpersonal focus: attraction to opposite-sex parent, identification with same-sex parent	**Initiative vs. Guilt** Child uses his/her senses and power to explore physical world and imagine a fantasy world. Conscience is developed as child starts to respond to an inner voice. Guilt arises when child undertakes activities that are in conflict with goals of others. Positive outcome is seen in direction and purpose.
6–11 years	**Conventional: Interpersonal Concordance Orient.** Behavioral decisions based on desire to gain approval from others; judgments made based on intentions. **Conventional: Law and Order Orientation** Behavioral decisions based on laws and respect for authority; laws take precedence over personal wishes.	**Latency** Primary body zone: none Activities: social relationships, mastery over impulses Major conflict: none Interpersonal focus: identification with same-sex peers and powerful heroes	**Industry vs. Inferiority** Child works toward completion of activities and tasks and achieving a sense of accomplishment and mastery. He/she becomes a rule-learner and works cooperatively and competitively with others. Inferiority arises when more is expected than the child can achieve. Positive outcome is seen in sense of competence.
12–18 years	**Postconventional: Social Contract Legalistic** Morality based on personal values; people must work to change laws that are not moral or just. **Postconventional: Universal Ethical Principle** Morality based on internalized ideals and conscience rather than social rules; universal principles of what is just.	**Genital** Primary body zone: genitals Activities: sexual maturity and expression Major conflict: separation from family Interpersonal focus: successful extrafamilial relationships	**Identity vs. Role Confusion** Child becomes pre-occupied with physical appearance, how he/she is seen by others, role he/she plays, and how his/her concepts and values mesh with those of peers and society. Role confusion occurs when child is unable to solve conflicts between concept of self and society. Positive outcome is seen in sense of fidelity to values and other people.

Figure 2-2   Developmental Theory

Source: Adapted from Dixon & Stein (1992), pp. 15–25 and Murray & Zentner (1993), pp. 159–166.

PRINCIPLE 1: Growth and development are orderly and sequential and proceed along a predictable course governed by the maturing brain. Monitoring the sequence of a child's developmental milestones characterizes developmental maturation.

PRINCIPLE 2: The pace of growth and development is specific for each child. This is a key principle when providing anticipatory guidance to parents regarding acquisition of developmental milestones. It is critical to understand that children mature at different rates; some children demonstrate early motor skills, while others acquire early language skills.

PRINCIPLE 3: Development occurs in a cephalocaudal, or head-to-toe, direction, and proximodistal development proceeds from the body's midline to the periphery. For example, a baby first develops head control, then trunk control (sitting), and finally control of the lower extremities (walking). Second, primitive reflexes (such as the Moro, grasp, and rooting reflexes) are normally present in the term infant and diminish over the next 4 to 6 months. The postural reflexes (such as the positive support, plantar, propping, and parachute reflexes) emerge at 3 to 8 months.

PRINCIPLE 4: Developmental abilities become increasingly integrated, organized, and differentiated. The infant's cry is different when hungry than when ill, and the school-age child responds in a specific way to the teacher in a classroom. Simple skills and behaviors become integrated, organized, and differentiated as the child matures.

Stages and age ranges of human development are as follows:

Stage	Age
Infant	Birth to 1 year
Toddler	1 to 3 years
Preschooler	3 to 6 years
School age	6 to 12 years
Adolescent	12 to 19 years

Infants (Birth to 1 Year)

Perceptual–motor development are two aspects of growth that function together in allowing children to become aware of their surroundings. Children gain information through their senses (i.e., taste, sound, touch, sight, and smell), and as they develop they learn to organize and interpret their perceptions. The child's weight will double by 6 months and triple by 1 year.

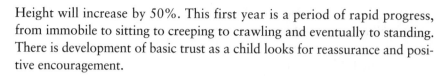

Height will increase by 50%. This first year is a period of rapid progress, from immobile to sitting to creeping to crawling and eventually to standing. There is development of basic trust as a child looks for reassurance and positive encouragement.

Toddlers (1–3 Years)

The toddler stage is characterized by growth, *locomotive skills, fantasy, language development*, and *self-control*. During this stage, toddlers learn to walk, talk, solve problems, and relate to others. The characteristic behavior of this developmental stage is *activity*. Children learn to gain control over their bodily movements and learn to integrate sensory information.

One major task for the toddler is learning to be independent, which is why toddlers want to do things for themselves, have their own ideas about how things should happen, and use "no" many, many times. This period is also referred to as "the terrible twos," a period of frustration for the child as well as the parent. Toddlers often display frustration through temper tantrums because they do not have the language skills to express themselves. The focus of play becomes increasingly symbolic. The child moves from reality (using blocks to build a tower) to object fantasy (pretending to be a robot). They are bursting with energy and ideas, need to explore their environment, and begin defining themselves as separate people. They want to be independent and yet they are still very dependent. They have difficulty separating themselves from their parents and other people who are important to them. Usually between 2.5 and 3 years of age, children begin to take an interest in toilet training, and by age 3 years they are ready to be known as preschoolers. By this age, most children are toilet trained, although they may not be fully trained until 4 or 5 years. They gradually begin taking an active interest in the world around them. *Remember that all toddlers are different and reach the various stages of development at different times.*

Preschoolers (3–6 Years)

During this period, children become slimmer as the lower body lengthens. They no longer have the protruding stomach, round face, and disproportionately short limbs and large head that are characteristic of the toddler. Preschoolers gain 4.5 lbs. per year and add almost 3 inches in height. The average weight and height are pretty much the same, approximately 40 lbs. and 42 inches. The brain has attained 90% of its adult weight. Concentration improves, and they have increased language and memory, and thus an increased desire and capacity to learn. Their motor skills improve to hopping, standing on one foot, kicking a ball and throwing a ball overhand, and going up and down stairs without support. Their fine motor skills improve to using a fork and spoon, coloring, and drawing. This developmental period is characterized by psychosocial and behavioral development that progresses to preschool readiness. It is during the end of this period that they recognize letters and learn to read.

School-Age Children (6–12 Years)

During the early part of this period, girls and boys are approximately the same in size, but toward the end of the school-age years, girls are beginning to surpass boys in both height and weight. There are major increases in strength and improvements in coordination, although muscles are still functionally immature as compared with those of the adolescent. With these changes comes a growing sense of competence and interest in participating in sports, gymnastics, and other physical activities. During this period, the school environment has significant impact on development and relationships. *The major developmental achievement of this period is the development of concrete operational thought and self-efficacy—the knowledge of what to do and the ability to do it.* As cognitive skills grow, children mature in their ability to understand the world and those around them. Children become more independent as their affections change from family to teachers and peer groups. At the same time, their need for positive relationships enforces their sense of self-esteem and self-worth.

Adolescents (12–19 Years)

Adolescence is the transition between childhood and adulthood and is one of the most dynamic stages of development. It is accompanied by dramatic physical, cognitive, social, and emotional changes. During this period, children undergo rapid changes in body size and shape, physiology, and social parameters. The transition from childhood to adulthood is controlled by hormones in conjunction with social structure.

There are three distinct periods of adolescence: early, middle, and late. Each period is characterized by biologic, psychological, and social issues. These three stages are experienced by most teens, although the age at which each stage is reached varies from child to child. These different rates of maturation are dependent upon physical development and hormone balance.

Medical History

The health history of the pediatric patient is similar in many ways to that of the adult, although the child's development as well as social and cognitive skills are key elements that are always taken into consideration. The following is an outline for a complete initial pediatric health history.

SUBJECTIVE INFORMATION

This information is received directly from the parent or in conjunction with the patient, and it is written in the patient's own words. It is a description and interpretation of the child's current situation based on the child's developmental level, cultural background, past experiences, and emotional attitude. This information establishes why the child has come for a visit and includes the name of the historian, if other than the mother, and the primary language spoken.

Chief Complaint

The chief complaint is the reason for the visit (e.g., well-child care, routine yearly physical exam, or sick visit). Often included in the chief complaint are the parental concerns," which focus on questions that the parents or child has at this visit. These concerns may be approached by asking, "What are you worried about the most?" or "Why does that worry you?" or "What brings you here today?" If specific issues are brought up, questions associated with them need to be addressed (history of present illness, or HPI). They include identification of the following:

- Date of onset
- Chronology
- Symptoms and signs, and their intensity
- Associated manifestations
- Interference with ADLs
- Measures that alleviate or exacerbate the problem
- Medications currently being used or used in the past to treat the problem
- Past history of the problem
- Whether anyone else in the child's family or environment has this problem
- Most importantly, the parent's opinion of what is going on or what he or she thinks is wrong with the child

Remember, the parent is, in most cases, the most familiar with the child and usually has a good sense of when something is wrong, when the child is not acting as usual, or when something is developing. Parents will often comment that their child just is not him or herself, but they "cannot identify what is wrong." The child may be more quiet than usual or less interactive, or the child's appetite may be slightly off.

Interval History

What has happened since you last saw the child? For example, have there been any accidents that required emergency department visits, illnesses that required hospitalization or extended school absenteeism, or exposure to communicable disease? An interval history can also focus on psychosocial issues, such as the death of a family member, pet, or relative. It may also address a change in the household, such as a divorce or marriage, or a change in family structure.

Past Medical History

IMMUNIZATIONS: This information is usually recorded in an immunization booklet.

Included is the date of the most recent purified protein derivative (PPD) test (for TB) and the response. Lead levels are also recorded in this booklet, as well as height and weight.

ACCIDENTS: Ask about accidents or injuries, when they occurred, and the treatment required and/or sequelae.

HOSPITALIZATIONS: Ask about admittance to the hospital as well as the reason and length of time hospitalized.

ILLNESSES: Illnesses include communicable diseases, chronic illnesses (e.g., asthma, diabetes), and psychiatric illnesses. Note age of onset, treatment, complications, and special testing.

ALLERGIES: Ask about drug, food, and environmental allergens and the reaction the child experiences. For example, does the child have a peanut allergy, develop urticaria, carry an EpiPen, or have environmental allergies?

MEDICATIONS: Ask about any prescribed medications, including dose, frequency, and time last taken. Also consider over-the-counter medications and homeopathic remedies.

PRENATAL HISTORY: Consider the age of the mother, her pregnancy history (gravida, para, abortus), maternal illnesses during pregnancy, and the presence of elevated blood pressure, glycosuria, proteinuria, and bleeding during pregnancy. Also consider the mother's history of infections (type and treatment), swelling of hands and feet, nausea, vomiting, excessive or inadequate weight gain, chronic illnesses, and medications (including prenatal vitamins and iron supplements). Ask about prenatal smoking (amount and frequency), alcohol intake (amount and frequency), and use of street drugs, such as cocaine, heroine, or cannabis (amount and frequency). Was the pregnancy planned? What was the mother's attitude toward pregnancy? The father's? Document prenatal care, including provider and regularity of prenatal care, special tests done during pregnancy, and prenatal caution and preparation.

LABOR AND DELIVERY: Determine the mother's attitude toward her labor and delivery experience. Ask about the onset of labor, how long it took, how it progressed, the degree of discomfort, supportive persons available, medications given during labor, anesthesia used, fetal monitoring, rupture of membranes, type of delivery (e.g., breech, vertex, cesarean section), use of forceps, episiotomy, and use of special equipment.

POSTNATAL HISTORY: Document the infant's weight and length, and status at birth (Apgar score). Ask if there were any problems with the baby at birth (special care nursery) and if the mother saw and held the baby immediately. Consider both the mother's and the infant's hospital course. *Mother:* history of fever, infections, engorgement, heavy bleeding. *Infant:* history of infection, jaundice, respiratory problems (blue spells), patterns of crying, feeding concerns, type of feeding, concerns with breast-feeding. Ask if the baby went home from the hospital with the mother, and try to determine the mother's perception of the infant.

FAMILY HISTORY: Determine the family's genogram, including age of parents and grandparents (on both sides) and the medical history of parents, grandparents, siblings, aunts, uncles, and first cousins. Look specifically for cardiac disease, hypertension, cancer, alcohol abuse, mental retardation or cognitive impairment, psychiatric illness, sickle cell disease, birth defects, diabetes, renal problems, thyroid problems, and attention-deficit disorder (ADD) or attention-deficit/hyperactivity disorder (ADHD).

SOCIAL HISTORY: Consider the child's living arrangements, the number of people living in the house, the child's primary caregiver, the family situation and dynamics, other children in the home, the size of the home, the physical environmental (e.g., neighborhood type, street type), the child's health insurance, parents' employment, education of parents, plans for mother to return to school or work, day-care arrangements, emotional support from family, the father's involvement with the baby, and any social agencies involved with the family.

Activities of Daily Living

Obtain a description of a typical day for the child.

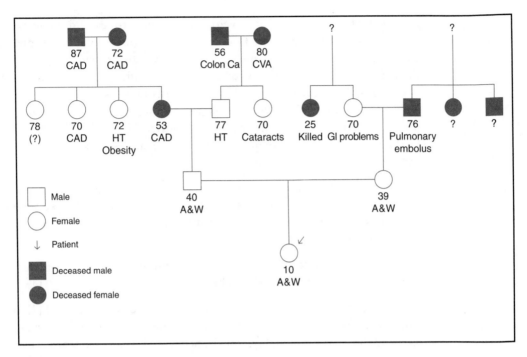

Figure 2-3 Genogram

NUTRITION: Is the child breast- or bottle-feeding (amounts and frequency), using a breast pump, spitting up, consuming other liquids (e.g., water, juice)? Is the child eating solids (types and amounts), and what is the frequency and method of introducing food? Is the child given a bottle at bedtime? *For older children*, obtain a 24-hour recall of the usual diet, including breakfast, lunch, dinner, and snacks. Consider milk, soda, and junk food intake; method of feeding; use of utensils; appetite; history of problems or sensitivities; allergies; favorite and least favorite foods; and school diet.

SLEEP: What is the child's bedtime hour and awakening hour? Does the child sleep in a crib, in his or her own room, with the mother (and if so, who else besides the mother and baby sleep in the room)? Determine whether the child receives a bottle during the night, and if so the frequency and purpose; whether the child naps during the day, and if so the frequency and duration; and whether the child experiences night terrors, nightmares, or otherwise difficult bedtime.

ELIMINATION: Ask about bowel movements, consistency, frequency, character, constipation, use of laxatives, toilet training, diapers, urine frequency, enuresis, and encopresis.

DEVELOPMENT: Ask about developmental milestones and when were they were achieved (e.g., held head erect, rolled over, sat without support, crawled, stood, walked alone, spoke in single words or sentences). Obtain the parental impression of growth and development, specific milestones in comparison with the child's siblings, concerns about sibling rivalry, and child's temperament. The Denver Developmental Screening Test (DDST) is used for infants, toddlers, and preschool children. The M-CHAT (Modified Checklist for Autism in Toddlers) is currently being used in many states to test for autism spectrum disorders.

SCHOOL: Document the child's grade in school, achievements, attendance, and whether he or she gets along with peers. Does the child like school or have issues with teachers or other students? Are there concerns about ADD/ADHD?

SPORTS: Document team participation, interest in sports, and extracurricular activities in school and after school.

PERSONALITY AND BEHAVIOR: Ask the parent to describe the child ("How would you describe your child?"), and ask about the method of discipline used and the child's personality, moods, behavioral issues, and temperament.

Screenings

Consider the following notes when screening:

- Height and weight are plotted on the growth chart for routine health visits. Evaluate the parents, keeping in mind that tall parents tend to have tall children.
- Head circumference is measured until 2 years of age and plotted on the growth chart for routine health visits. Always check the parents' head if the child's head circumference is above or below the normal percentile. Ask the parent if he or she has concerns about the child's head size, explaining that if the parent has a large head, the child may have a large head as well.
- Vision screen is performed yearly.
- Hearing screen is performed yearly.
- Lead screen is monitored yearly until 6 years of age. It may be done more frequently if there are specific concerns.
- Hematocrit is performed yearly.
- TB screen (PPD test) is planned if the child meets established criteria.

Review of Systems

The ROS is a thorough checklist of questions about recent symptoms and the child's health status since his or her previous physical examination, generally within the past year. In pediatrics, the ROS is asked of the accompanying parent; in school-age children and adolescents, the questions should be addressed to the child as well. If the parent or child states that some symptoms are present, it is helpful to elicit additional information to explore the problem further and determine a chief complaint. This information includes duration, frequency, intensity, time course, other specifics about the symptom(s), associated factors, and results of treatment.

It is helpful when introducing this part of the history to preface your ROS by stating that you will be asking many questions of both the parent and the child to find out how the child has been within the past year.

GENERAL HEALTH AND GROWTH: Ask the parent how he or she would describe the child's usual state of health. What is the parent's assessment of the child's growth and development, weight loss or gain, and general energy level, and has the child had any illnesses within the past month?

SKIN: Assess for dry or oily skin, rashes, diaper rash, birthmarks, mottling, urticaria, hives, pruritus, bruising, petechiae, pallor, lesions, changes in skin pigmentation, acne, sun protection.

HAIR AND NAILS: Assess for changes in appearance and texture of nails, nail biting, changes in amount and texture of hair, alopecia, or hirsutism.

HEAD: Ask about headaches (and frequency), head injury, and dizziness.

EYES: Assess for strabismus, diplopia, pain, redness, discharge, eyeglasses/ contact lenses, date of previous vision screening, history of infection, pruritus, tearing, cataracts, ability to see the board at school, problems reading, and whether sitting too close to the television.

EARS: Ask about ear infections (and frequency), tympanostomy tubes, discharge (and character), cerumen, the parent's or child's method of cleaning the ears, tinnitus, and concerns about hearing problems.

NOSE AND SINUSES: Ask about the frequency of colds, discharge (and character), epistaxes, allergies, mouth breathing, and snoring.

MOUTH AND THROAT: Assess the frequency of sore throats, presence of tonsils, presence of sores on the tongue or mucous membranes, teeth brushing, presence of dental caries, date of previous dental exam, orthodontia, difficulty swallowing, hoarseness, use of pacifier, thumb sucking, and drooling.

NECK: Assess for stiffness or difficulty in movement and swollen or tender glands.

RESPIRATORY: Is there a history of croup, asthma (triggers and frequency), shortness of breath, wheezing, chronic cough, pneumonia, upper respiratory infection (frequency)?

CARDIOVASCULAR: Assess for congenital heart problems, history of heart murmurs, exercise intolerance, dyspnea on exertion, palpitations, high blood pressure, and coolness or cyanosis in extremities.

GASTROINTESTINAL: Assess for abdominal pain; diarrhea; vomiting; pica; food intolerance; stool pattern, frequency, color, and characteristics; constipation; encopresis; history of pinworms or parasites; rectal bleeding or itching; flatus; colic; and painful defecation.

GENITOURINARY: Ask about toilet training, enuresis, urinating in straight stream, polyuria/oliguria, urine color, history of urinary tract infections, dysuria, and urgency.

FEMALE GENITALS: Has young girl noted genital itching, vaginal discharge (color and odor), or rash? Screen for sexual abuse of the preadolescent/adolescent: knowledge of pubertal changes, menarche (date and age, interval, duration, amount), dysmenorrhea, date of most recent menses, history of STDs, contraception, most recent gynecologic exam (if appropriate).

MALE GENITALS: Has young boy reported penis or testicular pain, testes descended bilaterally, discharge from penis, hernia, hydrocele or swelling in scrotum, or history of phimosis? Screen for sexual abuse of the preadolescent/adolescent: knowledge of pubertal changes, changes in testicular or penis size, nocturnal emissions, history of STD or STD screen, use of contraception.

MUSCULOSKELETAL: Assess for bone or joint pain, swelling, tenderness, redness, and weakness. Assess limitation of range of motion, gait strength and coordination, posture, feet (positioning), muscle tone, balance, and walking or crawling. Screen for scoliosis.

NEUROLOGIC: Is there a history of seizures, numbness, or tingling? (Appropriate attainment of developmental milestones, decline in developmental milestones.) (Behavioral issues are covered under ADLs.) If new onset of headaches, needs detailed history. Are there changes from the child's normal behavior?

HEMATOLOGIC: Assess for anemia, pallor, unusual bleeding, frequent epistaxes, blood in stool, easy bruising, enlarged lymph nodes, transfusions (and dates), and exposure to radiation or toxic agents.

ENDOCRINE: Are there changes in weight or growth pattern?

- Thyroid: masses in neck (goiter) sweating, heat or cold intolerance, changes in activity level, skin texture, changes in bowel habits
- Diabetes mellitus: polyphagia, polydypsia, polyuria, enuresis, weight loss, change in temperament
- Pituitary: growth pattern changes (especially growth rate), delayed sexual maturation or precocious puberty

PSYCHOLOGICAL: Assess for changes in mood or affect; difficulty in relationships with family, peers, or authority figures; depression; irritability; sleep disturbance; unusual eating behavior; phobias; hostility; destructive behavior; change in school performance; and enuresis or encopresis in previously continent child.

References

Cech, D., Martin, S. (2002). *Functional movement development across the life span.* Philadelphia: WB Saunders.

CDC website CDC.gov/nhanes/growthcharts

Potts, N., Mandleco, B. (2007). *Pediatric nursing.* (2nd Ed.). Australia: Thomson Delmar Learning.

Resources

Ball, J.W., Bindler, R. (2008). *Pediatric nursing,* (4th ed.). Upper Saddle River, NJ: Prentice Hall.

Bickley, L., (2003). *Bates guide to physical examination and history taking,* (8th ed.). New York: Lippincott.

Bright Futures. (2001). Education Center of the American Academy of Pediatrics (3rd ed.).

Burns, C., Dunn, A., Brady, M., Starr, N., Blosser, C. (2001). *Pediatric primary care: A handbook for nurse practitioners,* (3rd ed.). St Louis, MO: Saunders.

Colyar, M. (2003). *Well-child assessment for primary care providers.* Philadelphia: EA Davis Company.

Dixon, S., Stein, M. (2000). *Encounters with children, pediatric behavior and development* (3rd ed.). St. Louis, MO: Mosby.

Goldbloom, R. (2003). *Pediatric clinical skills,* New York: Churchill Livingston.

Hoekelman, R., Adam, H., Nelson, N. Weitzman, M. (2001). *Primary Pediatric Care,* St. Louis, MO: Mosby.

Jarvis, C. (2004). *Physical examination & health assessment,* 5th ed. St. Louis, MO: Elsevier.

Assessment Techniques and Vital Signs

Physical Examination

The physical examination is an evaluation of the body and its functions using the assessment techniques of inspection, palpation, percussion, and auscultation.

The following is a description of physical assessment techniques used in the assessment of each body system.

Assessment Techniques

A good rule of thumb, particularly when examining a young child, is to progress from the least intrusive area to the most intrusive. For example, listen to the lung sounds first and save the ear exam for last. Although assessment that causes discomfort or fear should be performed last, particularly when examining a toddler or even a fearful school-age child, the best approach is "seize the opportunity" and obtain that part of the exam to get what you can at the moment. This means that if you have a sleeping baby, listen to the heart and lungs while the patient is quiet. If the parent is holding the toddler on his

TABLE 3-1   SUMMARY OF AGES AND STAGES DEVELOPMENTAL THEORIES

Stage/Age	Piaget's Cognitive Stages	Freud's Psychosexual Stages	Erikson's Psychosocial Stages	Kohlberg's Moral Judgment Stages
1. Infancy Birth to 1 year	**Sensorimotor** (birth to 2 years): begins to acquire language Task: Object permanence	**Oral:** pleasure from exploration with mouth and through sucking Task: Weaning	**Trust vs. Mistrust** Task: Trust Socializing agent: Mothering person Central process: Mutuality Ego quality: Hope	**Preconventional Level:** 1. **Morality Stage:** Avoid punishment by not breaking rules of authority figures
2. Toddler 1 to 3 years	**Sensorimotor** continues **Preoperational** (2 to 7 years begins): use of representational thought Task: Use language and mental images to think and communicate	**Anal:** control of elimination Task: Toilet training	**Autonomy vs. Shame and Doubt** Task: Autonomy Socializing agent: Parents Central process: Imitation Ego quality: Self-control and willpower	
3. Preschool 3 to 6 years	**Preoperational** continues	**Phallic:** attracted to opposite-sex parent Task: Resolve Oedipus/ Electra complex	**Initiative vs. Guilt** Task: Initiative and moral responsibility Socializing agents: Parents Central process: Identification Ego quality: Direction, purpose, and conscience	2. **Individualism, Instrumental Purpose, and Exchange Stage:** "Right" is relative, follow rules when in own interest

TABLE 3-1 SUMMARY OF AGES AND STAGES DEVELOPMENTAL THEORIES *(continued)*

Stage/Age	Piaget's Cognitive Stages	Freud's Psychosexual Stages	Erikson's Psychosocial Stages	Kohlberg's Moral Judgment Stages
4. School Age 6 to 12 years	**Preoperational** continues **Concrete Operations** (7 to 12 years) begins: engage in inductive reasoning and concrete problem solving Task: Learn concepts of conservation and reversibility	**Latency:** identification with same-sex parent Task: Identify with same-sex parent and test and compare own capabilities with peer norms	**Industry vs. Inferiority** Task: Industry, self-assurance, self-esteem Socializing agents: Teachers and peers Central process: Education Ego quality: Competence	**Conventional Level:** **3. Mutual Expectations, Relationships, and Conformity to Moral Norms Stage:** Need to be "good" in own and others' eyes, believe in rules and regulations
5. Adolescence 12 to 18 years	**Formal Operations** (12 years to adulthood): engage in abstract reasoning and analytical problem solving Task: Develop a workable philosophy of life	**Genital:** develop sexual relationships Task: Establish meaningful relationship for lifelong pairing	**Identity vs. Role Confusion** Task: Self-identity and concept Socializing agents: Society of peers Central process: Role experimentation and peer pressure Ego quality: Fidelity and devotion to others, personal and sociocultural values	**4. Social System and Conscience Stage:** Uphold laws because they are fixed social duties

(continues)

TABLE 3-1 SUMMARY OF AGES AND STAGES DEVELOPMENTAL THEORIES *(continued)*				
Stage/Age	Piaget's Cognitive Stages	Freud's Psychosexual Stages	Erikson's Psychosocial Stages	Kohlberg's Moral Judgment Stages
6. Young Adult 18 to 30 years	**Formal Operations** continue		**Intimacy vs. Isolation** Task: Intimacy Socializing agent: Close friends, partners, lovers, spouse Central process: Mutuality among peers Ego quality: Intimate affiliation and love	**Postconventional Level:** **5. Social Contract or Utility and Individual Rights Stage:** Uphold laws in the interest of the greatest good for the greatest number; uphold laws that protect universal rights
7. Early Middle Age 30 to 50 years			**Generativity vs. Stagnation** (30 to 65 years) Task: Generativity. Socializing agent: Spouse, partner, children, sociocultural norms Central process: Creativity and person-environment fit Ego quality: Productivity, perseverence, charity, and consideration	
8. Late Middle Age 50 to 70 years			**Generativity vs. Stagnation** continues	
9. Late Adult 70 years to death			**Ego Integrity vs. Despair** (65 years to death) Task: Ego integrity Socializing agent: Significant others Central process: Introspection Ego quality: Wisdom	**6. Universal Ethical Principles Stage:** Support universal moral principles regardless of the price for doing so

Source: Ball, Jane W.; Bindler, Ruth C.; Cowen, Kay J., Child Health Nursing: Partnering With Children and Families, 2nd ©2010. Printed and Electronically reproduced by permission of Pearson Education, Inc., Upper Saddle River, New Jersey.

or her lap, approach the child slowly, letting the child explore your stethoscope, and then start from a distal point, gradually moving more proximal (i.e., start on the leg or arm and gradually move closer to the area to be auscultated). Often, allowing the child to hold the diaphragm of the stethoscope and putting your hand over the child's allows you to move from location to location. This provides the child with some control, decreases the child's fear, and allows you to listen to lung and cardiac sounds.

The goal of your examination is to increase the comfort level of the child, which in turns allows you to perform a more comprehensive exam. Although you are doing a routine examination, your patient does not consider it routine. During this time, focusing on developmental principles and approaches is important. If one approach does not work, try something else. Remember, when performing a physical exam, the child's developmental stage as well as social and cognitive skills are more meaningful than the child's exact chronological age. For example, a child who is prepubescent or in the early stages of puberty, when his or her body is changing, has a strong sense of modesty. Allow the child to decide whether their parent should be present during the exam. A younger adolescent may feel more comfortable and secure with a parent in the room, whereas an older adolescent prefers the independence of being examined without a parent present.

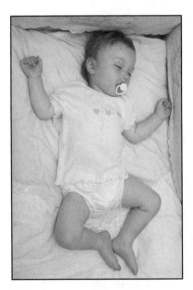

Figure 3-1   Proximdistal growth

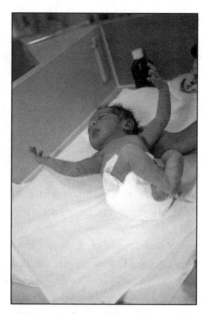

Figure 3-2 The Moro Reflex

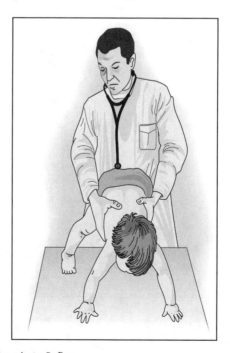

Figure 3-3 The Parachute Reflex

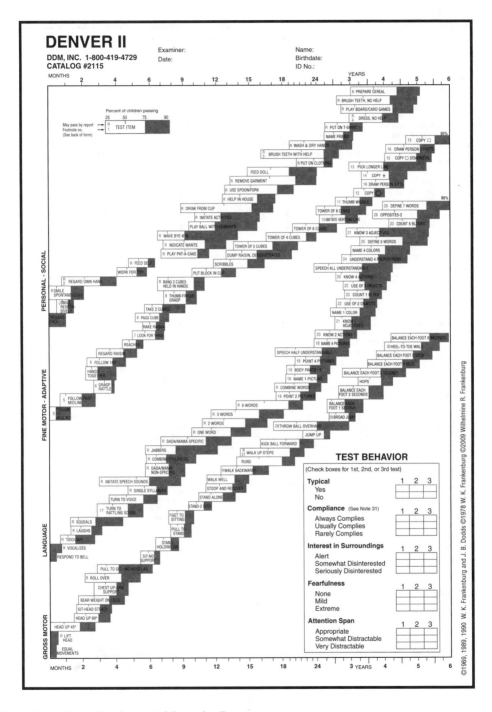

Figure 3-4 Denver Developmental Screening Test

DIRECTIONS FOR ADMINISTRATION

1. Try to get child to smile by smiling, talking or waving. Do not touch him/her.
2. Child must stare at hand several seconds.
3. Parent may help guide toothbrush and put toothpaste on brush.
4. Child does not have to be able to tie shoes or button/zip in the back.
5. Move yarn slowly in an arc from one side to the other, about 8" above child's face.
6. Pass if child grasps rattle when it is touched to the backs or tips of fingers.
7. Pass if child tries to see where yarn went. Yarn should be dropped quickly from sight from tester's hand without arm movement.
8. Child must transfer cube from hand to hand without help of body, mouth, or table.
9. Pass if child picks up raisin with any part of thumb and finger.
10. Line can vary only 30 degrees or less from tester's line.
11. Make a fist with thumb pointing upward and wiggle only the thumb. Pass if child imitates and does not move any fingers other than the thumb.

12. Pass any enclosed form. Fail continuous round motions.
13. Which line is longer? (Not bigger.) Turn paper upside down and repeat. (pass 3 of 3 or 5 of 6)
14. Pass any lines crossing near midpoint.
15. Have child copy first. If failed, demonstrate.

When giving items 12, 14, and 15, do not name the forms. Do not demonstrate 12 and 14.

16. When scoring, each pair (2 arms, 2 legs, etc.) counts as one part.
17. Place one cube in cup and shake gently near child's ear, but out of sight. Repeat for other ear.
18. Point to picture and have child name it. (No credit is given for sounds only.)
    If less than 4 pictures are named correctly, have child point to picture as each is named by tester.

19. Using doll, tell child: Show me the nose, eyes, ears, mouth, hands, feet, tummy, hair. Pass 6 of 8.
20. Using pictures, ask child: Which one flies?...says meow?...talks?...barks?...gallops? Pass 2 of 5, 4 of 5.
21. Ask child: What do you do when you are cold?...tired?...hungry? Pass 2 of 3, 3 of 3.
22. Ask child: What do you do with a cup? What is a chair used for? What is a pencil used for?
    Action words must be included in answers.
23. Pass if child correctly places <u>and</u> says how many blocks are on paper. (1,5).
24. Tell child: Put block **on** table; **under** table; **in front of** me, **behind** me. Pass 4 of 4.
    (Do not help child by pointing, moving head or eyes.)
25. Ask child: What is a ball?...lake?...desk?...house?...banana?...curtain?...fence?...ceiling? Pass 5 of 8, 7 of 8.
    of use, shape, what it is made of, or general category (such as banana is fruit, not just yellow). Pass 5 of 8, 7 of 8.
26. Ask child: If a horse is big, a mouse is ___? If fire is hot, ice is ___? If the sun shines during the day, the moon shines during the ___? Pass 2 of 3.
27. Child may use wall or rail only, not person. May not crawl.
28. Child must throw ball overhand 3 feet to within arm's reach of tester.
29. Child must perform standing broad jump over width of test sheet (8 1/2 inches).
30. Tell child to walk forward, ⬤⬤⬤⬤➔ heel within 1 inch of toe. Tester may demonstrate.
    Child must walk 4 consecutive steps.
31. In the second year, half of normal children are non-compliant.

OBSERVATIONS:

Figure 3-4 Denver Developmental Screening Test *(continued)*

If the patient chooses to have his or her parent wait in the waiting room, reassure the parent that he or she may come back in as soon as the exam is over. If your patient is a 2-year-old and is looking at you with apprehension, reassure both the child and the parent that the child can sit on the parent's lap. This makes both the child and parent happy, as there is usually less crying and the child is more comfortable.

Four assessment techniques will be reviewed: inspection, palpation, percussion, and auscultation.

Inspection

Inspection is the first assessment technique used. It is considered concentrated watching with careful scrutiny of the patient as a whole, incorporating observation, appearance, symmetry, behavior, and size, shape, and color. Inspection begins the moment you meet your patient. It takes time and conscious observation to note the patient's appearance, symmetry of both sides of the body, and behavior. Inspection also may include respiratory status, skin tone, and odor. For example, if a child has streptococcal pharyngitis, the classic odor is easily recognized by the well-trained provider. Inspection of the patient should be unhurried. Pay attention to detail and take time when looking at each area of the child's body, noting gait, stance, behavior, speech, clothing, and interaction with the parent and with you. This information is very telling in the overall assessment.

Palpation

Palpation follows inspection and is defined as the "act of touching a patient in a therapeutic manner to elicit specific information." Touching the patient allows you to assess temperature, moisture, texture, rigidity, or spasticity of skin. It also allows you to assess organ size and location, swelling, and the presence of tenderness, lumps, or masses. When palpating, there are two distinct approaches: light and deep palpation.

Light palpation is used first to detect subtle characteristics and is performed in a delicate, gentle manner using the pads of the fingers. It adjusts the patient to being touched and to the feel of your hands. It is important to warm your hands before placing them on the patient and to have short fingernails for professionalism and also to avoid hurting the child.

Deep palpation is performed following light palpation to assess the position and size of organs (as well as masses), their mobility, and their consistency.

The following guidelines will help you with palpation:

(a)

(b)

(c)

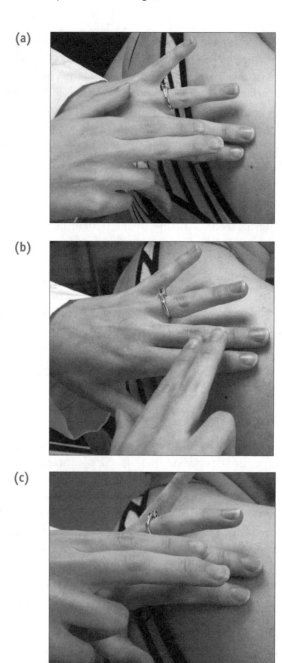

Figure 3-5 Percussion of the Posterior Thorax

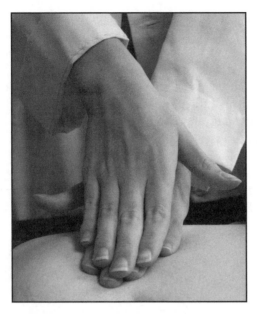

Figure 3-6 Palpation of Abdomen

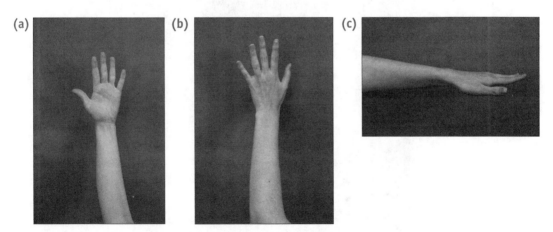

Figure 3-7 Parts of the Hand Used in Palpation
(a) Palmar surface; (b) Dorsal surface; (c) Ulnar surface

- Keep the fingers of your dominant hand together. Place the finger pads lightly on the skin over the area that is to be palpated. The hand and forearm will be on a plane parallel to the area being assessed.
- Depress the skin 1 cm in light, gentle circular motions.
- Keep the finger pads on the skin, and let the depressed body surface rebound to its natural position.
- Using a systematic approach, move the fingers to an adjacent area and repeat the process.
- Continue to move the finger pads until the entire area being examined has been palpated.
- If the patient has complained of tenderness in any area, palpate this area last. (Estes & Schaefer, p. 234.)

(a)

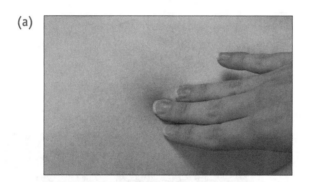

(b)

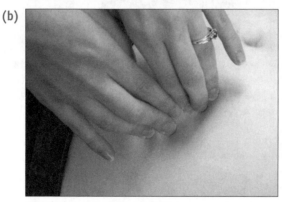

Figure 3-8 (a) Liver Palpation; (b) Hooking the Liver

Percussion

Percussion is the technique of tapping the patient's skin with short, sharp strokes using the middle finger of your dominant hand. Percussion can be difficult or awkward for new practitioners, but keeping your nails short and your hands relaxed helps to perfect this new skill. When percussing, the action is primarily in the wrist. The middle finger of your nondominant hand is pressed firmly against the skin. The middle finger of your dominant hand is used to tap briskly to the distal interphalangeal joint of the finger that is pressed firmly on the patient's skin. It is important to flex the tapping finger so that you are using the tip and not the pad of your finger. You percuss two to three times at each location. Remember, in children the body wall, such as the abdomen, may be thin with minimal muscle mass and or adipose tissue, so you do not have to be too forceful. If you are percussing an athletic adolescent, you may have to percuss a little stronger to produce adequate vibrations.

The sound waves produced are diagnostic of normal and abnormal findings, and indicate the density of the tissue being percussed. The waves are evaluated based on intensity, pitch, quality, and duration. The areas of the body most frequently percussed are the thorax and the abdomen. Percussion sounds are interpreted according to the sounds produced: *dullness*, *flatness*, *resonance*, hyperresonance, and *tympany*.

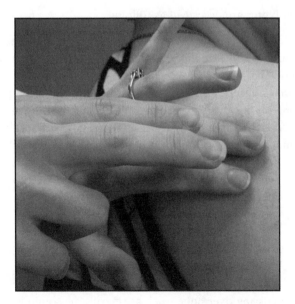

Figure 3-9   Percussion Technique: Tapping the Interphalangeal Joint.

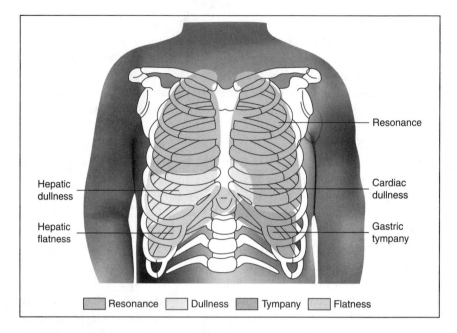

Figure 3-10 Example of Areas of Percussion

Source: This article was published in Mosby's Guide to Physical Examination, 6th edition, Seidel, Ball, Dains, and Benedict. Percussion technique, page 23. Copyright Elsevier (2006).

Percussion Notes are described as follows:

- *Tympanic* is described as intensity of loud, with a high pitch, moderate duration, drum-like quality, and heard best over the gastric bubble or in emphysematous lungs.
- *Resonant* is described as intensity of loud, with a low pitch, a long duration, a hollow quality and heard best over healthy lung tissue.
- *Dull* is described as soft to moderate intensity, with moderate to high pitch, moderate duration, thud like quality and heard best over the liver.
- *Flat* is described as soft with high pitch, short duration, very dull quality, and heard best over muscle.

Some of the common sounds associated with percussion are described as follows:

- When percussing over an organ, such as the liver, the sound produced is dull.
- When percussing over bone, such as the rib, the sound is flat.

- When percussing over an air-filled cavity, such as the lung, the sound is resonant.
- When percussing over the gastric air bubble in the upper stomach, the sound is tympanic.

Auscultation

Auscultation is the act of listening to sounds produced by the body. Sounds of importance are those of the thorax or lungs, the sounds produced in the abdominal viscera, and the sounds produced by the cardiovascular system. Most stethoscopes used today are acoustic ones that do not amplify body sounds and instead block out environmental sounds. The stethoscope has two listening heads, the bell and the diaphragm. The diaphragm is flat and transmits high-pitched sounds such as breath sounds and normal heart sounds. The bell is a concave cup that transmits low-pitched sounds such as certain heart murmurs and bruits.

When auscultating, a great deal of concentration is required, particularly when listening to the rapid heart sounds of an infant. It may be helpful to close your eyes, and be sure the room is quiet when focusing on specific body sounds. When using the diaphragm, place it firmly against the skin area to be

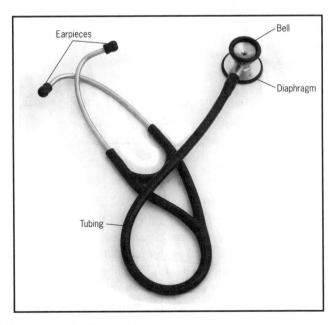

Figure 3-11 Acoustic Stethoscope

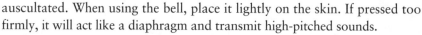

auscultated. When using the bell, place it lightly on the skin. If pressed too firmly, it will act like a diaphragm and transmit high-pitched sounds.

If you are purchasing a new stethoscope, the fit and quality are important. The slope of the earpiece should point forward toward your nose. This matches the natural slope of your ear canal and efficiently blocks out environmental sound. In addition, the earpieces should fit snugly. You can adjust the tension with different rubber or plastic earplugs until you achieve the most comfort. The tubing should have an internal diameter of 4 mm (0.125 in) and should be about 36 to 46 cm in length. The longer the tubing, the more distorted may be the sound.

The Assessment

After completion of the medical history and physical examination, both the subjective and objective assessments of the child are considered and a diagnosis is made based on these findings. If after your history and physical exam your diagnosis is a well child, the assessment is "well-child examination." If there are other age-specific medical problems, they should be listed under the assessment.

- *EXAMPLE*: Well-child examination: 2-year-old without problems
- *EXAMPLE*: Well-child examination: 5-year-old with problems
  - ➤ Dental caries
  - ➤ Eczema

The Plan

In a well-child visit, anticipatory guidance appropriate for each age would be included under the plan.

Measurement

Growth: Height and Weight

In pediatrics, serial somatic growth factors, which include height, weight, and head circumference are the most important indicators of a healthy child. Recognizing growth disorders as early as possible allows for better long-term prognosis and overall growth potential. Underlying diseases such as growth hormone deficiency (GHD) gastrointestinal disease, and hypothyroidism place a child at risk for growth disorder. Proper evaluation includes routine weight and height and plotting growth measurement on the growth chart. This provides you, as well as the parent, with a documented picture of the child's growth progress, and early recognition of abnormal growth. Deviation or abnormal growth patterns are often early warning signs of a pathologic process.

Safety in Infancy (0–1)

- Sleeping on back
- Smoke-free home, smoke detectors
- Water safety: buckets, bathtubs, and pools

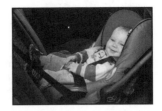

Safety in Early Childhood (1–5)

- Sunscreen and sun exposure
- Safe playgrounds and yards
- Car seats/booster seats/seat belts in back

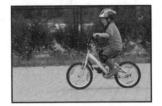

Safety in Middle Childhood (5–10)

- Dealing with strangers
- Fire safety
- Storing and locking guns

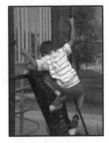

Safety in Adolescence (11–21)

- Alcohol, tobacco, and other drugs
- Safe dating, parties
- Physical, emotional, and sexual abuse

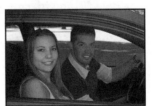

Figure 3-12 Examples of Anticipatory Guidance

Source: Adapted from Bright Futures Guidelines (3rd ed.). American Academy of Pediatrics, (AAP).

The use of growth charts was developed in 1977 by the National Center for Health Statistics (NCHS) as a tool specifically for health professionals to monitor children's growth. Serial recordings of growth are an indication of growth over time, and normal growth progresses along a certain percentile. In 2000, the CDC updated and revised the NCHS growth charts to be more reflective of height and weight of American children. The revised growth charts include body mass index (BMI) charts for children ages 2 to 20 years.

What is most important in recording a child's height, weight, and head circumference is that the child continues along a steady percentile over serial visits. Children should have periodic growth assessments at well-child visits. Infants should be weighed and measured at 2, 4, 6, 9, 12, 18, and 24 months during the first 2 years. Children older than 2 years should be monitored at least annually. Weight is additionally monitored during sick visits. If there is concern regarding either increased or delayed growth, measurements should be monitored more closely.

An important consideration is that growth variants are based on genetics and familial tendencies. An example of this is *constitutional growth delay* (CDG), which presents as a child that appears normal except for their short stature and often delayed puberty. Once puberty is reached, a normal growth spurt occurs and final adult height and sexual maturation occur. Questioning the parent about his or her own growth pattern while growing up can be reassuring to the child as he or she can see that they will attain normal growth, or that similar to their parent.

Figures 3-13 through **3-18** offer examples of growth charts.

Body Mass Index

In 1994, an expert committee of the American Academy of Pediatrics (AAP) developed guidelines for overweight adolescents and recommended that BMI be used routinely to screen for overweight in adolescents. In 1997, a committee on the assessment and treatment of childhood obesity concluded that BMI should be used to screen for childhood obesity. Eventually, the CDC and the AAP recommended the use of BMI to screen for overweight and obesity in children and adolescents ages 2–19 years.

For children, BMI is used to screen for obesity, overweight, healthy weight, or underweight. However, BMI is not a diagnostic tool. For example, a child may have a high BMI for age and sex, but to determine if excess fat is a problem, you would need to measure skin-fold thickness, evaluate diet activity, take a family history, and perform other appropriate health screenings. For children and teens, BMI is specific to age and sex, and is referred to as BMI for age (CDC, 2009).

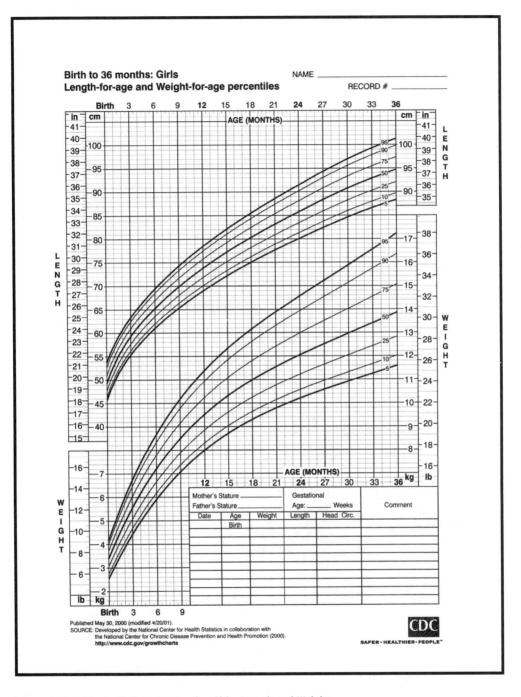

Figure 3-13 Chart, Birth to 36 Months: Girls, Length and Weight

Source: Developed by the National Center for Health Statistics in collaboration with the National Center for Chronic Disease Prevention and Health Promotion (2000). http://www.cdc.gov/growthcharts.

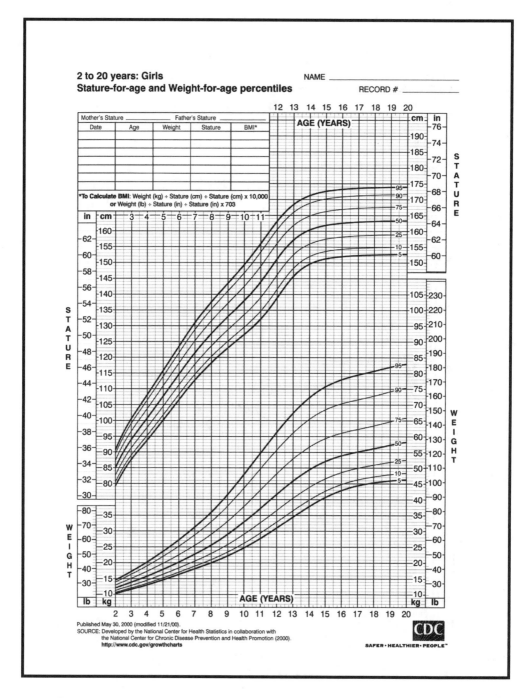

Figure 3-14 Chart, 2 to 20 Years: Girls' Stature for Age and Weight for Age Percentiles

Source: Developed by the National Center for Health Statistics in collaboration with the National Center for Chronic Disease Prevention and Health Promotion (2000). http://www.cdc.gov/growthcharts.

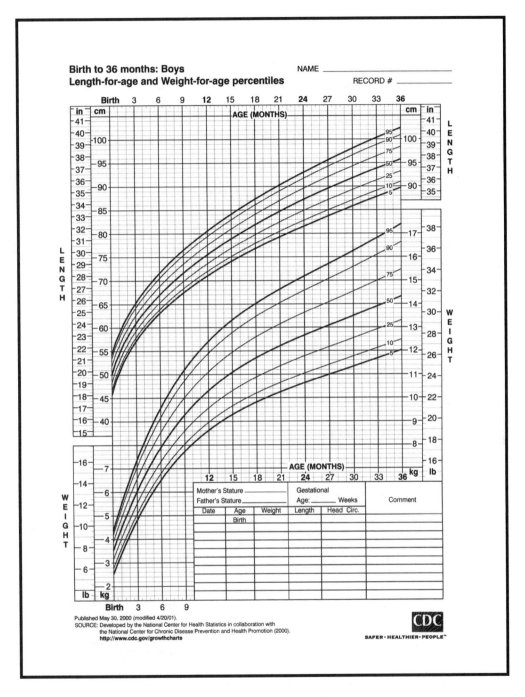

Figure 3-15   Chart, Birth to 36 Months: Boys, Length for Age Weight for Age Percentiles

Source: Developed by the National Center for Health Statistics in collaboration with the National Center for Chronic Disease Prevention and Health Promotion (2000). http://www.cdc.gov/growthcharts.

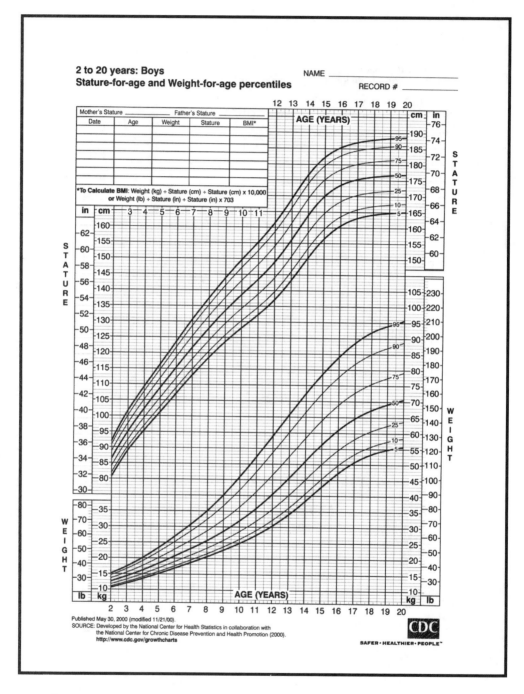

Figure 3-16 Chart, 2 to 20 Years: Boys' Stature for Age and Weight for Age Percentiles

Source: Developed by the National Center for Health Statistics in collaboration with the National Center for Chronic Disease Prevention and Health Promotion (2000). http://www.cdc.gov/growthcharts.

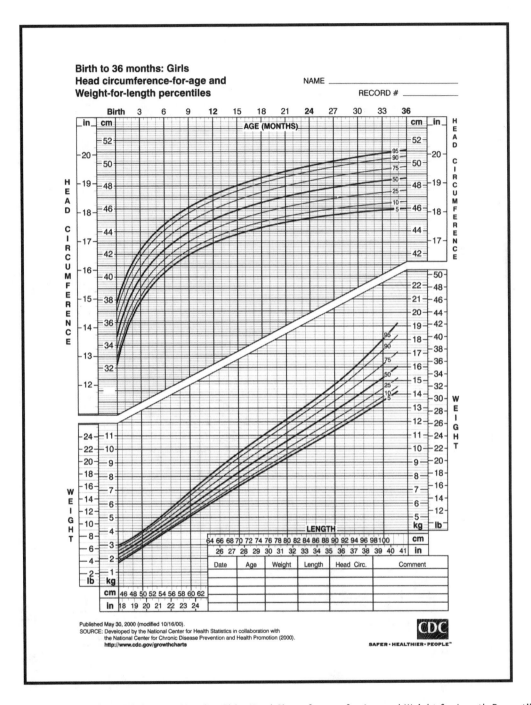

Figure 3-17 Chart, Birth to 36 Months: Girls, Head Circumference for Age and Weight for Length Percentiles

Source: Developed by the National Center for Health Statistics in collaboration with the National Center for Chronic Disease Prevention and Health Promotion (2000). http://www.cdc.gov/growthcharts.

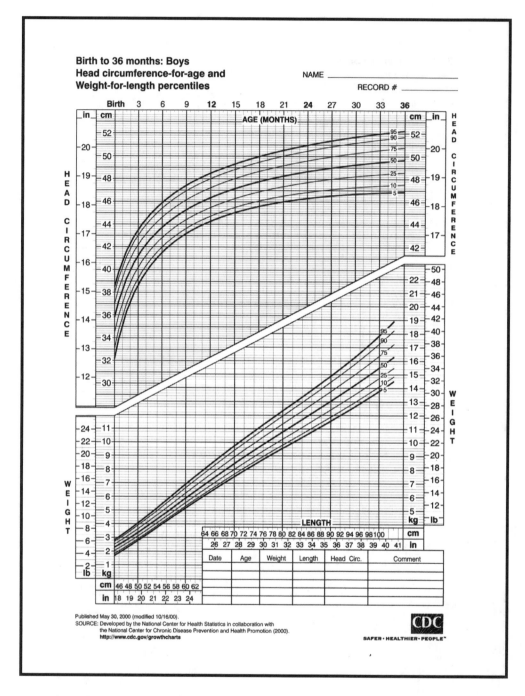

Figure 3-18 Chart, Birth to 36 Months: Boys, Head Circumference for Age and Weight for Length Percentiles

Source: Developed by the National Center for Health Statistics in collaboration with the National Center for Chronic Disease Prevention and Health Promotion (2000). http://www.cdc.gov/growthcharts.

After the BMI is calculated for children and teens, the BMI number is plotted on the appropriate BMI-for-age growth charts (for either girls or boys) to obtain a percentile ranking. Percentiles are the most commonly used indicator to assess the size and growth patterns of individual children in the United States. The percentile indicates the relative position of the child's BMI number among children of the same sex and age. The growth charts show the weight status categories used with children and teens (underweight, healthy weight, overweight, and obese) (CDC, 2009).

The child's weight status is described as follows:

1. Overweight if he or she has a BMI above the 95th percentile for his or her age
2. At risk of becoming overweight if he or she has a BMI between the 85th and 95th percentile for his or her age
3. Underweight if he or she has a BMI below the 5th percentile for his or her age

If the BMI percentile is at or greater than the 90th percentile, you may wish to discuss anticipatory guidance with your patient to encourage a healthy life style including dietary choices and physical exercise. BMI-for-age weight status categories and the corresponding percentiles are shown in **Table 3-2** (CDC, 2009).

Calculate the BMI as follows:

$$BMI = [weight \div (height \times height)] \times 703$$

Again, in this BMI formula, the child's weight is in pounds and height is in inches. Calculate BMI by dividing weight by height squared and multiplying by a conversion factor of 703.

If you are using the metric system to calculate BMI, use kilograms and meters for the child's weight and height. The formula is weight divided by height squared.

TABLE 3-2   BMI-FOR-AGE WEIGHT STATUS CATEGORIES AND THE CORRESPONDING PERCENTILES

Weight Status Category	Percentile Range
Underweight	Less than the 5th percentile
Healthy weight	5th percentile to less than the 85th percentile
Overweight	85th to less than the 95th percentile
Obese	Equal to or greater than the 95th percentile

Source: CDC Growth chart. National Center for Health Statistics in collaboration with National Center for Chronic Disease Prevention and Health Promotion, May 2002.

Infant Weight

Infants are weighed on infant scales with the child clothed only in a dry diaper, or no diaper at all. Always check calibration of the scale by setting the weight at zero, and note the beam balance. Weigh to the nearest 10 gm or 0.5 oz.

Child Weight

By age 2 or 3 years, when children are able to stand up on their own, they can be weighed on an upright scale. The child is weighed in his or her underwear or lightweight clothing to maintain modesty, and without shoes. Weight is read to the nearest 0.1 kg or 0.25 lb.

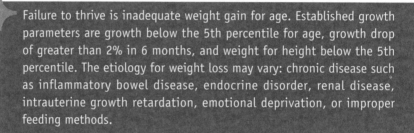

Failure to thrive is inadequate weight gain for age. Established growth parameters are growth below the 5th percentile for age, growth drop of greater than 2% in 6 months, and weight for height below the 5th percentile. The etiology for weight loss may vary: chronic disease such as inflammatory bowel disease, endocrine disorder, renal disease, intrauterine growth retardation, emotional deprivation, or improper feeding methods.

Serial recordings of weight are important so that an established pattern can be observed. If a child experiencing diarrhea is weighed, you may notice a decline in weight. This should be taken into consideration, and periodic follow-up weight checks are encouraged once the child is well to ensure that the previous weight is regained.

Infant Length

This measurement is assessed most accurately by using a horizontal measuring board. Place the infant in a supine position. Hold the infant's head in midline against the headboard. Because the infant's legs are normally flexed, extend them by holding the knees together and gently pushing them down until the legs are flat on the table, straight at the knees, and place the footboard against the bottom of the infant's feet.

Child Length

A child's body length is measured in a supine position until 2 years of age, at which point the child is able to stand on his or her own. By 2 to 3 years of age, the child's height is measured by standing the child against the

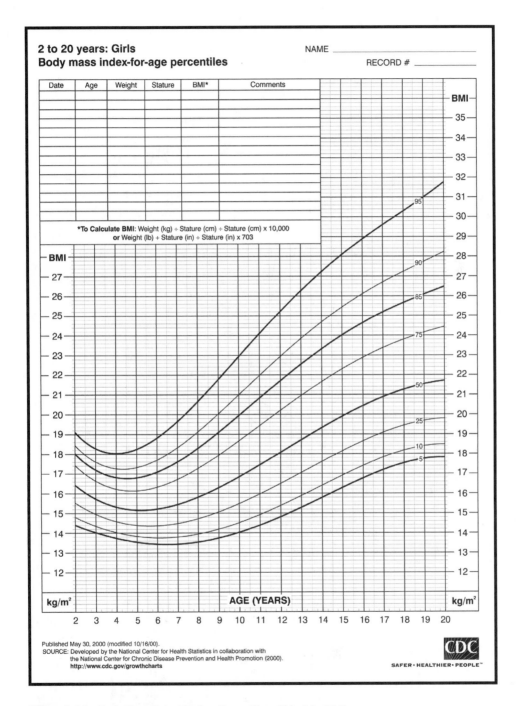

Figure 3-19   Body Mass Index for Age Percentiles: Girls 2 to 20 Years

Source: Developed by the National Center for Health Statistics in collaboration with the National Center for Chronic Disease Prevention and Health Promotion (2000). http://www.cdc.gov/growthcharts.

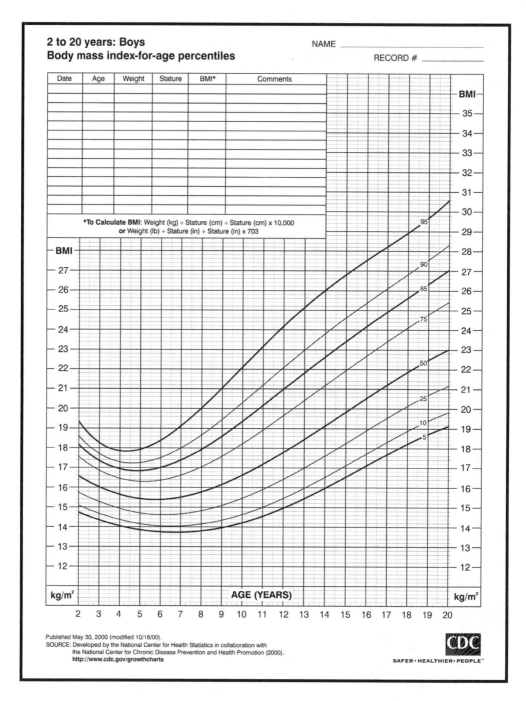

Figure 3-20 Body Mass Index for Age Percentiles: Boys 2 to 20 Years

Source: Developed by the National Center for Health Statistics in collaboration with the National Center for Chronic Disease Prevention and Health Promotion (2000). http://www.cdc.gov/growthcharts.

pole on the platform scale and positioning the headpiece directly on the crown. A child may feel more comfortable standing against the wall rather than against the measuring pole on the scale. You can obtain a more accurate measurement by using a freestanding measuring device or one that is mounted on the wall such as a stadiometer. Have the child stand erect with the heels, buttocks, and shoulders just touching the wall, looking straight ahead. The outer canthus of the eye should be at the same horizontal plane as the external auditory canal while positioning the headpiece. Position the headpiece at the crown placing it directly on the scalp. Plot the stature reading the nearest 0.5 cm or 0.5 in. You can also hold a book on the child's head at a right angle to the wall and measure just below the book. For visual explanation, see **Figure 3-21**.

Head Circumference

Measurement of the infant's head circumference is performed at each health maintenance visit from birth to age 2 years. After age 2 the major portion of brain growth has slowed with the brain achieving two-thirds its adult size. The average head circumference for full term newborns ranges between 32.5 and 37.5 cm with a mean of 33 to 35 cm. It is then monitored yearly until age 6 years. Head circumference is performed by circling the head with a cloth tape measure at the occipital protuberance and the supraorbital prominence in order to find the point of largest circumference. Measure the head three times, taking the largest value (Hoekelman, 2001, p. 62). In head circumference, a series of measurements is more significant than a single measurement, as it demonstrates the rate of head growth. Remember, measuring head circumference is measuring growth of the brain. The brain grows to 80% of its adult volume during the first 2 years of life.

Macrocephaly is abnormally large head size (97th percentile, or 2 standard deviations above the mean). It may be due to hydrocephalus secondary to increased intracranial pressure, or genetic disorders. A large head also may be due to a familial condition with normal brain growth. Microcephaly, or small head, is two standard deviations below the mean for age and gender. Early closure of cranial sutures, also referred to as craniosynostosis, can be due to a variety of genetic syndromes.

(a)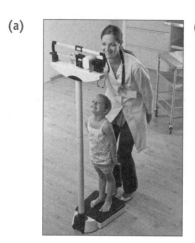

(b)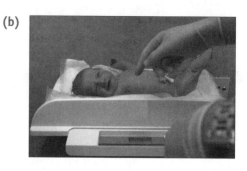

(c)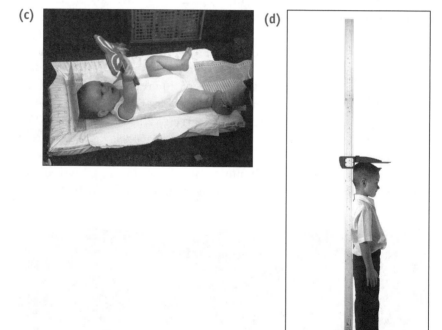

(d)

Figure 3-21   (a) Weight Measure; (b) Platform Scale; (c) Measure Mat, Infant; (d) Height

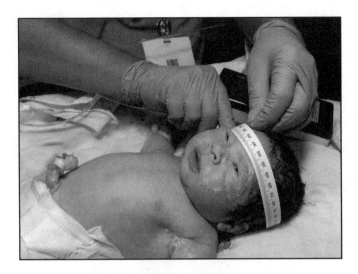

Figure 3-22   Appropriate Placement of the Measuring Tape to Obtain the Head Circumference

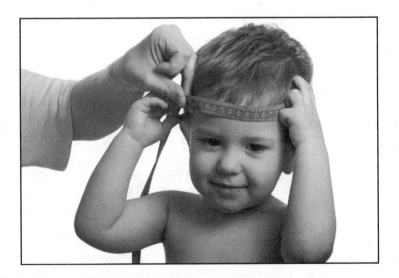

Figure 3-23   Appropriate Placement of Measuring Tape on Toddler's Head

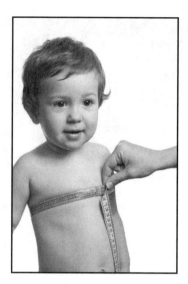

Figure 3-24 Measurement of Toddler's Chest Circumference

Chest Circumference

In newborns the chest circumference is compared with the head circumference. The chest circumference normally equals the head circumference for the first year of life, after which time it exceeds the head circumference (Hoekelman, 2001, p. 62). Chest circumference is measured by encircling the tape around the chest at the nipple line. This measurement is used in the assessment of growth abnormalities.

Vital Signs

Blood Pressure

Blood pressure measurement is done much the same as in an adult. Select the blood pressure cuff that is wide enough to cover two-thirds of the upper arm. A narrower cuff falsely elevates the blood pressure reading, as in an adult. Blood pressure readings are part of the physical examination of every child older than 3 years of age. An AAP study (2004) brought attention to the role of hypertension in the current epidemic of obesity in children, underscoring the need for intervention. The study indicated that the "the strong association of high blood pressure with obesity and the marked increase in the prevalence of childhood obesity indicate that both hypertension and prehypertension are becoming a significant health issue in the young."

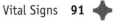

The AAP guidelines recommend therapeutic lifestyle changes, such as weight reduction, regular physical activity, and restriction of sedentary behavior, to help prevent increases in blood pressure.

A crying, anxious child may have elevations in systolic pressure of 30 to 50 mm Hg. Always repeat readings at the end of the visit. A trick is to leave the cuff on during the exam and then repeat the reading at the end of the exam. Use the disappearance of the Korotkoff sound for the diastolic reading in children just as in adults.

TABLE 3-3 GIRLS' SYSTOLIC BLOOD PRESSURE BY AGE AND HEIGHT
(Normal SBP is less than the prehypertensive result.)

Age	BP Classification	Systolic BP (mmHG)						
3	**Height (cm)**	91	92	95	98	100	103	105
	Prehypertension	100	100	102	103	104	106	106
	Stage 1 HTN	104	104	105	107	108	109	110
	Stage 2 HTN	116	116	118	119	120	121	122
4	**Height (cm)**	97	99	101	104	108	110	112
	Prehypertension	101	102	103	104	106	107	108
	Stage 1 HTN	105	106	107	108	110	111	112
	Stage 2 HTN	117	118	119	120	122	123	124
5	**Height (cm)**	104	105	108	111	115	118	120
	Prehypertension	103	103	105	106	107	109	109
	Stage 1 HTN	107	107	108	110	111	112	113
	Stage 2 HTN	119	119	121	122	123	125	125
6	**Height (cm)**	110	112	115	118	122	126	128
	Prehypertension	104	105	106	108	109	110	111
	Stage 1 HTN	108	109	110	111	113	114	115
	Stage 2 HTN	120	121	122	124	125	126	127
7	**Height (cm)**	116	118	121	125	129	132	135
	Prehypertension	106	107	108	109	111	112	113
	Stage 1 HTN	110	111	112	113	115	116	116
	Stage 2 HTN	122	123	124	125	127	128	129
8	**Height (cm)**	121	123	127	131	135	139	141
	Prehypertension	108	109	110	111	113	114	114
	Stage 1 HTN	112	112	114	115	116	118	118
	Stage 2 HTN	124	125	126	127	128	130	130

(continues)

TABLE 3-3 GIRLS' SYSTOLIC BLOOD PRESSURE BY AGE AND HEIGHT *(continued)*
(Normal SBP is less than the prehypertensive result.)

Age	BP Classification	Systolic BP (mmHG)						
9	*Height (cm)*	125	128	131	136	140	144	147
	Prehypertension	110	110	112	113	114	116	116
	Stage 1 HTN	114	114	115	117	118	119	120
	Stage 2 HTN	126	126	128	129	130	132	132
10	*Height (cm)*	130	132	136	141	146	150	153
	Prehypertension	112	112	114	115	116	118	118
	Stage 1 HTN	116	116	117	119	120	121	122
	Stage 2 HTN	128	128	130	131	132	134	134
11	*Height (cm)*	136	138	143	148	153	157	160
	Prehypertension	114	114	116	117	118	119	120
	Stage 1 HTN	118	118	119	121	122	123	124
	Stage 2 HTN	130	130	131	133	134	135	136
12	*Height (cm)*	143	146	150	155	160	164	166
	Prehypertension	116	116	117	119	120	120	120
	Stage 1 HTN	119	120	121	123	124	125	126
	Stage 2 HTN	132	132	133	135	136	137	138
13	*Height (cm)*	148	151	155	159	164	168	170
	Prehypertension	117	118	119	120	120	120	120
	Stage 1 HTN	121	122	123	124	126	127	128
	Stage 2 HTN	133	134	135	137	138	139	140
14	*Height (cm)*	151	153	157	161	166	170	172
	Prehypertension	119	120	120	120	120	120	120
	Stage 1 HTN	123	123	125	126	127	129	129
	Stage 2 HTN	135	136	137	138	140	141	141
15	*Height (cm)*	152	154	158	162	167	171	173
	Prehypertension	120	120	120	120	120	120	120
	Stage 1 HTN	124	125	126	127	129	130	131
	Stage 2 HTN	136	137	138	139	141	142	143
16	*Height (cm)*	152	154	158	163	167	171	173
	Prehypertension	120	120	120	120	120	120	120
	Stage 1 HTN	125	126	127	128	130	131	132
	Stage 2 HTN	137	138	139	140	142	143	144
17	*Height (cm)*	152	155	159	163	167	171	173
	Prehypertension	120	120	120	120	120	120	120
	Stage 1 HTN	125	126	127	129	130	131	132
	Stage 2 HTN	138	138	139	141	142	143	144

TABLE 3-4   BOYS' SYSTOLIC BLOOD PRESSURE BY AGE AND HEIGHT
(Normal SBP is less than the prehypertensive result.)

Age	BP Classification	Systolic BP (mmHG)						
3	*Height (cm)*	**92**	**94**	**96**	**99**	**102**	**104**	**106**
	Prehypertension	100	101	103	105	107	108	109
	Stage 1 HTN	104	105	107	109	110	112	113
	Stage 2 HTN	116	117	119	121	123	124	125
4	*Height (cm)*	**99**	**100**	**103**	**106**	**109**	**112**	**113**
	Prehypertension	102	103	105	107	109	110	111
	Stage 1 HTN	106	107	109	111	112	114	115
	Stage 2 HTN	118	119	121	123	125	126	127
5	*Height (cm)*	**104**	**106**	**109**	**112**	**116**	**119**	**120**
	Prehypertension	104	105	106	108	110	111	112
	Stage 1 HTN	108	109	110	112	114	115	116
	Stage 2 HTN	120	121	123	125	126	128	128
6	*Height (cm)*	**110**	**112**	**115**	**119**	**122**	**126**	**127**
	Prehypertension	105	106	108	110	111	113	113
	Stage 1 HTN	109	110	112	114	115	117	117
	Stage 2 HTN	121	122	124	126	128	129	130
7	*Height (cm)*	**116**	**118**	**121**	**125**	**129**	**132**	**134**
	Prehypertension	106	107	109	111	113	114	115
	Stage 1 HTN	110	111	113	115	117	118	119
	Stage 2 HTN	122	123	125	127	129	130	131
8	*Height (cm)*	**121**	**123**	**127**	**131**	**135**	**139**	**141**
	Prehypertension	107	109	110	112	114	115	116
	Stage 1 HTN	111	112	114	116	118	119	120
	Stage 2 HTN	124	125	127	128	130	132	132
9	*Height (cm)*	**126**	**128**	**132**	**136**	**141**	**145**	**147**
	Prehypertension	109	110	112	114	115	117	118
	Stage 1 HTN	113	114	116	118	119	121	121
	Stage 2 HTN	125	126	128	130	132	133	134
10	*Height (cm)*	**130**	**133**	**137**	**141**	**146**	**150**	**153**
	Prehypertension	111	112	114	115	117	119	119
	Stage 1 HTN	115	116	117	119	121	122	123
	Stage 2 HTN	127	128	130	132	133	135	135
11	*Height (cm)*	**135**	**137**	**142**	**146**	**151**	**156**	**159**
	Prehypertension	113	114	115	117	119	120	120
	Stage 1 HTN	117	118	119	121	123	124	125
	Stage 2 HTN	129	130	132	134	135	137	137

(continues)

TABLE 3-4 BOYS' SYSTOLIC BLOOD PRESSURE BY AGE AND HEIGHT *(continued)*
(Normal SBP is less than the prehypertensive result.)

Age	BP Classification	Systolic BP (mmHG)						
12	*Height (cm)*	140	143	148	153	158	163	166
	Prehypertension	115	116	118	120	120	120	120
	Stage 1 HTN	119	120	122	123	125	127	127
	Stage 2 HTN	131	132	134	136	138	139	140
13	*Height (cm)*	147	150	155	160	166	171	173
	Prehypertension	117	118	120	120	120	120	120
	Stage 1 HTN	121	122	124	126	128	129	130
	Stage 2 HTN	133	135	136	138	140	141	142
14	*Height (cm)*	154	157	162	167	173	177	180
	Prehypertension	120	120	120	120	120	120	120
	Stage 1 HTN	124	125	127	128	130	132	132
	Stage 2 HTN	136	137	139	141	143	144	145
15	*Height (cm)*	159	162	167	172	177	182	184
	Prehypertension	120	120	120	120	120	120	120
	Stage 1 HTN	126	127	129	131	133	134	135
	Stage 2 HTN	139	140	141	143	145	147	147
16	*Height (cm)*	162	165	170	175	180	184	186
	Prehypertension	120	120	120	120	120	120	120
	Stage 1 HTN	129	130	132	134	135	137	137
	Stage 2 HTN	141	142	144	146	148	149	150
17	*Height (cm)*	164	166	171	176	181	185	187
	Prehypertension	120	120	120	120	120	120	120
	Stage 1 HTN	131	132	134	136	138	139	140
	Stage 2 HTN	144	145	146	148	150	151	152

Incorrect cuff size is the most common explanation for elevated blood pressure readings. Hypertension, levels that exceed the range for age and gender, should be fully evaluated to determine the etiology. Additional risk factors associated with hypertension are diabetes and cholesterol disorders, history of preterm infants, low birth weight, history of congenital heart disease, or difficult or prolonged hospital stay (AAP, 2004).

Temperature

Temperature in children can be measured via four routes: oral, rectal, tympanic, and axillary. The route chosen is based on the child's age, development, and medical condition.

Oral Temperature

An oral temperature is generally reserved for the older child, from 5 to 6 years or older. It can be used when children are old enough to cooperate and keep their mouth closed and the thermometer under their tongue.

Rectal Temperature

The rectal temperature is the most accurate and can be taken in children of all ages, although in children 5 years and older an oral or tympanic temperature is appropriate and less invasive. In a young child with diarrhea, an alternative route should be considered. The rectal temperature normally measures higher in infants and toddlers, with an average of 37.8°C (100°F). Rectal temperature is preferred at this age when there is question of a febrile illness. Rectal temperature in infants and children measures higher then in adults. The average rectal temperature for a child is 37.8°C or 100°F. It generally does not fall below 99.0°F until after 3 years of age.

The procedure for taking the temperature rectally is as follows:

- Put a small amount of lubricant, such as petroleum jelly, on the end of the thermometer.

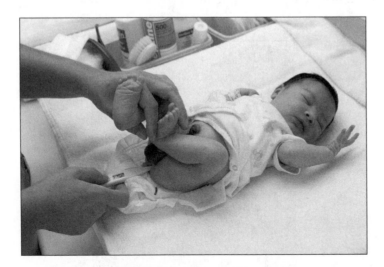

Figure 3-25 Rectal Temperature

- Place the child prone on a firm surface, or have the parent hold the child prone on his or her lap. Hold the child by placing your palm against his or her lower back, just above the bottom.
- You can also place the child in a supine position and bring the feet together up toward the chest.
- With the other hand, gently insert the thermometer through the anal sphincter to a depth of approximately 1 inch, or 2 to 3 cm. Deeper insertion into the colon risks rectal perforation.

Tympanic Temperature

Tympanic (ear) thermometers are another option for toddlers and pre-schoolers who are resistant to the rectal route or not cooperative enough for the oral route. However, while these thermometers give quick results, they must be placed correctly in the child's ear to be accurate. Too much earwax can cause the reading to be incorrect.

Axillary Temperature

Although the least invasive and easily accessible means of measuring temperature, axillary temperature is generally the least accurate, as noted by Cusson et al. (Jarvis, 2004, p. 166). The procedure is as follows:

- Have the parent hold the child on his or her lap with the child's arms wrapped around (hugging) the parent.
- Place the tip of the thermometer well into the axilla.
- Hold the child's arm close to his or her body.

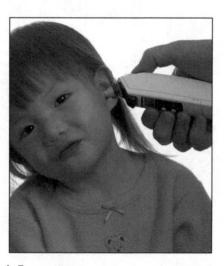

Figure 3-26 Tympanic Temperature

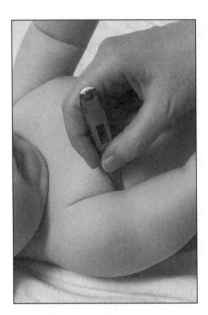

Figure 3-27   Axillary Temperature

> ➤ In infants, birth to 3 months, temperature greater than 38°C
>   (100°F) requires further evaluation, as this may be an indication
>   of serious illness.
> ➤ Parents who wrap the child in blankets will note increased skin
>   temperature, although core temperature may remain normal.
> ➤ Young children can spike high temperatures (up to 104°F) with
>   minor illnesses or infections.

Pulse

In infants and toddlers, palpation of an apical rate is the most reliable.
There is greater fluctuation in heart rate in infants and children than in
adults due to illness, crying, or physical activity. In older children, palpate
the radial artery. In both cases, count the pulse for a full minute to take
into account irregularities. See **Table 3-5**.

> An elevated heart rate or tachycardia is indicative of fever, anxiety,
> dysrhythmia, congestive heart failure, or medication. A decreased
> heart rate or bradycardia may be due to drug ingestion, hypoxia, or
> intracranial or neurologic conditions (Bickley, 2003, p. 661).

TABLE 3-5	AVERAGE HEART RATE OF INFANTS AND CHILDREN	
Age	Beats/Minute	Average
Newborn	100–170	140
1 year	80–170	120
3 years	80–130	110
6 years	70–115	100
10 years	70–110	90
14 years	60–110	89–90
18 years	60–100	72

Respirations

In an infant, it is helpful to watch the abdominal movement, as the infant's respirations are more diaphragmatic than thoracic. Again, as with measuring the pulse, illness, crying, or physical activity can cause fluctuations in the respiratory rate. See **Table 3-6**.

Guideline for cutoffs for defining tachypnea:
- Infants 0–2 months: > 60/min
- Infants 2–12 months: > 50/min
- Children > 12 months: > 40/min

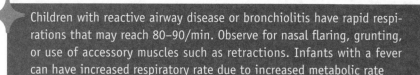
Children with reactive airway disease or bronchiolitis have rapid respirations that may reach 80–90/min. Observe for nasal flaring, grunting, or use of accessory muscles such as retractions. Infants with a fever can have increased respiratory rate due to increased metabolic rate

General Considerations Related to Vital Signs

Overall, when taking a young child's vital signs, consider the following tips: Have small toys available to distract the child, and have a clip-on toy (such as a teddy bear) attached to your stethoscope. A finger puppet works wonders in distracting a small child, as does a colorful Band-Aid on your finger. Singing or whistling also acts as a means of distraction.

TABLE 3-6 AVERAGE RESPIRATORY RATE OF INFANTS AND CHILDREN		
Age	Resting Respiratory Rate	Average
Newborn	30–50	40
1 year	20–40	30
3 years	20–30	25
6 years	16–22	19
10 years	16–20	18
14 years	14–20	17
18 years	16–20	18

> ## Red Flags

- When plotting weight parameters, an unexplained change of 2% or more, either above or below those previously recorded, warrants further investigation.
- When plotting height parameters, below-average or above-average parameters, without explanation (such as familial tendency), require further investigation.
- Head circumference that is falling off the established curve for the child, either above or below, requires further investigation.
- When plotting vital signs, those outside of established criteria should be further assessed.

Suggested Documentation for Vital Signs, Height, Weight, and Head Circumference

Document the following:

- Temperature, indicating method
- Pulse
- Respirations
- Blood pressure
- Height, weight, and head circumference, which are plotted on the appropriate growth chart
- BMI, which is calculated and plotted on the appropriate chart

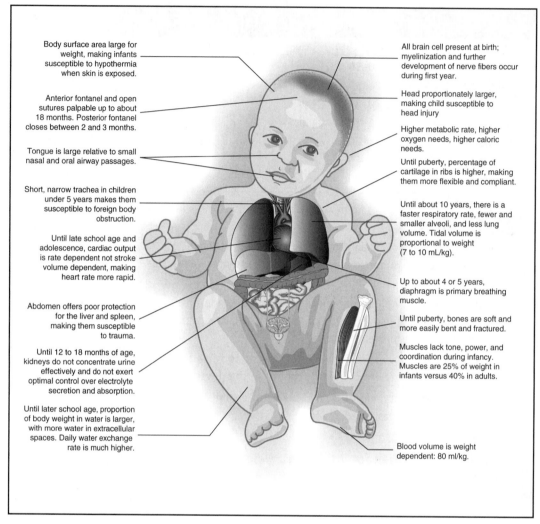

Body surface area large for weight, making infants susceptible to hypothermia when skin is exposed.

Anterior fontanel and open sutures palpable up to about 18 months. Posterior fontanel closes between 2 and 3 months.

Tongue is large relative to small nasal and oral airway passages.

Short, narrow trachea in children under 5 years makes them susceptible to foreign body obstruction.

Until late school age and adolescence, cardiac output is rate dependent not stroke volume dependent, making heart rate more rapid.

Abdomen offers poor protection for the liver and spleen, making them susceptible to trauma.

Until 12 to 18 months of age, kidneys do not concentrate urine effectively and do not exert optimal control over electrolyte secretion and absorption.

Until later school age, proportion of body weight in water is larger, with more water in extracellular spaces. Daily water exchange rate is much higher.

All brain cell present at birth; myelinization and further development of nerve fibers occur during first year.

Head proportionately larger, making child susceptible to head injury

Higher metabolic rate, higher oxygen needs, higher caloric needs.

Until puberty, percentage of cartilage in ribs is higher, making them more flexible and compliant.

Until about 10 years, there is a faster respiratory rate, fewer and smaller alveoli, and less lung volume. Tidal volume is proportional to weight (7 to 10 mL/kg).

Up to about 4 or 5 years, diaphragm is primary breathing muscle.

Until puberty, bones are soft and more easily bent and fractured.

Muscles lack tone, power, and coordination during infancy. Muscles are 25% of weight in infants versus 40% in adults.

Blood volume is weight dependent: 80 ml/kg.

Figure 3-28 Anatomic and Physiologic Characteristics of the Child

Case Study: Fever of Unknown Origin

A mother brings her 2-month-old daughter to your office with a 48-hour history of irritability and fever. The mother reports that the child's fever was as high as 102°F, rectally. She denies any other symptoms such as cough, rhinorrhea, vomiting, or diarrhea. The mother reports that she gave the child Tylenol the night before, but none today, and that the child is not taking her bottle.

On examination, you observe the following:

- Vital signs: normal except for rectal temperature, which is 39.1°C (102.4°F)
- Her physical exam is normal, without source for the fever.

Questions

1. What are key factors to consider in your clinical judgment and observation?
2. What is the rationale for your clinical approach based on the age of this child?
3. What are the guidelines for treatment of a child 3 months or younger with a fever of unknown origin?

Answers

1. Key factors to consider are (1) the child's age, (2) height of temperature, (3) severity of illness, (4) presence of a focus of infection, and (5) white cell count.
2. The neonate or young infant may not have the characteristic signs of serious infection (temperature can be high or low). Consider the following: Localizing features may be absent; the child can deteriorate rapidly; the neonate may be infected with organisms from the birth canal; young infants with fever, especially those under 3 months of age, need rapid assessment and investigation and admission to a hospital.
3. The guidelines include full blood count, blood cultures, urine culture, lumbar puncture for examination of cerebrospinal fluid, and chest x-ray.

References

American Academy of Pediatrics. (2004). Hypertension. *Pediatrics. 114(2), 555–576.*

Bickley, L. (2003). *Bates' guide to physical examination and history taking* (8th ed.). New York: Lippincott Williams & Wilkins.

Centers for Disease Control and Prevention. (2009). Clinical growth charts. Retrieved June 9, 2010, from http://www.cdc.gov/growthcharts/clinical_charts.htm

Hoekelman, R., Adam, H., Nelson, N., & Weitzman, M. (2001). *Primary pediatric care.* St. Louis, MO: Mosby.

Jarvis, C. (2004). *Physical Examination & Health Assessment* (5th ed.). St. Louis, MO: Elsevier.

Resources

Ball, J.W., Bindler, R. (2008). *Pediatric nursing* (4th ed.). Upper Saddle River, NJ: Prentice Hall.

Bright Futures. (2001). *Education center of the american academy of pediatrics.*

Burns, C., Dunn, A, Brady, M., Starr, N., Blosser, C., (2000). *Pediatric primary care: a handbook for nurse practitioners,* (3rd ed.). St. Louis, MO: Saunders.

Cech, D., Martin, S. (2002). *Functional movement development across the life span.* Philadelphia, PA: Saunders.

Colyar, M. (2003). *Well-child assessment for primary care providers.* Philadelphia: EA Davis Company.

CDC website CDC.gov/nhanes/growthcharts

Dixon, S., Stein, M. (2000). *Encounters with children, pediatric behavior and development* (3rd ed.). St. Louis, MO: Mosby.

Goldbloom, R. (2003). *Pediatric clinical skills.* New York: Churchill Livingston.

Henry, J.J. (1992). Routine growth monitoring and assessment of growth disorders. *Journal of Pediatric Health Care,* 6(5), 291–301.

Potts, N., Mandleco, B. (2007). *Pediatric nursing.* (2nd ed.). Australia: Thomson Delmar Learning.

Sorof, J.M., Lai, D., Turner, J., Poffenbarger, T., Portman, R.J. (2004). Overweight, ethnicity, and the prevalence of hypertension in school-aged children. *Pediatrics. 113(3), 475–482.*

Newborn Assessment

Rosemarie A. Fuller

Introduction

The ability to perform a comprehensive physical assessment of the newborn is an integral part of nursing care. This assessment provides a baseline from which variations and abnormalities may be identified. Performing a physical assessment quickly and efficiently is a skill that takes much practice. A well-organized, consistent approach assures that all required areas of the assessment are included. The purpose of this chapter is to review techniques and skills used in a comprehensive assessment of the newborn. Fetal development, normal variations, and abnormalities requiring further examination will also be discussed.

Definitions

Newborn: A child less than 1 month of age.

Gestational age: The number of completed weeks of pregnancy. Gestational age is further defined as follows:
- Full-term: Between 38 and 42 weeks
- Preterm: Less than 37 weeks
- Postdates: Greater than 42 weeks
- Late preterm infant (LPTI): Between 35 and 37 weeks. This classification came about in 2005 to identify those infants who,

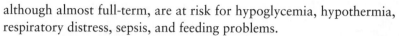

although almost full-term, are at risk for hypoglycemia, hypothermia, respiratory distress, sepsis, and feeding problems.

➤ The AWHONN Near-Term Infant Initiative: A conceptual framework for optimizing care for near-term infants (Medoff-Cooper, Bakewell-Sachs, Buus-Frank, Santa-Donato, & Near-Term Infant Advisory Panel, 2005).

Postnatal age: The number of days or weeks after delivery. A preterm baby at 35 weeks who was born 4 weeks ago now has a *postnatal* age of 1 month.

Corrected gestational age: The gestational age plus postnatal age. This calculation is used in assessing developmental milestones in a preterm infant up to 2 years of age to compensate for delays due to prematurity. The baby in the previous example, born at 35 weeks and now 1 month old, has a *corrected* gestational age of 39 weeks.

Newborns are also described in terms of intrauterine growth:

SMALL FOR GESTATIONAL AGE (SGA) OR INTRAUTERINE GROWTH RESTRICTION (IUGR): Newborns who fall under the 10th percentile for growth. This condition may be caused by maternal illness, smoking, placental problems, or multiple gestation and is further categorized as symmetrical and asymmetrical. *Asymmetrical* growth retardation is so called because while the infant's weight is less than the norm, the head circumference is within normal limits, indicating brain sparing. In this situation, the condition causing the low birth weight occurred later in pregnancy after sufficient brain growth. The causative factor in *symmetrical* growth retardation occurred early in pregnancy, resulting in suboptimal weight as well as suboptimal brain growth.

LARGE FOR GESTATIONAL AGE (LGA): Newborns above the 90th percentile for growth.

APPROPRIATE FOR GESTATIONAL AGE (AGA): Newborns between the 10th to 90th percentiles for growth.

See **Table 4-1** for a description of problems associated with classification categories.

Developmental Considerations

When performing a newborn assessment, it is helpful to keep the infant warm, unclothed, and in a well-lit environment. Newborns are also less able to habituate to stimuli when compared with older children and adults. This means that each time they are touched, spoken to, or handled, their

TABLE 4-1   PROBLEMS ASSOCIATED WITH CLASSIFICATION CATEGORIES

Classification	Potential Problems	Causes
SGA/IUGR	Hypothermia Hypoglycemia Birth asphyxia Polycythemia	Low body fat and brown fat stores; faster metabolic rate; increased production of RBCs to increase oxygen-carrying capacity
LGA	Hypoglycemia Respiratory distress Birth trauma Hyperinsulinemia Retained birth fluid	Adequate stores of glucose but ineffective utilization; cesarean section; diabetes in pregnancy; surfactant reduced
Preterm	Hypothermia Hypoglycemia Respiratory distress	Low stores of glucose or brown fat; insufficient surfactant

SGA, small for gestational age; IUGR, intrauterine growth retardation; LGA, large for gestational age; RBCs, red blood cells

Source: Reprinted from The Journal of Pediatrics, 119: 3, Ballard, J.L, Khoury, J.C., Wedig, K., Wang, L., Eilers-Walsman, B.L., and Lipp, R., New Ballard Score, expanded to include extremely premature infants, 417–423, 1991, with permission from Elsevier.

reactions do not attenuate, requiring increased metabolism of oxygen and glucose. An examiner who uses gentle touch and responds to the infant's cues assists the newborn to regulate responses at the lowest metabolic cost. By beginning with the least invasive techniques, such as observation and auscultation, and moving to the more invasive techniques, the examiner can use opportunities as they arise to complete the examination.

Thermoregulation

A normal temperature in the newborn is controlled by the hypothalamus. Stimuli from the skin are processed by the hypothalamus, and temperature is then regulated through metabolism, muscle tone, and vasomotor activity. One method the newborn uses to maintain temperature is the metabolism of brown fat, a vascular type of fat tissue that surrounds the newborn scapulae, adrenals, and perihilar area. When metabolized, brown fat generates heat, which is conducted through blood vessels to warm the newborn. The amount of brown fat present is determined by gestational age, so the more preterm it is, the less brown fat is available for heat production. This type of heat production is called nonshivering thermogenesis. In general, newborns are able to maintain a normal temperature when stable; however, if stressed, the infant undergoes heat loss through a physiologic cascade called cold stress. Cold stress increases metabolism, use of glucose and oxygen, and breakdown of brown fat. The consequence of these effects is hypoglycemia, release of fatty acids, hypoxia, anaerobic metabolism, and lactic acid buildup. Lactic acid exacerbates metabolic acidosis, resulting in pulmonary vasoconstriction, decreased surfactant production, and respiratory distress.

Heat is lost in the newborn through four mechanisms:

- *EVAPORATION*: Heat lost through the conversion of a liquid to a gas. Evaporation includes insensible losses from breathing and sweating. The maturity of the stratum corneum layer of the skin is a major factor that impacts this type of heat loss. Keratin is a protein layer that protects the epithelium and is relatively water impermeable. Maturity of the keratin layer is directly related to gestational age so that the more preterm the infant, the greater the transdermal water that will be evaporated and the greater the resultant heat lost. Damage to the skin also interrupts the skin barrier, allowing evaporative loss.
- *CONDUCTION*: Heat loss from the newborn due to contact with a cold surface. Characteristics such the temperature gradient between the cold surface and the newborn and the size of the areas in contact determine the degree of heat lost in this way.
- *CONVECTION*: Heat loss from the newborn due to air drafts. The diameter of the newborn's extremities affects this type of loss. The decreased muscle tone and limb flexion, reduced body fat, and smaller extremities make the preterm baby more vulnerable to heat loss through convection.
- *RADIATION*: Heat loss from the newborn due to solid surfaces that are not in contact. For example, a newborn's crib or isolette could be affected by a cold outside window. The size of the surfaces and the distance between them impact the degree of heat loss.

Prevention of Heat Loss

Heat loss can be prevented by placing the infant on a prewarmed surface with prewarmed blankets and maintaining ambient room temperature of at least 75°F. Keeping the newborn away from drafts, windows, and cold walls reduces the effects of radiation and convection (Kattwinkel, 2007).

Obtaining a History

One of the most important ways of anticipating problems in the delivery room and beyond is by obtaining a comprehensive history that includes maternal health history, prenatal history, and circumstances of delivery. Additional components of the interview process and health history are included in this chapter.

Health History

The health history includes a review of maternal medical and surgical history, injuries and hospitalizations, allergies, and chronic conditions. Information regarding medications, immunizations, and drug and alcohol use should also be noted. Because immunization schedules change so frequently, they will not be discussed here; however, a current schedule for immunizations may be obtained from the CDC (www.cdc.gov). A prenatal history includes circumstances around past and current pregnancies and complications of labor and delivery. Newborn information to obtain includes gestational age, birth order in multiple pregnancies, birth weight, Apgar scores, postnatal problems (if any), age, and weight at discharge.

Particularly important information to document is a history of congenital abnormalities. Minor congenital defects are present in about 15% of infants. Major defects, seen in about 2–5% of infants, are responsible for about 20% of all infant deaths. There are four causes of defects:

- *MALFORMATIONS* occur in the first 3–6 weeks of gestation, during structural formation.
- *DISRUPTIONS* occur after formation of fetal structures and include amniotic band syndrome.
- *DEFORMATIONS* result from mechanical forces, mainly on the musculoskeletal system, and include positional abnormalities of the feet or facies.
- *SYNDROMES* are defined as three or more defects that occur consistently together and have an identifiable cause, such as a chromosomal or genetic factor.

Factors that may cause defects in the infant include exposure to environmental teratogens, chemicals, medications, infectious diseases, or other maternal illnesses.

Maternal Infections

TOXOPLASMOSIS: If this is the mother's first toxoplasmosis infection, the fetus is more likely to be infected. Intracranial calcifications and chorioretinitis are seen. If the cysts of toxoplasmosis are latent, the newborn may experience subclinical illness.

RUBELLA: The risk of malformations is increased the earlier in the pregnancy the exposure to this virus occurs and depends on the organ systems developing at the time. Fetal loss, cataracts, congenital deafness, patent ductus arteriosus (PDA), ventricular septal defect (VSD), and atrial septal defect (ASD) occur from early exposure to the rubella virus.

CYTOMEGALOVIRUS: Unlike with many illnesses, maternal immunity does not protect the fetus from this virus and most mothers are asymptomatic. Fetal loss frequently occurs after early pregnancy exposure; chorioretinitis, microcephaly, and hepatosplenomegaly occur in the fetus after late exposure.

SYPHILIS: Increasing in incidence, syphilis results in congenital deafness and mental retardation in the newborn.

HERPES SIMPLEX: If the exposure to this virus occurs during pregnancy, the sequelae are more serious and include microcephaly, retinal and eye abnormalities, and hepatosplenomegaly. If the exposure occurs at birth, conjunctivitis or pneumonia may occur during the first 2 to 3 weeks of life. The virus causes shingles in adults through what is termed retro-axonal flow, meaning the virus follows nerve pathways during latency. When stressed, the adult will develop classic grouped vesicles along those dermatomes.

HIV: Passive immunity is conferred to the fetus for approximately the first 6 months of life. Antibodies identified after that time indicate infection in the newborn. Less than 30% of newborns born to HIV-positive mothers develop active infection.

PARVOVIRUS: This virus causes red cell hemolysis and nonimmune hydrops in the fetus.

VARICELLA: This virus causes a typical skin rash, chorioretinitis, encephalitis, and cardiac abnormalities.

Maternal Medications, Drugs, and Alcohol

ANTICONVULSANT MEDICATIONS: Maternal use of anticonvulsants such as Dilantin produce a wide variety of malformations, including cardiac, cranial, and midfacial abnormalities.

ANTIHYPERTENSIVES: Maternal use has been implicated in growth retardation and renal abnormalities.

COCAINE: Maternal use may result in fetal loss, renal abnormalities, and gastrointestinal (GI) abnormalities. Cocaine is a potent vasoconstrictor that decreases circulation and oxygenation to the fetus.

ALCOHOL: Maternal ingestion results in a typical facial appearance—flat nasal bridge and midface, flat philtrum, and small upper lip—as well as mental retardation. Fetal alcohol syndrome (FAS) is well documented in these newborns.

SMOKING: Maternal smoking decreases circulation to the fetus and contributes to IUGR.

Maternal Medical Conditions

ASTHMA: This condition contributes to IUGR. It may result in polycythemia and jaundice in the newborn in response to the hypoxia seen in this condition.

CARDIAC DISEASE: Polycythemia and jaundice may result, and there is a 15% risk of cardiac disease in the fetus/newborn.

DIABETES: This condition contributes to LGA infants as well as polycythemia, birth trauma, and congenital cardiac abnormalities.

THYROID DISEASE: The fetus produces its own thyroid hormones at about 10 weeks. Hypothyroidism in the fetus is not detected until birth due to passage of maternal thyroid hormones. Hyperthyroidism in the mother may result in preeclampsia, preterm birth, or IUGR.

HYPERTENSION: The effects of hypertension depend on severity, management, and gestational age; IUGR is the most frequent finding.

AUTOIMMUNE DISEASE: Heart block in the fetus/newborn may result.

IDIOPATHIC THROMBOCYTOPENIA (ITP): Intracranial hemorrhage in the newborn may result.

Genogram

A genogram is used to identify possible familial disorders and may be presented in written or graphic form (**Figure 4-1**). A sample genogram showing the information to include follows:

- Paternal grandmother: deceased, 89, CHF
- Paternal grandfather: deceased, 85, CVA
- Maternal grandmother: alive and well, 82
- Maternal grandfather: deceased, 52, MVA
- Mother: alive, 68, HTN
- Father: alive, 69, HTN
- Sister: alive, 45, HTN
- Brother: alive and well, 40
- Patient: alive and well, 38
- Husband: alive and well, 44
- Son: alive and well, 5
- Daughter: alive and well, 3

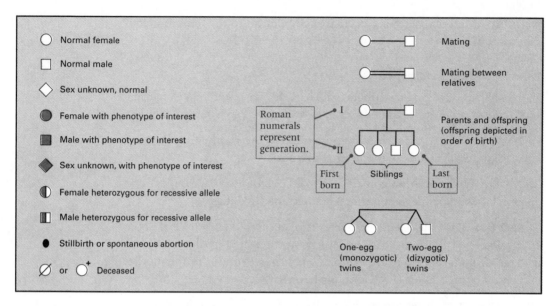

Figure 4-1   Genogram

Psychosocial History

This part of the history includes information regarding religious beliefs, relationships and support systems, psychiatric history, and treatment. Important to include, particularly in the assessment of the pregnant adolescent, is a history of risk factors. This information may be obtained with the help of the acronym **HEADSSS**:

> H—home life and family situation
>
> E—employment and education history
>
> A—activities, such as sports participation
>
> D—drugs, alcohol, and tobacco use
>
> S—social activities
>
> S—sexual activities
>
> S—suicidal ideation and depression

Techniques of Assessment in the Newborn

Several techniques are used in the newborn examination: *observation, auscultation,* and *palpation*. Percussion, a common technique in examining older children and adults, is rarely used in newborns due to limitations of the size of the baby and the fact that it can be a painful procedure. When examination of the abdomen or lungs is needed, an x-ray is less invasive and provides high-quality information.

Transillumination is used to identify the presence of misplaced air or fluid. The skull may be transilluminated to detect hydrocephalus, the chest for evidence of pneumothorax (or extra pulmonary air), and the scrotum for the presence of a hydrocele. To perform this technique, the room should be darkened. A transilluminator, flashlight, or other light source is placed over the area to be examined. Light will be transmitted through the skin, producing a corona of light around the source or a red glow as light is conducted through the tissues. A corona greater than 2 cm on the chest is consistent with pneumothorax; hydroceles will produce a glowing of the testicular sac.

Observation

Observation is usually the first of the techniques used. The newborn should be observed in a warmed environment, unclothed and in adequate light, ideally while asleep or quietly alert. Muscle tone, color, respiratory effort, any obvious abnormalities, responsiveness to the environment and examiner, self-consoling behavior, and family interactions should be documented. Findings on initial observation guide the examiner toward focused history or examinations.

Auscultation

The best stethoscope available should be used, with a chest piece appropriate to the age and size of the child. The earpieces should be inserted facing backward and slightly downward, directed toward the examiner's tympanic membrane. The diaphragm is used to assess *high*-pitched, more superficial sounds, while the bell is used to assess *deeper* sounds. Auscultation is usually performed when the newborn is quiet, prior to palpation to avoid stimulating the newborn and inaccurately increasing bowel sounds.

When auscultating *breath sounds*, comparison is made alternating between the right and left chest, anteriorly and posteriorly. *Heart sounds* should be assessed in the following areas:

- *AORTIC AREA*: second intercostal space, right sternal border
- *PULMONIC AREA*: second intercostal space, left sternal border
- *MITRAL AREA*: between the fourth and fifth intercostal spaces, at the midclavicular line
- *TRICUSPID AREA*: between the fourth and fifth intercostal spaces, at the lower left sternal border

Bowel sounds are auscultated over all four quadrants, noting quality, frequency, and pitch of sounds.

A normal heart rate for a newborn is between 140 and 160 beats per minute. Due to unopposed sympathetic nervous innervation, preterm infants have higher heart rates, reaching 180 beats per minute.

A normal respiratory rate is between 40 and 60 breaths per minute. Respirations will increase with crying, fever, respiratory distress, hypercapnia (elevated CO_2 levels), and certain metabolic conditions.

Palpation

In the newborn, gentle palpation is performed to assess skin texture, pulses, capillary refill, organ size, and abnormalities. It is important to compare sides for equality when palpating. Hands should be warmed and gloves worn during this part of the examination.

Measurements of the Newborn

Size Measurements

Head circumference, length, and abdominal and chest circumferences are obtained initially in the newborn as a basis of comparison for growth. The head circumference should be measured around the widest part of the brow and the occiput. Length may be difficult to measure directly due to head molding and flexor tone in the extremities. This measurement is commonly taken by marking the crown and heel of the infant on a blanket or sheet. The distance between the marks is then measured.

Chest circumference is measured at the level of the nipples and is compared with the head circumference, particularly when microcephaly or macrocephaly is a concern. There is normally a 2-cm difference between the head and chest circumferences, the head being the larger of the two measurements. The distance between the nipples may also be measured and is usually one-quarter of the chest circumference.

Temperature Measurement

In infants, a rectal temperature is the closest to the core temperature. Temperature is measured while the infant is supine with legs held securely in a flexed position. Tympanic membrane temperatures are fast, but the newborn's auditory canal is more horizontal compared with older children and may give variable readings.

Blood Pressure Measurement

Blood pressure measurement may be obtained in the newborn period by using an appropriate-sized cuff. Newborn blood pressure cuffs come in sizes 1–4. An appropriate cuff size is 25% wider than the diameter of the limb. The air-filled bladder of the cuff should encircle the extremity without overlapping. Blood pressure averages vary based upon gestational age and postnatal age (University of Virginia Patent Foundation, 2007).

Assessment of the Newborn's Head, Eyes, Ears, Nose, and Throat (HEENT)

Fetal Development

The head, eyes, ears, nose, and throat begin to develop by weeks 3–4 of gestation. Neural crest cells, which arise from the fore-, mid-, and hind brain, are essential in the development of these structures, as well as in the formation of pulmonary and cardiac outflow tracts, so that any defect that occurs during this stage of development impacts many organ systems.

The central nervous system (CNS) begins to form in week 3 from a section of tissue called the neural plate. This plate folds, becoming the neural tube. One end of the newly formed neural tube becomes the brain; the remainder becomes the spinal cord. Primitive neural cells, axons, and dendrites begin to form. Glial cells, which provide support, differentiate into astrocytes and myelin sheaths. These sheaths are vital to the speed of conduction of sensory input. Sensory and motor neurons arise from neural crest cells at around weeks 3–4 of gestation when the neural plate folds. Sensory neurons in the newborn are not fully myelinized, slowing conduction of input.

Assessing the Head

Observation

Observe the hair for color, thickness, and distribution, and the scalp for bruising, swelling, or asymmetry. Scalp lacerations may occur during an operative delivery or when fetal scalp electrodes or fetal scalp blood sampling has been performed. The size and location, as well as any bleeding, should be noted. These lacerations usually heal without intervention. Fat necrosis in the scalp is an area of hair loss and thickening of the underlying scalp due to intrauterine pressure. Aplasia cutis is a defect in scalp tissue development and may be a normal variation or associated with trisomy 13.

The presence of whorls in the hair is assessed. Due to rapidity of brain growth, one or two whorls are formed at about week 16 of gestation. Abnormal hair growth or whorls are also associated with abnormal brain growth and mental retardation. Head shape is often distorted after birth. Pressure from delivery on the presenting part of the head may cause scalp swelling, a condition called *caput succedaneum*. This swelling will resolve in several days and crosses suture lines. *Cephalhematoma* is caused by subperiosteal bleeding and is a result of trauma during birth. This condition does not cross suture lines, is usually found on the parietal bones, and may take several weeks to months to resolve. Subgaleal bleeding is a rare but emergent condition that occurs most commonly after forceps delivery. Bleeding occurs above the periosteum, presents as a boggy mass under the scalp, is accompanied by scalp bruising, and crosses suture lines. The swelling may be noted immediately after birth in severe cases or may develop 12–72 hours after delivery. If progression is slow, the entire periosteal area may be affected, with symptoms of hemorrhagic shock. The prognosis is usually good; however, treatment for any shock as well as assessment and treatment of jaundice may be required.

In newborns, lymph nodes and the thyroid gland are not usually palpated, although on occasion enlarged axillary lymph nodes may be found in infants. The most common mass in the neck is a cystic hygroma noted laterally over the clavicles. This type of growth may compromise respirations if enlarged and generally requires surgical removal. Masses found high in the neck or along the sternocleidomastoid muscle are thyroglossal duct cysts or branchial cleft cysts.

The face is observed for symmetry of features and movement. The presence of a cord around the neck, called a *nuchal cord*, may produce scleral hemorrhages and facial petechiae. These resolve in several days. Pressure placed on the head or face in utero or congenital malformations may distort facial features. Excess skin, or webbing, of the neck may be noted in several congenital abnormalities such as Down syndrome.

Cranial shape may be affected by position in utero or from early fusion of the cranial bones at the suture lines. The shapes that result from craniosynostosis include:

- *BRACHYCEPHALY*: Closure of the coronal sutures, producing a wide skull.
- *PLAGIOCEPHALY*: Closure of the sutures on one side, producing an asymmetrical skull. Occipital plagiocephaly is seen particularly in growing preterm or full-term infants due to supine positioning causing flattening of the occipital bone.
- *SCAPHOCEPHALY*: Closure of the sagittal sutures, producing a long, narrow skull.

■ *DOLICHOCEPHALY*: Elongation of the skull in the anterior–posterior plane, without fusion of the sutures. It is seen in preterm and full-term infants and is due to side-lying positioning.

Many newborns exhibit jitteriness, which is normal and should be differentiated from seizure activity. Normal jitteriness is stimulus sensitive and may be stopped by gently grasping the extremities involved. Seizure activity may be subtle, such as swimming motions of the arms, cycling of the legs, sucking, blinking, or apnea. Tonic–clonic seizures may also be noted and usually progress in severity. An electroencephalogram (EEG) is helpful in identifying seizure activity. Benign myoclonic jerking is not considered a seizure; it occurs as a single jerk in sleep, does not progress, and is not supported by history of birth trauma or perinatal distress.

Some newborns may exhibit a temporary weakness of muscles of the face or extremities due to traction or pressure on nerves during delivery.

Palpation

Palpate and measure the anterior and posterior fontanelles. The anterior fontanelle is diamond shaped, may be slightly full and soft when the baby is supine, and closes by around 18 months. The posterior fontanelle is triangular shaped, smaller, and closes by about 2–3 months of age; it may be audible when there are vascular abnormalities in the brain.

Palpation of the occipital bone will sometimes elicit a type of crepitus produced by softening of the bone due to in utero pressure or may be associated with hydrocephalus; this softening is called craniotabes.

Auscultation

Rarely, bruits in the temples or neck may be auscultated in the newborn and may indicate the presence of a vascular malformation in the brain.

Assessing the Mouth

Observation

Observe the mouth for color of the mucous membranes. A mild circumoral cyanosis is normal in the first 24–48 hours, but should resolve after the transition period.

Teeth begin to develop from dental buds at about 7 weeks. Occasionally natal teeth are seen, which are soft and not well anchored; they must be removed by a pediatric dentist to avoid aspiration. The palate is formed by the fusion of midfacial tissue at about week 7 of gestation. Failure of fusion of this tissue results in a cleft lip and palate, jaw defects, and other midline defects as well as brain abnormalities. Newborns may have variations in the shape of their palate, which may interfere with nursing by altering the ability to generate negative pressure for sucking. Common palate shapes are the *bubble palate*, in which a round arch is felt just behind the upper gum line, an *arched palate*, and a *grooved palate*, seen in newborns who have been orally intubated for ventilation purposes.

Newborns may have small firm white nodules on either the gums or the palate. These *Epstein pearls* are a normal variation and often occur in conjunction with milia. Young babies may also have thrush, a fungal infection characterized by the presence of fixed plaques on the cheeks and tongue. These may be mistaken for milk curds and may be removed with gentle cleansing.

The tongue begins to develop at about 4 weeks. At this point, it is joined to the floor of the mouth before it is freed. If this process does not occur, ankyloglossia, or tongue tie, is seen.

Observe the newborn for the presence of secretions. Excess secretions may be due to polyhydramnios, a condition that exists when there is an abnormality of the upper GI system, preventing amniotic fluid from being swallowed so that it accumulates to an excess degree. In renal conditions in which there is minimal urine made, a condition called oligohydramnios, or minimal amniotic fluid, is seen.

Assessing the Eyes

The eye begins to develop at about 22 days of gestation. The formation of the optic cup around this time allows development of the inverted retina found in all vertebrates. By the end of week 9 of gestation, the lens, optic nerve, cornea, and sclera have begun to form.

Observation

Observe for abnormalities of the sclerae and irises, as well as abnormalities of the lids, nasolacrimal ducts, eyebrows, and alignment of the eyes. Inspect the conjunctivae by pulling down gently on the lower lids. Ptosis, or drooping of the eyelids, is common and should resolve in several days. Gentle eversion of the upper and lower lids may also be needed. Scleral hemorrhages and swelling of the eyelids are common after birth and resolve in several days. Strabismus, or crossing of the newborn's eyes, and nystagmus, a rapid back and forth movement of the eyes, are signs of incoordination of the musculature of the eyes and resolve in several weeks. *The newborn will not produce tears for 3–4 months, so any discharge should be noted.*

The position of the palpebral fissures, the eye openings, should be noted. An upward slant of the fissures is seen is termed a Mongolian slant and is associated with Down syndrome. Epicanthal folds are vertical folds located next to the nares and at the inner canthus of the eye; if present, they are also associated with Down syndrome.

Because the nasolacrimal ducts are not completely patent, a whitish discharge may be seen after birth and may be cleansed with warmed water. Brushfield spots are white flecks that occur in the iris surrounding the pupil. If found, these may be associated with Down syndrome. A coloboma is a keyhole-shaped defect of the lids, iris, retina, or optic disc. It occurs during week 7 of gestation when a structure in the eye called the choroid fissure fails to close.

The pupils are assessed for equality of size, shape, and response to light, and presence of the red reflex. The mnemonic PERLA (pupils are equally reactive to light and accomodation) is used to describe pupillary light response. This assessment is best accomplished when the baby is in a quiet, alert state, in a slightly darkened room, and with the eyes open.

To assess the pupils and red reflex, an ophthalmoscope is used. An examiner with refractive errors may need to remove his or her glasses; however, contact lenses may be left in place. Begin by selecting the large, round white circle of light (the other beams are used for specialized examinations). Turn the lens disc to "0" diopters. To assess the baby's *right* eye, the ophthalmoscope is held in the examiner's *right* hand. The ophthalmoscope is held about 10–15 inches from the baby's eye in the frontal plane. While looking through the aperture, a red reflection of light coming from the pupil should be elicited. In babies with a darker complexion, however, the red reflex may appear pale or gray. While assessing the red reflex, the corneal light reflection should be assessed to confirm that it falls in the same place on both eyes. Often, a subtle strabismus may be found by identifying asymmetry of the corneal light reflex.

 Red Flags

- Corneal haziness is seen in relation to glaucoma.

- Inability to elicit a red reflex or visualization of a dull white or gray pupil may indicate retinoblastoma or cataracts.

- Be alert for inability to elicit focusing and following on a brightly colored object and inability to follow as it is moved slowly through the baby's line of vision.

- Be alert for purulent eye drainage. When accompanied by mild to moderate lid edema, injected (reddened or hyperemic) sclerae may indicate an infection. Mild symptoms are characteristic of chemical conjunctivitis. Purulent drainage seen in the first week of life, especially with moderate to severe lid swelling, may indicate gonococcal, bacterial, or chlamydial infection. Clear drainage is seen in viral or allergic conjunctivitis.

Assessing the Ears

The external ear, which collects sound; the middle ear, which conducts it; and the inner ear, which converts sound to impulses in the brain, begin to develop from paired pharyngeal pouches at about 22 days. Because these structures develop so early, ear defects are almost always seen in major chromosomal abnormalities.

Observation

The pinnae are observed for normal formation and for pitting or tags. The position of the ears is evaluated by drawing an imaginary line from the inner canthus (corner of the eye) to the outer canthus and extending this line to the top of the ear. The upper third of the ear should fall above this line. Some newborns' ears may be rotated slightly backward, which gives them the appearance of being low set, a finding consistent with several genetic abnormalities. Rotated ears are considered "pseudo" low set, and may be a normal variation.

Skin tags in front of the ears may be found. As an isolated finding, they may be a normal variation; however, they are also seen in conjunction with renal abnormalities. Because the ears, kidneys, and umbilical cord develop at the same time, often ear tags or pits will be accompanied by a renal defect and a two-vessel cord.

Sensorineural hearing loss may be identified as early as 6 months if there is no response to loud sounds. Babies with this type of hearing loss babble normally until about 6 months, when speech should become more imitative and speech delays become more obvious. In newborns, response to a loud sound should elicit a startle response. If further assessment is needed, an auditory evoked potential examination will identify hearing loss.

Visualizing the tympanic membrane in a newborn may be complicated by the presence of vernix in the canal; however, assessment of the presence of the membrane is important baseline information to obtain. To view the tympanic membrane, use an otoscope with the smallest-sized speculum. To examine the *right* tympanic membrane, the otoscope is held in the examiner's *right* hand, grasped between the thumb and fingers. In newborns and infants up to about 2 years, the ear canal is horizontal, so it may be helpful to apply gentle *downward* traction on the pinnae, compared with the upward traction exerted in the older child. The otoscope is gently inserted just inside the ear canal, aiming downward and toward the newborn's nose.

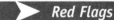 **Red Flags**

Be alert for the following:

- Inability to elicit a response to a loud sound
- Malformations of the pinnae

- True low-set ears that are not rotated
- Ear tags or pits

Assessing the Nose and Sinuses

The frontal and sphenoid sinuses do not begin to develop until about 2 years of age. Along with the ethmoid and maxillary sinuses, they continue to grow until reaching their mature size during adolescence.

Observation

The nares are observed for formation, discharge, and flaring, a sign of respiratory distress seen particularly in the newborn period. The examiner may note choanal atresia, wherein either one or both of the nasal passages are narrowed, limiting breathing through the nasal passages. The condition is identified when a small-sized catheter cannot be passed easily through one or both nares.

A flattened nasal bridge and small philtrum (the vertical groove between the upper lip and external nasal septum), as well as small palpebral fissures and upper lip, are associated with FAS. This condition is often accompanied by IUGR, tone and feeding problems, and neurologic involvement.

Palpation

Patency is assessed by gently occluding one nostril, then the other.

Normal Variations in the Newborn

Newborns may have some transplacentally acquired maternal hormones that cause swelling of the nasal mucosa. This condition is normal, and suctioning should be avoided unless there is discharge, as it may increase the swelling. Saline nasal drops are often helpful.

As mentioned previously, newborns are sometimes born with neonatal teeth. These teeth are often quite soft and generally need to be removed by a pediatric dentist to prevent aspiration. A newborn may have variations in the shape of the palate, which may interfere with nursing by altering the baby's ability to generate negative pressure for sucking. Common palate shapes are the *bubble palate*, in which a round arch is felt just behind the upper gum line; an *arched palate*; and a *grooved palate*, seen in newborns who have been orally intubated for ventilation purposes.

Newborns may also have small, firm white nodules on either the gums or the palate. These Epstein pearls are a normal variation and often occur in conjunction with milia.

Young babies may also have thrush, a fungal infection characterized by the presence of fixed plaques on the cheeks and tongue. These plaques may be mistaken for milk curds, which may be removed with gentle cleansing.

Ankyloglossia, or tongue tie, is identified by an inability to extend the tongue past the gum line along with a heart-shaped indentation at the tip of the tongue. This condition should be referred to a pediatric oral surgeon for correction to allow normal breast- or bottle-feeding as well as the normal development of speech later in childhood. In the older school-age child, enlarged tonsils are a normal finding, unless accompanied by odor or exudate.

 Red Flags

- Nasal flaring, especially if accompanied by audible grunting and retractions, may be seen, particularly during the winter in respiratory syncytial virus (RSV) infection.
- Check for obstruction of one or both nares, cleft lip and/or palate, and cyanosis of the lips and/or oral mucosa.

Assessment of the Newborn's Cranial Nerves

CRANIAL NERVE I: Smell may be difficult to assess, but strong scents, such as an alcohol pad, may be placed near the newborn's nares and should elicit a grimace.

CRANIAL NERVES II, III, IV, AND VI: The baby's ability to focus and follow is assessed with a brightly colored object. Rods and cones, the structures in the eyes that enable color discrimination, are not mature in the newborn until about 6 months, so babies are relatively unable to discern pastel colors. Primary colors such as bright red and blue, black, and white are preferred when testing vision.

CRANIAL NERVES V, IX, XII: Rooting, sucking, and swallowing are assessed by placing a gloved finger next to the newborn's mouth and observing as the baby turns to and attempts to latch onto the finger. Sucking is measured by the strength of the suck and the burst pattern. While feeding, most babies suck 5–6 times then pause to hold their breath and swallow. This suck–swallow coordination is important to note as a mechanism to protect the airway from aspiration. The ability of the tongue to extend past the gum line is an important component of latching on and generating negative pressure while sucking. A baby without this ability is considered to have ankyloglossia, tongue tie. If severe enough, this condition may need correction as the child gets older to prevent speech impairment.

CRANIAL NERVE VII: Grimacing and facial symmetry may be assessed during other parts of the examination. Blinking is assessed by lightly tapping on the forehead between the eyes, a technique termed glabellar tap.

CRANIAL NERVE VIII: The baby's ability to become alert to a sound and attend to voices or sounds is assessed by placing the baby supine on a flat surface and producing a sound or speaking to the baby while standing to the side. The child should turn toward the sound.

Assessment of the Newborn's Reflexes

PALMAR GRASP: A finger placed in the baby's hand should elicit a grasp. This reflex is extinguished by about 2 months.

STEP: While holding the baby upright, gently brush the bottoms of the baby's feet with the edge of the examining surface. This maneuver should elicit lifting of one leg and extending of the other. This reflex extinguishes at about 2–4 months.

ROOT: As described earlier in the chapter, the rooting reflex is demonstrated by placing a gloved finger next to the newborn's mouth and observing as the baby turns to and attempts to latch onto the finger. This reflex extinguishes by 3–4 months.

MORO: The Moro reflex is identified by an upward, inward movement of the arms and is extinguished by 4–6 months. This reflex may be tested in several ways:

1. The examiner holds the baby with a hand under the head and a hand under the buttocks. Carefully, but quickly, the hand holding the head is dropped by about 1–2 inches and returned to a level position.

2. The newborn's arms may be held in flexion for several seconds then gently, but quickly, extended and released. This maneuver elicits an arm recoil followed by the Moro reflex.

3. Gently shake the surface the newborn is lying on, for example the mattress or open crib.

ATONIC NECK REFLEX (ATNR): As the baby's head is turned to either the right or the left side, the baby should extend the arm and flex the leg on the side he or she is facing, with flexion of the arm and extension of the leg on the opposite side (the so-called fencing position). This reflex is extinguished by 4–6 months.

PLANTAR GRASP: Pressure is applied just behind the baby's toes, on the bottom of the foot. The toes should curl inward. This reflex extinguishes by about 10–12 months, prior to, and allowing, the development of walking.

BABINSKI: The sole of the foot is stroked from heel to toes, which, unlike with older children and adults, should elicit an *upward* fanning of the toes. After 2 years, the toes should flex inward.

Red Flags

- Seizures may be subtle in the newborn and consist of rhythmic sucking, bicycling, or swimming movements.
- Be alert for diminished power or tone.
- A bulging fontanelle can indicate increasing intracranial pressure.
- Be alert for premature closure of any of the sutures in a newborn (craniosynostosis).
- Increasing head circumference of greater than 2% is seen in relation to increased intracranial pressure.
- A depressed fontanelle is seen in relation to dehydration.

Assessment of the Newborn's Respiratory System

Fetal Development

The lungs develop from the foregut during the first 5 weeks of gestation, termed the *embryonic period*. Arteriovenous connections between the developing heart and lungs are beginning to form, which will provide perfusion to lung tissue. Formation will continue after birth until full lung growth is reached at about 8 years of age.

The lungs begin to develop at about 3–7 weeks' gestation, termed the *embryonic stage*. During the *pseudoglandular stage*, from 5 to 17 weeks' gestation, the major airways and lymphatic system form. During the *canalicular stage*, from 16 to 26 weeks' gestation, conducting airways and vascularization develop. A less stable form of surfactant is dominant at this time.

During the *terminal sac stage*, at 24–38 weeks' gestation, the conducting airways and alveoli begin to mature and enlarge, and type I and II alveolar cells produce a more stable form of surfactant. Adequate ventilation is determined by respiratory reflexes, chemical receptors, compliance of the chest wall and lung tissue, and pulmonary resistance. Pulmonary resistance is in part determined by the presence of surfactant.

Surfactant is a detergent-like substance that lines the alveoli and decreases surface tension, allowing air entry and gas exchange. Its main function is to stabilize alveoli during exhalation to prevent collapse. Phospholipids are critical in the formation of surfactant, and levels of these chemicals may be measured in amniotic fluid in pregnancy to determine maturity of the fetal lungs. Surfactant production and maturity is facilitated by steroids, thyroid hormones, and catecholamines, such as caffeine. Physiologic stress also has a maturational effect on surfactant. Maternal diabetes, however, has a negative effect on surfactant production, but it is unknown whether the effect is from elevated glucose or insulin levels.

The newborn has a higher anterior larynx; a larger, stiffer glottis; and a more acute glottic angle compared with older children. The cricoid cartilage is the narrowest part of the hour glass–shaped larynx, and the trachea lacks cartilaginous support for several months after birth. Although the newborn's airway is only 50% smaller than an adult's, resistance is 5–6 times greater. In addition, the newborn's rib cage is softer and more pliable, offering little resistance to recoil. These factors combine to place the newborn at risk of airway compromise and collapse.

Fetal Circulation and the Transition Period

The fetal lungs, filled with amniotic fluid, receive about 10% of circulation prior to birth. In utero, there are three vascular connections that shunt the remaining 80% of blood flow away from the lungs. These shunts are described as follows:

PATENT DUCTUS ARTERIOSUS (PDA): This shunt connects the aorta with the pulmonary artery. In utero, the pulmonary vasculature is constricted and the systemic vasculature is relaxed to facilitate blood flow away from the lungs. This produces a gradient that causes blood to flow across the PDA from right to left. After birth, when pulmonary vascular resistance decreases and systemic vascular resistance increases, blood flows from left to right across the PDA. This may be a temporary condition, resolving within several days while transition occurs. The stimulus for the PDA to close is elevated oxygen levels, so if a newborn is hypoxic due to cardiac or respiratory illness, the PDA may remain open, resulting in increased flow to the right ventricle and lungs. Pulmonary symptoms, including crackles, may occur if the condition is not corrected.

PATENT DUCTUS VENOSUS (PDV): This connection at the level of the liver shunts blood directly into the vena cava.

PATENT FORAMEN OVALE (PFO): This connection at the level of the atrial septum shunts blood directly from the right to the left atrium, bypassing the right ventricle and its tricuspid valve.

The umbilical cord contains three vessels: two muscular arteries on one plane and a less muscular vein. When viewing the cord after birth when it has been cut, it gives the appearance of a face, with the arteries appearing as the eyes and the vein appearing as the mouth.

Nutrients and oxygen are picked up from the placenta, then circulate through the umbilical vein to the fetus. At the level of the liver, the majority of blood flows through the PDV into the inferior vena cava. Entering the right atrium, the majority of blood is shunted across the PFO, through the left atrium, across the mitral valve, and into the left ventricle. A small amount of blood flows from the right atrium, across the tricuspid valve into the right ventricle, and from there across the pulmonic valve to the lungs.

Blood flows from the left ventricle across the aortic valve into the aorta. The PDA also shunts blood into the aorta from the pulmonary artery. Blood then flows into the two umbilical arteries and back toward the placenta. By definition, an artery carries oxygenated blood *away* from the heart and a vein carries deoxygenated blood *towards* the heart. There are two places (occasions/occurrences?) in which arteries carry blood, which is *deoxygenated* and veins carry blood which is *oxygenated;* the first is in the umbilical vessels - the umbilical arteries carry deoxygenated blood and the umbilical vein carries oxygenated blood. The other place where this occurs is after birth when in the pulmonary artery carries *deoxygenated* blood towards the lungs, and the pulmonary veins carry *oxygenated* blood back toward the heart.

With delivery of the head and chest, and clamping of the cord, elastic recoil on the chest generates negative pressure, which fills the alveoli with air. Most lung fluid is expelled during contraction and at birth; the remainder is reabsorbed after birth. After birth, pulmonary vascular resistance decreases, blood flow to the lungs increases, and a higher blood oxygen level is achieved in the newborn's blood.

Interpreting X-rays

X-rays are obtained to provide information about structures and abnormalities in the organs and bones. X-rays penetrate the body and are absorbed based on the density of the tissue: The lighter the structure appears, the denser the tissue. Bones, then, would appear to be white; solid tissue such as the liver would appear gray, and air-filled cavities such as the lungs and stomach would appear almost black.

In assessing an x-ray, it is helpful to develop a systematic approach, beginning with the quality of the examination. Position, degree of penetration, lung expansion, and artifact should be included when evaluating quality.

POSITION: The newborn chest x-ray should be taken with the infant positioned supine on a level surface. The view taken in this position is called an anteroposterior (AP) view. If the baby's body is rotated to the right or left, it is difficult to assess the lungs and heart size. Cross-table lateral x-rays, in which the baby is supine but lifted up on a surface of blankets, and lateral decubitus x-rays, in which the baby is positioned on either the right or left side, are also commonly taken. Both of these views are used to assess air and fluid levels in the chest or abdomen, such as would be seen with pneumothorax or free abdominal air.

DEGREE OF PENETRATION: The degree of penetration is determined by over- or underexposure of the x-ray. A lighter-appearing x-ray is underexposed; a darker-appearing x-ray is overexposed. Both of these conditions make it difficult to assess lung fields.

X-rays should be taken during inhalation to view the lung fields when *fully expanded*. Normally, the newborn's lungs are expanded to the level of the eighth to ninth ribs. Lungs may be underexpanded in surfactant deficiency, if the newborn is underventilating due to illness, or if the x-ray is taken during exhalation. Lungs may also be overexpanded, such as during mechanical ventilation or in conditions of air trapping.

ARTIFACT: Artifact should be identified. Indwelling ports or catheters should be clearly identified. It is helpful to view every other part of the x-ray prior to examining the desired area. Fractured clavicles and long bones may be missed when evaluating lungs, and skin folds may be confused with a collapsed lung edge unless clearly appreciated.

Observation

Assessment in the immediate newborn period is vital in recognizing the successful achievement of the transition phase and the presence of respiratory distress. Onset of symptoms may be noted immediately after delivery, or may appear later. The newborn should be observed at rest. The respiratory rate should be between 40 and 60 breaths per minute, with occasional pauses of less than 20 seconds, followed by a slightly faster rate. This pattern, termed periodic respirations, is normal in the newborn and is differentiated from apnea, which lasts longer than 20 seconds and is frequently accompanied by a dip in the heart rate. Diaphragmatic breathing, in which the abdomen rises with each breath as the chest remains fairly stable, may also be seen during the newborn period.

Grunting, flaring, and retracting (GFR) indicate increased respiratory effort as the newborn uses accessory muscles to generate negative pressure in the chest. Unequal chest excursions are a sign of pneumothorax. Diaphragmatic breathing may also be seen during the newborn period in which the abdomen rises with each breath as the chest remains stable.

Respiratory rate will be elevated with crying, fever, respiratory distress, hypercapnia (elevated CO_2 levels) and certain metabolic conditions. Respiratory rate may be decreased in sleep, or after delivery following intrapartum administration of opioid pain medications. Signs of respiratory distress include grunting, flaring of the nares and retracting. Retracting is a term used to describe the use of accessory muscles to generate negative thoracic pressure during inspiration. Suprasternal, intercostal and substernal muscles may appear to indent as they are utilized to maximize each breath.

Auscultation

Breath sounds are of three types:

- *BRONCHIOLAR*: The loudest sounds, audible in the midchest over the larger airways
- *BRONCHOVESICULAR*: Softer sounds, audible over the smaller airways
- *VESICULAR*: The softest sounds, audible in the lung periphery

Abnormal sounds include crackles, wheezes, and rubs. Crackles are characterized as fine or coarse and indicate fluid or consolidation in the lung parenchyma. Stridor, associated with airway resistance, may be heard on inspiration, which is due to large airway obstruction, or on exhalation, which is associated with obstruction in the alveoli. Rubs are audible over the lungs or heart and indicate pleural or pericardial fluid.

Palpation

Using the heel of the hand over the chest, an examiner may identify fremitus, a crackling sensation noted when air is dissecting subcutaneously or when there are secretions in the larger airways.

 Red Flags

- Tachypnea may indicate pulmonary or cardiac disease.
- Unequal chest excursions or breath sounds due to spontaneous pneumothorax (sometimes noted in athletes) may occur spontaneously in the newborn period as a result of transthoracic pressures generated with the first cry after delivery.
- Intercostal retractions are a sign of increased work of breathing.
- Apnea is a cessation of breathing for greater than 20 seconds. This condition should be differentiated from periodic respirations in the newborn, which last less than 20 seconds and are a normal variation.

Assessment of the Newborn's Cardiac System

Fetal Development

The cardiovascular system is the earliest to develop, being complete by about 18 weeks' gestation. In response to the tremendous metabolic needs of the fetus. Cardiac development begins at about 18–19 days with the formation of a primitive heart tube and the ebb and flow circulation. This tube develops five segments; from the uppermost to the lowermost, they are called the truncus, bulbus cordis, primitive ventricle, primitive atrium, and sinus venosus. The aortic and pulmonary valves develop from the bulbotruncal segment, the mitral and tricuspid valves, and the sinoatrial (SA) junction from the atrioventricular (AV) canal. At about 23 days, the bulbotruncal area loops to the left and comes to rest against the primitive ventricle. If it loops to the *right*, a condition called dextrocardia results.

The atria develop at about week 5 of gestation from the sinus venosus, and simultaneously the ventricles form from the primitive ventricle. The pulmonary infundibulum, the portion of the upper right ventricle involved in tetralogy of Fallot, develops at about the same time from the bulbus cordis.

The heart at this point consists of a single AV canal. Endocardial cushions develop and partition the canal into right and left chambers. The atrial and ventricular septa form at about week 7 of gestation. ASDs and VSDs occur during this stage.

An outflow tract also begins to form during week 7, which will become the aortic arch and pulmonary trunk. This outflow tract spirals and differentiates to assume its final position. Transposition of the great vessels occurs when the outflow tract does not spiral appropriately.

Prior to the 30th week of gestation, the left ventricle dominates in size and mass because of the differences between pulmonary and systemic vascular resistance. However, as the lungs develop and pulmonary vascular resistance increases, the right ventricle becomes dominant. After birth it is common to see a mild physiologic right ventricular hypertrophy for several months.

Factors that impact the fetal and newborn heart include immature parasympathetic innervation (vagus) prior to birth and unopposed sympathetic nervous innervation, resulting in tachycardia in preterm infants. During maturation, with increasing peripheral nervous system innervation and influence of the vagus nerve, the fetal and newborn heart rate decreases to the normal range of 140–160 beats per minute.

The newborn heart contains fewer receptor sites and is therefore characterized by a blunted response to medications. The conical shape of the newborn heart minimizes stretch response to filling, and increased energy demands allow less reserve during stress.

Observation

The chest is observed for heaves, pulsations, and cyanosis. Cyanosis occurs when 5 g/daL (grams per decaliter) of hemoglobin is deoxygenated. In a polycythemic newborn, cyanosis may be present with a normal blood oxygen level because there are many more red blood cells available for oxygen-carrying capacity. In an anemic newborn, however, blood oxygen values may fall precipitously before cyanosis is present. Oxygen saturation describes the amount of oxygen that combines with hemoglobin in a sample of blood. The amount of available oxygen, hemoglobin, blood pH, and temperature are factors that determine saturation. Compared to adults, fetal hemoglobin, present for several weeks after birth, has a tendency to bind but not release oxygen as readily. Thus, although the blood is well oxygenated, less oxygen is available to the tissues. Factors that cause fetal hemoglobin to release oxygen are hypothermia, acidosis, and hypercarbia. This tendency is described by the oxyhemoglobin dissociation curve.

Palpation

Palpate the point of maximal impulse (PMI), the point at which the heartbeat feels the strongest. The normal position for the PMI in the newborn is about the fourth intercostal space, to the left of the sternal border. In newborns, the location of the PMI is shifted in cases of pneumothorax or dextrocardia, so this is good baseline information to obtain.

An active precordium may be an indication of cardiomegaly or a cardiac defect. Perfusion is assessed by applying pressure to produce blanching over an extremity or the trunk, then counting the number of seconds required for capillary refill to occur. In newborns, the normal time of 3–5 seconds may be exceeded due to vascular transition. This technique may not be accurate, however, in hypothermic babies. Pulses should be assessed in all four extremities to determine forcefulness and quality. In infants with coarctation of the aorta, pulses will be decreased in the lower extremities. Babies with transposition of the great vessels will demonstrate pulses greater in the right arm and leg compared with the left-sided extremities.

Auscultation

The *first heart sound* (S_1) results from closure of the mitral (left AV) valve and tricuspid (right AV) valve, and is best heard at the apex. The *second heart sound* (S_2) results from closure of the pulmonic and aortic valves and is heard best at the second intercostal space.

A murmur is caused by turbulence from blood flow across an abnormal valve or through a defect in a septum. Murmurs are graded from 1–6, and documented as the auscultated grade over 6—the maximum score possible. For example, a very faint murmur would be documented as 1/6:

- *GRADE 1*: Barely audible with a stethoscope
- *GRADE 2*: Quiet but easily heard
- *GRADE 3*: Louder than a 2
- *GRADE 4*: Loud, with a palpable thrill over the PMI

- *GRADE 5*: Audible with the stethoscope barely on the chest; thrill is palpable
- *GRADE 6*: Audible without a stethoscope, with a thrill

Several common murmurs may be audible in the newborn period. The first is the murmur of the PDA. This machinery-like murmur is audible at about the fourth intercostal space to the left of the sternal border. Another common murmur may be heard, grade 1–2/6, over the pulmonic area during the first few days of life. This is the murmur of transient peripheral pulmonic stenosis (PPS). Until pulmonary artery pressure decreases to normal, flow will be heard across the branch pulmonary arteries. This high-pitched, soft murmur is best heard at the second intercostal space, left sternal border. The transitioning pulmonary resistance may also result in a narrow, transient splitting of the S_2. A wider, persistent split S_2 is characteristic of an ASD.

The murmur of a VSD is harsh and may be soft or loud depending on the size of the defect.

In general, the smaller the defect, the more turbulence is produced and the louder the sound. A VSD murmur is audible at the fifth intercostal space, left sternal border.

A split S_2, grade 1–3/6, may be heard in the first few hours of life due to delayed closure of the pulmonic valve in response to hemodynamic adaptations after birth. A fixed, widely split S_2, however, is the hallmark of an ASD.

Electrocardiogram

Conduction originates in the right upper atrium of the heart, in the SA node. From here it moves down to the AV node and divides at the bundle branches to polarize the ventricles.

These events are depicted in the electrocardiogram (ECG). Depolarization of the atria is represented by the P wave. The PR interval, the isoelectric segment between the P wave and beginning of the QRS complex, represents impulse conduction through the atria to the bundle branches. The QRS complex represents ventricular depolarization. The ST segment, measured from the end of the QRS complex to the beginning of the T wave, represents repolarization of the heart.

Arrhythmias

The most common arrhythmias in the newborn are atrial premature contractions, bradycardia, and tachycardia. Premature contractions are beats that occur earlier than normal in a complex. Premature atrial contractions may be audible transiently and are characterized by *irregularly irregular* beats. Benign, these beats are commonly due to circulating catecholamines from birth, resolve spontaneously, and require no treatment.

Arrhythmias are identified by P waves that are not followed by a QRS complex or that are buried in the preceding T wave. Often there is a compensatory pause if the beat was initiated during repolarization, when the heart is refractory to impulse conduction.

Bradycardia, defined as slower-than-normal conduction, may be caused by vagal stimulation or by metabolic or congenital abnormalities. Bradycardia may produce escape beats that arise from atrial, junctional, or ventricular tissue. These beats will be seen in the P and QRS complexes and will be audible as an irregular rate.

Tachycardia, a faster-than-normal rate of 200–230 beats per minute, arises from the SA node. It is initiated from hyperthermia, sepsis, anemia, or medications. Supraventricular tachycardia originates in the atria and includes atrial flutter and fibrillation as well as Wolff-Parkinson-White syndrome. This condition is thought to be related to bands of connective tissue in the heart that did not degenerate during the fetal period. These bands create an abnormal pathway for conduction of an impulse and may require ablation to resolve.

Common Cardiac Defects in the Newborn

Acyanotic Lesions: Left-to-Right Shunt with Increased Pulmonary Flow

PDA

- PDA is caused by failure of the ductus arteriosus to close after birth.
- Left-to-right shunt results from increasing systemic and decreasing pulmonary vascular resistance.
- The murmur is characterized by a machinery-like sound, most audible at the fourth intercostal space to the left of the sternal border. It may radiate to the posterior chest.
- Symptoms are derived from the degree of pulmonary involvement.
- Symptoms include bounding pulses, active PMI, and wide pulse pressure.

VSD

- VSD is characterized by a harsh systolic murmur audible at the lower left sternal border of the fifth intercostal space.
- If the defect is a small one in the muscular portion of the septum, it may close spontaneously.
- If the defect is in the membranous portion, it usually requires surgical correction.
- There may be see signs of congestive heart failure and pulmonary hypertension due to increased cardiac load from pulmonary circuit and systemic requirements.

ASD

- ASD occurs commonly in the area of the foramen ovale.
- The murmur is audible in the pulmonic area.
- The examiner may also hear a *widely* split S_2 due to left-to-right shunting and delayed closure of the pulmonic valve.

Coarctation of the Aorta

- Coarctation of the aorta may present with a shocklike appearance.
- Symptoms result from left-to-right shunting, pulmonary involvement, and left-sided failure.
- It may present with cyanosis depending on where the coarctation occurs.
- Lower extremity blood pressures and pulses will be lower than upper extremity blood pressures.
- The examiner may hear a systolic murmur and a third heart sound ("Ken-tuck-*ee*").

Cyanotic Lesions: Right-to-Left Shunt

Transposition of the Great Vessels

- This condition occurs from failure of aortopulmonary root to spiral.
- Cyanosis is caused by separate pulmonary and systemic circuits.
- Duct-dependent lesions allow venous and arterial blood to mix.
- The heart outline is small and narrow on x-ray.

Tetralogy of Fallot

- This defect of the right ventricular pulmonary infundibulum involves the following:
  - ➤ VSD
  - ➤ Pulmonary stenosis
  - ➤ Overriding of the aorta
  - ➤ Right ventricular hypertrophy
  - ➤ Often PDA
- Systemic oxygenation depends on mixture across the VSD or PDA.
- Symptoms include cyanosis, tachypnea, hypotension, and decreased tone.
- Severity of symptoms depends on the degree of pulmonary stenosis.

▷ Red Flags

- Tachypnea at rest indicates cardiac disease.
- Unequal pulses may indicate coarctation (increased pulses in the upper extremities) or transposition of the great vessels (decreased right-sided pulses).
- Bounding pulses, especially in the palms, are indicative of PDA in the newborn.

- Hypertension is diagnosed if the systolic or diastolic blood pressures are greater than the 95th percentile for age and sex, after three measurements are taken on the same arm, with the same equipment and in the same position, at three different times.
- Wide pulse pressure greater than 20–30 mm Hg due to a low diastolic pressure may indicate cardiac disease.

Assessment of the Newborn's Gastrointestinal/Gastrourinary System

Fetal Development

The GI system begins to develop around week 4 of gestation from the foregut, midgut, and hindgut. The foregut differentiates into the trachea, esophagus, stomach, and duodenum. The midgut forms the intestinal loop, and the hindgut differentiates into the colon, anal canal, bladder, and urethra. The intestines are formed from the midgut at about week 5 of gestation. Due to rapid growth of the intestines, the abdomen becomes too small to contain them and they protrude into the umbilical cord, a condition termed physiologic umbilical herniation. At about week 10, the herniated loops return to the abdomen and assume their final positions in the abdominal cavity.

The permanent kidney begins to form at about week 5 of gestation, ascends from the pelvis into the abdomen, and is functional by the end of the first trimester. The bladder and collecting system form at about weeks 4–7.

The gonads form from primitive germ cells and migrate to the genital ridges at about week 5 of gestation. At this time, the gonads are undifferentiated, although the sex of the fetus has been determined from fertilization. The presence of the Y chromosome determines male morphology of the gonads. Testosterone and antimüllerian hormone (AMH) are produced, stimulating differentiation of the male gonads. Maternally and placentally acquired estrogen is involved in differentiation of the female gonads. External genitalia are distinguishable by the end of the first trimester. A deficiency of testosterone in the male, or the presence of testosterone in the female, will produce ambiguous genitalia that may present as enlarged clitoris, enlarged or rugated labia majora, or micropenis. The sex of the baby should not be identified unless definitive testing is done.

Although the exact cause is unknown, two of the most common causes of ambiguous genitalia are congenital adrenal hyperplasia (CAH), in which the adrenal glands produce an excess of male hormones, or maternal intake of drugs that have male hormone activity, such as progesterone, in early pregnancy.

Observation

The abdomen is observed for masses, musculature, formation of the genitalia, discharge, and hernias. The umbilical cord is evaluated for number of vessels, redness, color, and foul-smelling discharge. The location of the urethral meatal opening is identified, and the scrotal sac and testes are assessed. The testes, which are located in the abdomen during fetal life, descend into the scrotum by birth. If they are not palpable in the scrotum or inguinal canal, they are termed undescended testes and require surgical repair if they have not spontaneously resolved by 1 year of age.

Hydroceles, unilateral or bilateral scrotal enlargement, may be noted in newborns and are classified as either communicating or noncommunicating. During prenatal life, a segment of abdominal tissue, the processus vaginalis, loops through the inguinal ring into the scrotal sac bilaterally. This loop of tissue generally disintegrates. Sometimes when it does not, it leaves a pathway for abdominal contents (hernia) or fluid (hydrocele) to move into the scrotal sac. If the fluid can move freely through the loop, the size of the hydrocele will fluctuate and is termed a communicating hydrocele. This type of hydrocele will eventually need to be surgically repaired. If fluid is trapped in a small distal segment of the loop, the resulting hydrocele is termed noncommunicating; it will not change in size and does not require repair. A unilateral or bilateral bluish discoloration of the scrotum may be an indication of incarcerated hernia or testicular torsion and requires immediate evaluation.

The penis is assessed next. A chordee may be seen, which is a fibrotic band of tissue extending the length of the ventral surface of the penis. This band of tissue may cause a slight curvature of the penis. It may also be associated with ambiguous genitalia. The foreskin is examined and gently retracted. It will not retract the entire length of its surface, but inability to retract the foreskin in a newborn, termed phimosis, may interfere with urination and should be further evaluated. Malposition of the opening of the urethral meatus on either the lower or upper surfaces of the penile shaft, termed hypospadias and epispadias, requires further evaluation.

Palpation

Skin texture should be palpated for temperature and hydration, and the edges of the liver and spleen should be assessed. To palpate the liver edges in a newborn, place the middle and index fingers horizontally over the ribs on the right side. Run the fingers down the ribs to the rib edge (costal margin). A gentle, inward movement should locate the liver edge at 1 to 2 cm below the costal border. The liver edge should feel firm against the examining fingers. The spleen is assessed in the same way, but at the left costal border, although in the newborn period the spleen should not be palpable. Kidneys are not usually palpated in the newborn.

The diastasis rectus muscle edges, located longitudinally at either side of the abdomen, are not approximated in the newborn for several weeks, resulting in a midline bulge during crying. This bulge is often mistaken for a hernia but resolves without treatment.

Auscultation

Auscultate for bowel sounds and bruits over the major vessels of the abdomen.

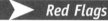 **Red Flags**

- Tracheoesophageal fistula (TEF) is a condition in which there is an abnormal connection between the trachea and the esophagus, allowing amniotic fluid from the stomach to pass into the trachea, causing choking and respiratory distress. There are five types of TEF. From the most common to the least common, they are as follows:
  - *Type L*: The lower segment of the esophagus is connected to the trachea, leaving a blind upper pouch.
  - *Type O*: There is no connection between the trachea and esophagus, but the esophagus has both an upper and lower blind pouch.
  - *Type H*: The esophagus is not divided, but a bridge, or H-type connection, exists between the esophagus and trachea.
  - *Type U*: The upper segment of the esophagus is connected.
  - *Type B*: Both upper and lower segments of the esophagus are connected.
- Bloody stools in the newborn may indicate volvulus, intussusception, bowel abnormalities, or necrotizing enterocolitis, a bowel infection. Formula intolerance may also produce minor blood in the stools.
- Be alert for signs of dysfunction: decreased or absent bowel sounds, distention, projectile vomiting, and absence of void or stool within the first 24 hours of birth.

Assessment of the Skin

Fetal Development

The newborn skin is a protective barrier that helps maintain thermoregulation, provides protection against infection and insensible water loss, and assists the newborn in receiving tactile stimulation. There are two layers of skin: the epidermis and the dermis. The epidermis, the topmost layer, contains the stratum corneum. Cells of this layer contain keratin, the tough protein layer that protects the underlying epithelium and is relatively water impermeable. Maturity of the keratin layer is directly related to gestational age.

The dermis lies beneath the epidermis and contains connective tissue that adheres the two layers. In newborns this adhesion is not as strong as in older babies and adults, which puts the newborn at risk for injury. The dermis of a full-term newborn is only 60% as thick as that of an adult. At birth, the newborn skin has an alkaline surface, but within days the pH of the skin falls to less than 5.0, creating an acid mantle. This acid mantle helps protect against organisms and infection. Other factors that put the newborn at risk for tissue injury include increased water content, increased permeability, and larger surface area (Association of Women's Health, 2007).

Rashes and skin abnormalities may be described using the following terminology:

- *MACULE*: A flat, nonpalpable, circumscribed area of discoloration. Mongolian spots are an example of macules.
- *VESICLE*: A small fluid-filled sac. Grouped vesicles are seen in herpes simplex.
- *PAPULE*: A solid, raised mass, usually less than 0.5 cm.
- *NODULE*: A papule that is larger than 0.5 cm.
- *PUSTULE*: A vesicle that contains purulent material.
- *WHEAL*: An erythematous raised area such as might be seen in an allergic reaction.
- *BULLA*: A larger fluid-filled vesicle.

Jaundice

Jaundice is a yellowish discoloration of the skin that is categorized as either physiologic or pathologic. In utero, the fetus produces an abundance of red blood cells to facilitate oxygen binding and carrying capacity. After birth, the excess red blood cells are hemolyzed, producing bilirubin. The bilirubin is bound to albumin, transported to the liver, conjugated, and excreted in the urine and stool. Several conditions that affect the level of serum bilirubin contribute to jaundice, including the following:

- *INCREASED PRODUCTION OF BILIRUBIN* occurs in bruising, polycythemia, blood group incompatibility, and sepsis.
- *DECREASED CLEARANCE* occurs when serum levels of albumin are low, medications are administered that compete for binding sites, or conjugation in the immature liver is delayed.

- *ENTEROHEPATIC CIRCULATION* is characterized by reabsorption of bilirubin from the bowel due to slow bowel transit time or late stooling.

Physiologic jaundice is a normal process occurring in virtually all newborns. This type of jaundice occurs at about the third day, has a slow rate of rise and does not exceed 12 mg/dl. The condition resolves spontaneously at about the end of the first week of life and is usually due to immature hepatic function or dehydration. Physiologic jaundice may occur later and last longer in preterm infants.

Pathologic jaundice is defined as jaundice that occurs in the first 24 hours after delivery, is characterized by a rapid rate of rise, and achieves levels greater than 15 mcg/mL. Pathologic jaundice, as the name indicates, may be anticipated by antepartal history and is associated with blood group incompatibility, excess red cell breakdown or sepsis. This type of jaundice requires treatment to resolve ranging from phototherapy to exchange transfusion.

The most common cause of pathologic jaundice is blood group incompatibility. In this condition fetal red cells have entered the maternal circulation through either a previous delivery when exposure occurred at birth, an amniocentesis, or some disruption of the placenta such as motor vehicle accident or hypertension. In this condition the chorionic villi are disturbed, allowing fetal cells to enter the maternal circulation. The mother then produces antibodies, which cross the placenta during the subsequent pregnancy, resulting in hemolysis of fetal red blood cells. The most antigenic reactions occur in blood group incompatibility such as an Rh negative mother carrying an Rh positive fetus, or a type O mother carrying a type A fetus. Maternal antibodies, which have been produced during an earlier pregnancy cross the placenta resulting in hemolysis of fetal red blood cells.

Jaundice is also associated with breastfeeding. Breastfeeding mothers in whom a let down response is not well established initially may note breastfeeding-*associated* jaundice, which resolves once the baby's intake improves. In rare cases a mother's breast milk may lack an enzyme required to metabolize bilirubin, resulting in true breast milk jaundice. This condition occurs around the tenth day of life, and usually does not require that the mother stop breastfeeding. In most cases supplementation with formula after breastfeeding is sufficient to resolve the jaundice.

Newborn skin is characterized by several normal variations:

- *MONGOLIAN SPOTS:* These bluish, flat, irregular macules are most often found on the buttocks, lower back, and upper thighs.

- *MILIA*: Pores may be filled with vernix, the thick, creamy white material found on the skin of a newborn, appearing as white, flat macules.
- *NEONATAL ERYTHEMA TOXICUM*: These lesions consist of a red base with a small raised pustule; they may be scattered over the body and are found singly or grouped.
- *PUSTULAR MELANOSIS*: These small, flat macules may be found on the trunk or extremities and usually result when the pustules of erythema toxicum rupture in utero.
- *CUTIS MARMORATA*: This marbled appearance of the skin mainly occurs when the baby is cool.
- *HARLEQUIN SIGN*: This sign of vascular immaturity can produce a demarcation between the right and left sides of the baby's body in which half the body is pale and the other half is ruddy.
- *ACROCYANOSIS*: This temporary mild cyanosis of the hands and feet is seen in the first few hours of life in response to vascular adaptations.

> ### Red Flags

Central cyanosis occurs when 5% or more of hemoglobin is deoxygenated. Babies with excess red blood cells (polycythemia) may appear cyanotic even with normal blood oxygen levels. Conversely, anemic babies may *not* demonstrate cyanosis even when hypoxic.

Assessment of the Musculoskeletal System

Fetal Development

The skeletal system develops from neural crest tissue forming connective tissue, mesenchyme, at about 4 weeks' gestation. This tissue migrates and differentiates into several types of skeletal cells. Limb buds begin to form at about 6 weeks, and at birth the central portion of the bone is ossified, while the ends of the bones, the epiphyses, remain cartilaginous.

Observation

The extremities, spine, and skull are assessed through observation. Skull shapes were discussed previously in the assessment of the head.

The hands and feet should be observed for polydactyly (extra digits), syndactyly (webbing of digits), or other abnormalities. The extremities should be assessed for strength, tone, and range of motion.

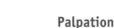

Palpation

The clavicles are palpated along their length for fractures, which are identified by crepitus over the area of injury.

Developmental dysplasia of the hips is assessed with the Ortolani and Barlow maneuvers. With the infant in the supine position, the examiner places his or her hands around the hip joint, with the middle fingers on the trochanters and thumbs against the inside of the groin. The Barlow test is performed by flexing the hips and *adducting* the thighs (applying pressure inward and downward). Then, with the hips still flexed, the thighs are abducted (turned outward), which constitutes the Ortolani maneuver. Normally, hearing no *clunk* of the hip joints is normal in the newborn until about 3 months, as neuromuscular maturity progresses in a cephalocaudal (head to toe) and proximodistal (inner to outer) fashion. After this point, it will be more difficult to assess for hip dislocation due to increased tone in the joints. Laxity in the *knee* joint of newborns may produce a *click*, which, because it may radiate, can be mistaken for a hip click. To identify the location of the click, the examiner places a finger over the knee joint while performing the hip assessment. The knee click can then be distinguished.

With the infant suspended over the examiner's hand, the spine is observed and palpated for intactness. An occult spina bifida will be appreciated at the lower end of the spine. Open neural tube defects such as meningocele are visible along the spine and require immediate evaluation.

Metatarsus adductus, an incurving of the feet in the newborn due to intrauterine position, is a normal finding and is distinguished from clubfoot in that the feet may be gently moved to an anatomically normal position.

Talipes equinovarus, or clubfoot, is a defect of the ankle and requires follow-up. The affected foot may *not* be moved to a normal anatomic position.

Gestational Age Assessment

The gestational age of a newborn, or the number of completed weeks of pregnancy, is important to calculate accurately and cannot be determined accurately from either the mother's menstrual history or the baby's weight. A careful gestational age assessment done after birth is accurate to approximately 2 weeks of the estimated gestational age. Once the gestational age has been assessed, it is plotted along with head and length measurements. This information is used to identify potential risk factors in the newborn and provides indirect information about the intrauterine environment.

Neuromuscular Maturity

Score	-1	0	1	2	3	4	5
Posture							
Square window (wrist)	>90°	90°	60°	45°	30°	0°	
Arm recoil		180°	140–180°	110–140°	90–110°	<90°	
Popliteal angle	180°	160°	140°	120°	100°	90°	<90°
Scarf sign							
Heel to ear							

Physical Maturity

							Maturity Rating	
Skin	Sticky, friable, transparent	Gelatinous, red, translucent	Smooth, pink; visible veins	Superficial peeling and/or rash; few veins	Cracking, pale areas; rare veins	Parchment, deep cracking; no vessels	Leathery, cracked, wrinkled	
Lanugo	None	Sparse	Abundant	Thinning	Bald areas	Mostly bald		
							Score	Weeks
Plantar surface	Heel-toe 40–50 mm: -1 < 40 mm: -2	> 50 mm, no crease	Faint red marks	Anterior transverse crease only	Creases anterior $2/3$	Creases over entire sole	-10	20
							-5	22
							0	24
Breast	Imperceptible	Barely perceptible	Flat areola, no bud	Stippled areola, 1–2 mm bud	Raised areola, 3–4 mm bud	Full areola, 5–10 mm bud	5	26
							10	28
Eye/Ear	Lids fused loosely: -1 tightly: -2	Lids open; pinna flat; stays folded	Slightly curved pinna, soft slow recoil	Well curved pinna, soft but ready recoil	Formed and firm, instant recoil	Thick cartilage, ear stiff	15	30
							20	32
							25	34
Genitals (male)	Scrotum flat, smooth	Scrotum empty, faint rugae	Testes in upper canal, rare rugae	Testes descending, few rugae	Testes down, good rugae	Testes pendulous, deep rugae	30	36
							35	38
							40	40
Genitals (female)	Clitoris prominent, labia flat	Clitoris prominent, small labia minora	Clitoris prominent, enlarging minora	Majora and minora equally prominent	Majora large, minora small	Majora cover clitoris and minora	45	42
							50	44

Figure 4-2   Ballard Standard Form

Source: From Ballard JL. New Ballard score, expanded to include extremely premature infants. J. Pediatr. 1991;119:417–423. Reprinted with permission.

Case Study:
Assessment of a Late Preterm Infant

You are a pediatric nurse practitioner with admission/discharge privileges at the local community hospital. The newborn nursery is a level-1 nursery, which means it provides care for normal newborns. You are asked to complete an admission assessment on the following newborn:

> B. B. Smith was born at 35 weeks to a 26-year-old G1 now P1 mother. All prenatal screens were negative. The pregnancy was complicated by mild gestational diabetes, well controlled with diet. Mother has no known drug allergies and was on prenatal vitamins throughout pregnancy. She was otherwise well.
>
> The baby was born by uncomplicated vaginal delivery with Apgar scores of 7 at 1 minute and 9 at 5 minutes. The mother wishes to breastfeed and would like a visit from the lactation consultant.

Questions

1. Based on the obstetric history, what findings in the newborn would you anticipate?
2. As you assess the newborn, you note a grade 1/6 machinery-like murmur audible at the fourth intercostal space, left sternal border. What type of murmur would this be, and what is the etiology?
3. Your examination reveals a normal newborn. The baby's temperature is 98.7°F, the blood glucose is 87, and the baby will be breastfeeding. What are your concerns, if any?

Answers

1. The baby was born at 35 weeks and 6 days, which classifies him as an LPTI. Findings that you may anticipate are temperature and blood glucose instability, potential for mild respiratory distress, feeding problems, and sepsis. The mother has gestational diabetes, which puts the infant at risk for LGA, blood glucose and temperature instability, feeding problems, and potential for birth trauma. In addition, the mother's blood type is O positive, which presents the potential for blood group incompatibility and jaundice.
2. This is most likely a PDA murmur, which is identified by the timing, quality, and location of the murmur. PDA is due to persistent fetal circulation and the reversal of blood flow from the aorta to the pulmonary artery due to increased left atrial pressure.

3. Due to the baby's late-preterm status, the potential for temperature instability, hypoglycemia, and sepsis would be a concern. A complete blood count with differential and blood cultures may be indicated. Temperature and blood glucose would need to be followed. The lactation consultant should be aware of the risk factors and should see the mother as soon as possible to assure adequacy of initial breastfeeding. Vitamin K and eye prophylaxis should be administered.

References

Association of Women's Health, Obstetric and Neonatal Nurses. (2006). *Hyperbilirubinemia: identification and management in healthy term and near-term newborn* (2nd ed.). Washington D.C.

Association of Women's Health, Obstetric and Neonatal Nurses. (2007). *Neonatal skin care: Evidence-based clinical practice guideline* (2nd ed.). Washington DC: Author.

Ballard, J.L., Khoury, J.C., Wedig, K., et al. (1991). New Ballard score, expanded to include extremely premature infants. *Journal of Pediatrics, 119,* 417–423.

Kattwinkel, J., et al. (Eds.). (2007). Perinatal Continuing Education Program, 2007. Book 2. Thermoregulation module. American Academy of Pediatrics and the University of Virginia Patent Foundation.

Medoff-Cooper, B., Bakewell-Sachs, S., Buus-Frank, M. E., Santa-Donato, A., & Near-Term Infant Advisory Panel. (2005). The AWHONN Near-Term Infant Initiative: A conceptual framework for optimizing health for near-term infants. *Journal of Obstetric, Gynecologic, and Neonatal Nursing, 34*(6), 666–671.

University of Virginia Patent Foundation. (2007). Perinatal Continuing Education Program, 2007. Book 2. Neonatal care. American Academy of Pediatrics and the University of Virginia Patent Foundation.

Resources

Battaglia, F.C., Lubchenko, L.O. (1967). A practical classification of newborn infants by weight and gestational age. *Journal of Pediatrics, 71,* 159–163.

Lubchenko, L.O., Hansman, C., Boyd, E. (1966). Intrauterine growth in length and head circumference as estimated from live births at gestation ages from 26–42 weeks. *Pediatrics,* 403–408.

MacDonald, M.G., Mullett, M.D., Seshia, M.K. (Eds). (2005) *Avery's neonatology: Pathophysiology and management of the newborn.* Philadelphia: Lippincott Williams and Wilkins.

Sadler, T.W. (2009). *Langman's medical embryology: North American edition* (11th ed.). Philadelphia: Lippincott Williams and Wilkins,.

Tappero, E.P, Honeyfield, M.E. (2009). *Physical assessment of the newborn.* (4th ed.). *NICU* Santa Rosa, CA: Ink.

Thureen, P., Hall, D., Deacon, J., Hernandez, J. (2004). *Assessment and care of the well newborn.* Philadelphia: WB Saunders.

Trotter, C., Carey, B. (2000) Radiology basics: Overview and concepts. *Neonatal Network, 19*(2), 35–47.

Examination of the Skin, Hair, and Nails

Anatomy and Physiology

The Skin

The skin—also called the integument, which means covering—includes the nails and hair as well as the glands. and comprises the largest organ of the body. It is composed of two distinct regions, the epidermis and the dermis. The epidermis, composed of epithelial cells, is the outermost protective layer. The underlying layer, the dermis, makes up the bulk of the skin and is a tough leathery layer composed of fibrous connective tissue. The dermis is vascularized, and nutrients reach the epidermis by diffusing through the tissue fluid from blood vessels in the dermis. The subcutaneous tissue is known as the hypodermis or superficial fascia. Technically, it is not considered part of the skin, although it shares some of the skin's protective functions. The hypodermis consists of mostly adipose tissue. It primarily anchors the skin to the underlying structures, such as muscles, and allows the skin to slide relatively freely over those structures. Because of its fatty composition, the hypodermis acts as a shock absorber and insulates the deeper body tissues from heat loss. It is the hypodermis that thickens markedly when one gains weight.

The epidermis consists of four distinct cell types and four distinct layers, except for the palms of the hands and soles of the feet, where there are five layers. The deepest layer of the epidermis is the *stratum germinativum*, or basal cell layer. It is composed of columnar-shaped cells. These cells undergo continuous mitosis to produce new cells that replace cells that are lost from the top layer of the epidermis. The stratum germinativum provides the skin with tone and creates pigment-producing melanocytes that filter ultraviolet light. The next layer is the *stratum spinosum*, which overlies the stratum germinativum. This layer consists of layers of polyhedral-shaped cells. The *stratum granulosum* overlies the stratum spinosum and is composed of cells that contain glycolipids that are a major factor in slowing water loss across the epidermis. The additional layer, the *stratum lucidum*, is found exclusively on the palmar and plantar surfaces. It contains dead keratinocytes and thickened plasma membranes, and it aids in the formation of keratin. The last layer is the *stratum corneum*, also known as the horny layer, which provides a waterproof barrier. This layer is in a continual state of desquamation, or shedding, as new skin cells are pushed up from the lower layers. A complete turnover of new cells occurs every 3 to 4 weeks. These cornified, or horny, cells are familiar as dandruff and flakes that slough off from dry skin.

The color of the skin is controlled by three pigments: *melanin, carotene*, and *hemoglobin*. The melanocytes of individuals with dark skin produce much more and darker melanin than those of fair-skinned individuals. Freckles and pigmented moles are examples of local accumulation of melanin. Melanocytes are stimulated to greater activity when a person is exposed to sunlight. Prolonged sun exposure causes a substantial melanin buildup that helps protect DNA from ultraviolet radiation. This melanin buildup is what causes darkening of the skin or a sun tan. Although melanin has protective effects, excessive sun exposure eventually damages the skin by causing clumping of elastin fibers, leading to leathery skin and altering the DNA skin cells, which eventually can lead to skin cancer.

Carotene is a yellow pigment found in such plants as carrots. It tends to accumulate in the stratum corneum and in fatty tissue of the hypodermis. When large amounts of carotene-rich food, such as carrots or sweet potatoes, are ingested, a yellow-orange tone can be seen where the stratum corneum is thickest, such as the palms and soles.

The oxygenated hemoglobin is reflected in the pinkish hue of fair-skinned individuals. Caucasian skin contains small amounts of melanin and the epidermis is transparent, thus allowing the hemoglobin color to show through. When hemoglobin is poorly oxygenated, such as in periods of cyanotic episodes or severe anemia, both the blood and skin of light-skinned people appear pale, cyanotic, or even gray in color.

The Glands

There are two groups of glands in the skin: the sebaceous glands and the sweat glands. The sebaceous glands are sebum-producing glands and are found all over the body except on the palms and soles. They are relatively small on the trunk and limbs but are large on the face, ne ck, and upper chest where they secrete sebum, an oily secretion. Sebum lubricates the hair and skin, preventing hair from becoming brittle and slowing water loss from the skin. The secretion of sebum is stimulated by hormones, especially androgens, which become activated during puberty. Acne is an example of active inflammation of the sebaceous glands.

The sweat glands are classified as two types: apocrine glands and eccrine glands. Apocrine glands are primarily located in the axillary and anogenital areas. They become active during puberty and are controlled by the sympathetic nervous system in association with pain and stress. The eccrine glands are distributed all over the body. Their main role is to assist in thermoregulation and to prevent overheating of the body. See **Figure 5-1**.

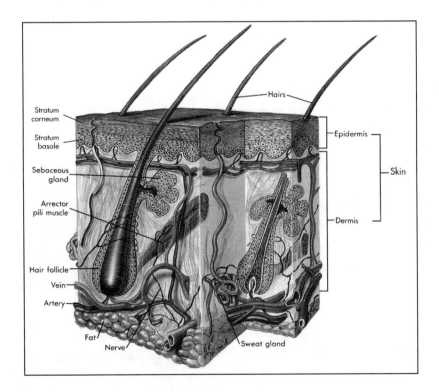

Figure 5-1 Skin Structure

The Nails

Nails are a scale like modification of the epidermis that form a clear protective covering on the dorsum of the distal part of the finger or toe. They are composed of hard keratin. Each nail has a free edge, a body portion, and a proximal or root embedded in the skin. The nail bed is the deeper layers of the epidermis that extends beneath the nail. The thickened proximal portion of the nail bed, called the nail matrix, is responsible for nail growth. The white crescent area called the lunula or "little moon" lies over the thickened nail matrix. See **Figure 5-2**.

The Hair

There are millions of hair follicles scattered over the body. They are classified as vellus or terminal. The vellus hair, also called body hair, of children and adult females is pale with a fine, fleecelike texture. The coarser hair of the eyebrows and scalp is terminal hair. During puberty, terminal hairs appear in the axillary and pubic regions of both sexes, and on the chest, arms, and legs of males. The terminal hairs grow in response to the stimulation of male sex hormones, androgens. Hair growth and density are influenced primarily by nutrition and hormones.

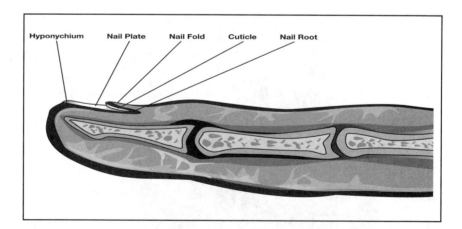

Figure 5-2 Structure of the Nail

Assessment Considerations: Subjective Information

The Skin

With any rash at any age, three questions to ask include:

- How long has your child had it?
- Does it itch?
- What have you used to treat it?

Infants
Skin considerations pertinent to the infant include:

- What is the child's feeding history? Is the child breast- or bottle-feeding? If on formula, what type?
- If eating solid foods, what foods have been introduced and when?
- Is the parent making the food or purchasing ready-made baby food?
- What is the child's diaper history, including type of diapers and creams or lotions used in the diaper area? Ask the parent what is used to clean the child's skin and how often the child's diaper is changed. If using cloth diapers, determine what type of detergent is used or whether any new detergents are being used.
- What types of clothing does the child wear, and how is clothing washed? Consider the types of soaps and/or detergents used as well as new clothing and/or bedding.
- What is the child's bathing frequency, and what soaps, lotions, and oils are used?
- Have over-the-counter treatments been used? If so, how effective have they been? Are they topical or systemic?
- Have prescription medications been used? If so, how effective have they been? Are they topical or systemic?
- Are there any systemic symptoms now, or were there before onset of the rash, such as fever, vomiting/diarrhea, cough, or nasal congestion?
- Has there been a prior incidence of a similar rash?
- Do any other family members or individuals in contact with the child have a similar rash?
- Does the parent apply sunscreen to the child when outside?
- Does the child have a history of medication, environmental, or food allergies?

School-Age Children

Skin considerations pertinent to the school-age child include:

- Does the child have a history of allergic disorders such as eczema, urticaria, pruritus, hay fever, asthma, or other chronic respiratory disorders?
- Are there pets in the house?
- Has the child had exposure to a communicable disease such as scarlet fever or varicella?
- Has the child had exposure to contagious skin conditions such as scabies, lice, or impetigo?
- What types of food does the child generally eat, including snacks?
- Has the child recently traveled into or out of the country?
- Has the child eaten anywhere other than the home, such as at a restaurant, recently?
- Has the child experienced dietary changes or been exposed to new foods?
- Has the child worn/used new clothing, bedding, or towels recently?
- Has the child been exposed to new detergents, lotions, creams, or soaps?
- Has the child had recent outdoor exposures, such as hiking, camping, or swimming?
- Does the child have new play areas?
- Are immunizations up to date?
- Does the child have a history of medication, environmental, or food allergies?
- Do other family members or children in school have a similar rash?

Adolescents

Many of the previous questions can apply to adolescents. Additional considerations include:

- Has the adolescent had recent exposure to drugs, environmental or occupational toxins, or chemicals?
- Is the adolescent involved in sports such as wrestling, football, or swimming?
- Does the adolescent have a history of acne and new medications, both topical and systemic?
- Does the adolescent use sunscreens?
- Does the adolescent have a history of tattoos or body piercing?

The Hair

Infants

- Has there been a change in the quality, texture, or distribution of the child's hair?
- Is there scaling on the scalp?
- Does the child have a history of systemic illness such as malnutrition, thyroid disease, or other chronic illness?

School-Age Children

- Has there been a change in the quality, texture, or distribution of the child's hair?
- Is there concern regarding infestation such as lice or nits?
- Does the child have a history of broken hair associated with fungal infections?
- Does the child chronically manipulate the hair?
- Has the child had recent exposure to new soaps, lotions, creams, or hair products?

Adolescents

- Has the adolescent recently applied chemicals such as dyes or straighteners to the hair?
- Has the adolescent had recent exposure to new cosmetics or skin products?

The Nails

Infants

- Has there been a change in the quality or texture of the nails?
- Does the child have a history of nail infections such as paronychia?
- Does the infant suck his or her thumb or fingers?
- Is there a history of systemic illness such as malnutrition, thyroid disease, or other chronic illness?
- How do you trim the child's nails?

School-Age Children

- Has there been a change in the quality or texture of the nails?
- Does the child bite his or her nails?
- Does the child have a history of nail infections such as paronychia?
- How are the fingernails and toenails cut?

Adolescents

- Has there been a change in the texture or quality of the nails?
- Does the adolescent bite his or her nails?
- Does the adolescent have a history of paronychia?
- How are fingernails and toenails cut?
- Does the adolescent use acrylic nails?

Family History

During the assessment, also consider the child's family history of skin, hair, and nail conditions. Is there a history of skin disorders or allergies such as eczema, psoriasis, hives, atopic dermatitis, hay fever, or specific food or environmental allergies? Is there a history of respiratory disorders such as asthma, or frequent upper respiratory infections?

Review of Systems

The systems review for skin, hair, and nails includes attention to any previous sensitivities or systemic problems such as endocrine, cardiac, or hematologic disorders. Also consider history of respiratory disorders with associated asthma, eczema, or allergies.

Assessment Considerations: Objective Information

Overview of the Skin Examination

Skin pigmentation varies based on the racial group, as does hair texture and the number of sweat glands. For example, rashes may be difficult to discern in children with darker skin. Assessment of cyanosis and pallor in African Americans may be best measured by examining the mucous membranes or the nail beds.

Table 5-1 provides a chart of skin variation based on the child's race.

As part of the assessment, the *inspection* of the skin describes the lesion based on characteristics such as location, quantity, grouping, shape, quality or morphology, color, and distribution. During inspection, assess the rash to determine if it is generalized, localized, and/or symmetrical. Note if the rash is on exposed areas of the skin or in flexor surfaces, such as in the crease of the elbow or knee. The shape of the rash may be described as round, oval, irregular, or coalesced. Measure the size of a lesion with a tape measure or small ruler, preferably in centimeters. Common objects are frequently used as a reference for size, including coins or household items such as a pea. Lesions should be measured in all dimensions (height, width, and depth), if possible. Assess the color in terms of hyperpigmented, hypopigmented, or erythematous. If there is exudate, note the amount and color.

TABLE 5-1	SKIN VARIATIONS BY RACE OF CHILDREN
Race	Characteristics (and Implications for Care)
African American	**Skin** Pallor best detected in nail beds or mucous membranes; cyanosis may appear deep blue or black on skin. Varying degrees of pigmentation from very light to deep black; pigmentation increases similar to Asians. **Implications for care:** May need to palpate rashes because of difficulty visualizing; erythema often seen as deep red or violet. Apocrine sweat glands more numerous than among Native Americans and Asians. Increased cutaneous melanin; protects against sun damage. Mongolian spots present in 90% of infants. **Implications for care:** Do not assume caregivers know what these are; explain that these spots are not uncommon in some races and tend to fade as the child gets older. Need to document because they can be misdiagnosed as bruises, common in child abuse. **Other** Pseudofolliculitis barbae: Papulopustules occur at hair follicles, caused by hair re-entering the skin. Seen almost exclusively in African American males. **Hair** Variety of textures; increased sebaceous secretions. Hair may spontaneously knot; rubbing can have a wooling effect. **Nail beds** Diffuse pigmentation of nail, especially in darker clients.
Asian	**Skin** Pallor is best detected in nail beds and mucous membranes. Pigmentation varies from brown to pale yellow-tinged. Pigmentation is very light at birth, darkens with age until 2 to 3 months old. Apocrine sweat glands fewer than in Caucasians and African Americans. Mongolian spots (blue-black hyperpigmentation found in the lumbosacral area) present in 90% of infants. **Implications for care:** See African American. **Hair** Sparse body hair; chest hair frequently absent in adolescent males. Color very dark; usually deep brown to black. Texture may be fine to coarse; generally straight but may be wavy. **Nail beds** Darker pigmentation may be present.

(continues)

TABLE 5-1 SKIN VARIATIONS BY RACE OF CHILDREN *(continued)*	
Race	**Characteristics (and Implications for Care)**
Caucasian	**Skin** Large variations in skin tones and degree of pigmentation. More apocrine sweat glands than among Asians and Native Americans. Decreased melanin leads to high risk for sunburn, and skin damage leading to higher incidence of skin cancer than in other races. **Implications for care:** Early skin cancer prevention education important for caregivers. Stress importance of routinely using sunscreen on children and infants older than 6 months. Freckles seen in fair-skinned school-age children with frequent exposure to the sun. **Other** Higher incidence of adolescent acne. **Hair** Wide variation in hair color and texture. Color ranges from blond to black; texture may be straight to very curly, thick to fine. **Nail beds** Pale to deep-pink pigmentation.
Hispanic American	**Skin** Pallor best detected in mucous membranes. Varying degrees of pigmentation. Largest percentage have tan to dark brown skin. Increases in pigmentation similar to Asians and African Americans. Mongolian spots present in 90% of infants. **Implications for care:** See African American. **Hair** Varying textures: wavy, curly, straight; mostly black or dark brown. **Nail beds** Deep pigmentation may be present.
Native American	**Skin** Pallor best detected in mucous membranes. Varying degrees of pigmentation; increased pigmentation similar to Asians, African Americans, and Hispanics. Fewer apocrine sweat glands than in African Americans and Caucasians. Mongolian spots present in 90% of infants. **Implications for care:** See African American. **Hair** Variations in texture may be coarse to fine; hair may be straight, wavy, or curly. **Nail beds** Deep pigmentation may be present.

Source: Potts/Mandleco. Pediatric Nursing, (2nd ed.). © 2007 Delmar Learning, a part of Cengage Learning, Inc. Reproduced by permission. www.cengage.com/permissions

Additionally, assess the hair, nails, and mucous membranes, noting texture, color, and presence and character of lesions. See **Figure 5-3** for examples of common lesions.

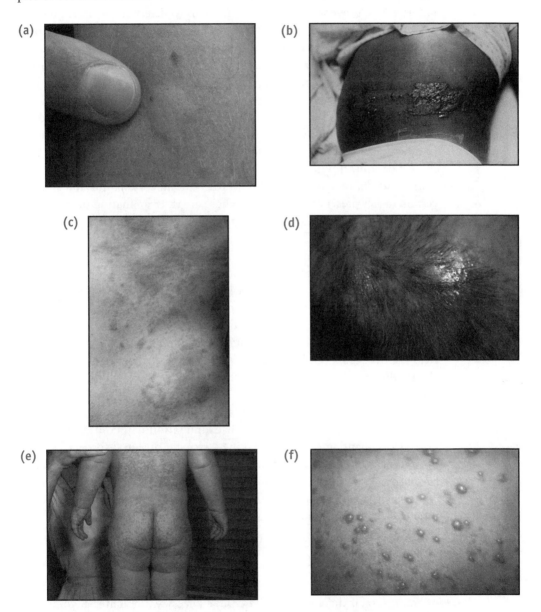

Figure 5-3 Arrangement of Lesions: (a) Insect Bites; (b) Herpes Zoster; (c) Poison Ivy; (d) Tinea Capitis; (e) Measles; (f) Molluscum Contagiosum (See Color Plate)

Palpation includes assessment of the lesion by using your hands and fingers to gather information. Because the palmar surface of your fingers and finger pads are more sensitive than the fingertips, use them when discriminatory touch is needed. Use your finger pads to determine warmth, tenderness, tone, texture, consistency, masses, fluid, and crepitus. Wearing gloves during palpation protects not only the provider but the patient as well.

Check with the parent regarding what treatments have been used, including over-the-counter or prescribed medications (e.g., medication prescribed for a previous skin rash). Also ask whether the child has taken any medication recently for another illness, such as a penicillin-based medication for an infection. Questions about travel outside of the United States or to other parts of the United States are helpful in pinpointing a specific type of rash or contact with certain environmental exposures.

In children, it is also helpful to always examine the palms and soles as certain rashes present with lesion on those areas. Examination of the mouth for blisters or mucocutaneous lesions is equally important.

Another means of assessing a rash or skin disorder, particularly if you think it is possibly due to a fungal infection, is to perform a potassium hydroxide (KOH) culture. This culture is done with a sample of a scale of skin or a hair shaft. The majority of tinea capitis in the United States is due to *Trichophyton tonsurans*, occurring more frequently in African American patients. *T. tonsurans* does not fluoresce on exposure to a Wood's lamp, therefore a KOH and/or fungal culture is necessary to confirm the diagnosis (Goldstein, 2009). Always ask the parent what he or she thinks caused the rash and whether anyone else in the home or close relatives have the same problem.

By the time you start the examination, you should have a general idea as to the differential diagnosis. Your examination will confirm the diagnosis. Good lighting is always vital in assessment of skin disorders. Equally important is having the child put on a hospital gown so you can examine the entire skin. Although the history may indicate a localized problem, a comprehensive examination of the skin can reveal other cutaneous manifestations that may be supportive of your diagnosis.

Skin Examination: Infants

Inspection of the newborn's skin starts with an overall assessment of the infant, noting if there is *vernix caseosa*, a cheesy white material composed of sebum and desquamated epithelial cells that cover the body. All newborns have some degree of *vernix caseosa* on their skin that acts as a protectant to keep the fetus's skin hydrated. See **Figure 5-4**.

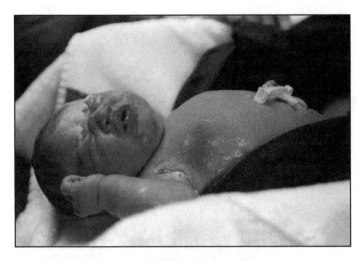

Figure 5-4   Vernix Caseosa

Some newborns also have edema of their hands, feet, and pubis that resolves within a few days. In the first few hours after delivery, the newborn's skin may appear very red. The more transparent the skin, the redder the color. After the first 12 to 24 hours, the newborn's skin develops a more gentle pink color, although skin color is partially determined by the subcutaneous fat content. The chubbier the baby, the less transparent the skin, and a softer pink color predominates.

On the newborn's skin, you may also notice *lanugo*, a fine, downy growth of hair that is particularly noted on the back and shoulders (**Figure 5-5**). Lanugo is often more prevalent on premature infants. This hair is lost within the first few weeks and has no relevance to scalp hair or thickness. The baby born with a lot of scalp hair may lose it within several months, and it will be replaced with new hair, often of a different color and texture.

Conditions occurring in the infant include:

PHYSIOLOGIC JAUNDICE or yellowish discoloration of the skin and eyes may be noted within the first 2 or 3 days of life and peaks at day 5. It may disappear by the end of the first week or possibly persist. If it persists, further testing is necessary. Physiologic jaundice is caused by the newborn's immature liver, which cannot adequately alter and remove the excess bilirubin.

ACROCYANOSIS is a bluish discoloration or cyanosis of the infant's hands and feet when exposed to cooler temperatures (**Figure 5-6**). It is caused by the instability of the peripheral circulatory system.

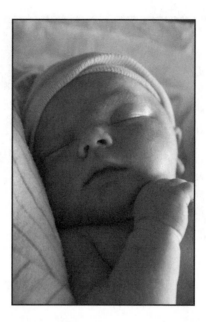

Figure 5-5 Lanugo

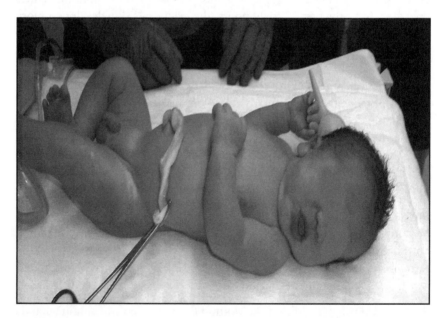

Figure 5-6 Acrocyanosis

CUTIS MARMORATA is a transient mottling, or lattice-like pattern noted on the extremities and trunk when the infant is exposed to cooler temperatures (**Figure 5-7**). It is due to vasomotor changes in the dermis and subcutaneous tissue.

ERYTHEMA TOXICUM is a benign self-limited asymptomatic skin condition that appears within the first 1–3 days of life. It presents as small eruptions of erythematous papules and vesicles. It initially appears on the face and may spread to the trunk. It is benign and requires no treatment.

HARLEQUIN COLOR CHANGE, or transient cyanosis, of one-half of the body is due to vascular instability. The lower half of the body becomes pink, and the upper half is pale.

MONGOLIAN SPOTS are irregular areas of deep blue pigmentation with the appearance of ecchymosis (**Figure 5-8**). They are caused by infiltration of melanocytes into the dermis. Usually found in the sacral and gluteal regions, these spots are seen predominantly in children of African American, Asian, or Hispanic descent. They may last for several years and eventually fade. Mongolian spots may be confused with bruising and/or signs of child abuse.

VASCULAR NEVI, or stork bites, are capillary hemangiomas (**Figure 5-9**). They are flat and of a deep pink color that blanches easily. They are usually found on the eyelids, nose, and nape of the neck.

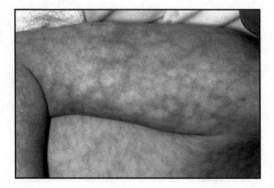

Figure 5-7   Cutis Marmorata (See Color Plate)

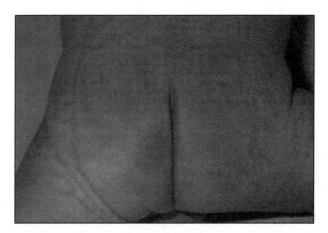

Figure 5-8 Mongolian Spots

MILIA are a common finding on the newborn (**Figure 5-10**). They are pinhead-sized, white, raised areas noted on the chin, nose, and forehead. They result from sebum retention in the openings of the sebaceous glands. They generally appear within the first few weeks and resolve spontaneously in several weeks.

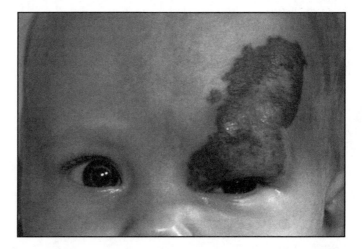

Figure 5-9 Capillary Hemangioma

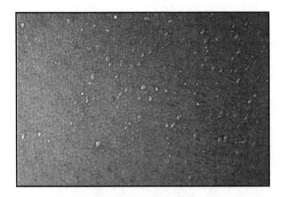

Figure 5-10   Milia (See Color Plate)

MILIARIA RUBRA refers to obstructed sweat ducts caused by a warm, humid environment. They present as tiny, irritated papules or vesicles with an erythematous base. This condition is often referred to as prickly heat and resolves in 1–2 weeks.

THRUSH, OR ORAL CANDIDIASIS, is a common oral lesion observed in the mouth of infants (**Figure 5-11**). It is characterized by white patches on the tongue or buccal mucosa following breastfeeding or antibiotic dosing. These patches may cause bleeding when removed. Thrush may resemble milk residue; however, milk residue can be easily removed with a swab.

More detail on the integumentary system of the newborn is included in Chapter 4.

Skin Examination: School-Age Children

When examining school-age children, explain what you are going to do and engage them in conversation appropriate for their age. Use terms that are easy to understand and be reassuring. Ask them to show you their rash, and ask them direct questions, such as, "Does it itch?" "Does it bother you?" and "Does it itch more at night?' Many rashes may bother a child more at night because of the warmth of the bedclothes and lack of other stimuli to occupy the child. Ask about any classroom pets or if they have been at a friend's house after school. Often, a parent is unaware of classroom pets or a child's after-school activities at a friend's house.

When examining school-age children, you will have better success gaining their cooperation by explaining things to them first and allowing them to tell you about the reason for their visit and about their rash. It is

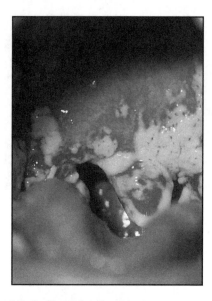

Figure 5-11   Oral Candidiasis (See Color Plate)

always helpful to examine the entire body in assessing a rash, and many children are modest, particularly as their bodies begin to change in early puberty. Explain to them that it is important for you to examine their whole body even though the rash is just on their arm or leg. Inform them that you will leave the room while they change into a hospital gown. Tell them they can leave their underwear on, but must remove their socks and shoes. If examining young children who are very reticent about allowing you to examine them, allow them to sit on their parent's lap.

An important consideration is that the rash may have looked different several days ago and has evolved over time. Questioning that helps in describing the initial presentation can narrow the differential diagnosis.

Skin Examination: Adolescents

In the examination of adolescents, it is important to speak to them in an adult manner, but to be sensitive to their evolving sense of body image and concept of physical appearance. Discuss with them their reason for the visit. Often a hospital gown is necessary for total inspection of the skin. Leave the room while you ask them to change, keeping in mind that modesty is of particular concern during the pubertal changes of adolescence.

The major changes during pubertal growth in the adolescent are hormonal and include growth and development of sebaceous and apocrine glands, increased production of sebum, growth of pubic and axillary hair, and seborrhea and dandruff in scalp hair. These changes, as well as exogenous cutaneous factors such as eczema, folliculitis, and bacterial and parasitic infections, contribute to the anxiety of adolescents and their obsession with body awareness.

Sensitivity during the history and while examining the skin of the adolescent is of particular importance when inspecting the face, chest, and back during the assessment of acne. Equal sensitivity is required when inspecting the genitalia for genital lesions such as genital warts. Close inspection of tattoos and body piercing is important in the assessment of cutaneous infections.

After examining the skin, remember to examine the oral mucosa as well as scalp, hair, and nails. Many cutaneous disorders present with lesions on the buccal mucosa or palatal petechiae associated with group A streptococcal pharyngitis (**Figures 5-12** and **5-13**). Some of the more common skin disorders seen during adolescence include acne vulgaris, pityriasis versicolor, folliculitis, tinea corporis, scabies, eczema, and hyperhidrosis and hirsutism specifically associated with polycystic ovary disease in adolescent females.

When identifying skin lesions, use the appropriate terminology based on characteristics of the lesion such as exudate, pattern of arrangement,

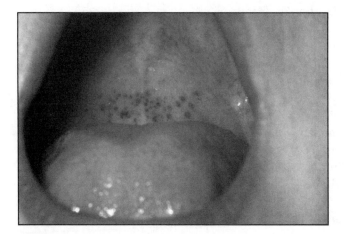

Figure 5-12   Paladial Petechiae

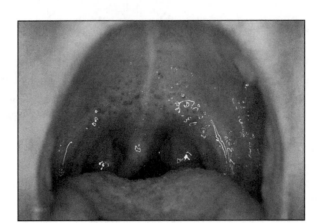

Figure 5-13 Palatal Petechiae Associated with Streptococcus Pharyngitis

location, and distribution. The following chart is helpful when describing cutaneous lesions (Seidel, Ball, Dains, & Benedict, 2006):

CHARACTERISTICS
- ➤ Size: measure all dimensions
- ➤ Shape or configuration
- ➤ Color
- ➤ Texture
- ➤ Elevation or depression
- ➤ Pedunculation

EXUDATES
- ➤ Color
- ➤ Amount
- ➤ Consistency

PATTERN OF ARRANGEMENT
- ➤ Annular (rings)
- ➤ Grouped
- ➤ Linear
- ➤ Diffuse

LOCATION AND DISTRIBUTION
- ➤ Generalized or localized
- ➤ Region of the body
- ➤ Patterns: dermatomal, flexor or extensor, random; relation to clothing lines or jewelry (e.g., finger rings)
- ➤ Discrete or confluent

Common Skin Abnormalities in Children

The following skin disorders are categorized according to bacterial infections, fungal infections, viral infections, infestations, and inflammatory disorders.

Bacterial Infections

IMPETIGO is a contagious bacterial infection caused by either *Staphylococcus* or *Streptococcus* species (**Figure 5-14**). It presents as moist vesicles with erythematous bases. The vesicles rupture to form thick, honey-colored crusts. Bullous impetigo is almost always caused by *Staphylococcus aureus*. This condition starts as small red macules and progresses to fragile bullae that rupture with exposure to form a scalded or shiny-red erosion of the skin. The lesions are annular in shape and usually discrete.

A FURUNCLE, OR BOIL, is a bacterial infection involving the soft tissue, namely the dermis and the subcutaneous tissue. It is characterized by painful areas of erythema, swelling, and warmth. It is an infection of the hair follicle in which purulent material extends through the dermis into the subcutaneous tissue where a small abscess forms (Goldstein, 2009). Today, with the concern of community-acquired methicillin-resistant *Staphylococcus aureus* (MRSA), it is prudent to culture draining inflamed lesions.

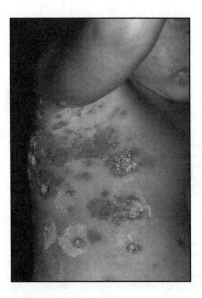

Figure 5-14   Bullous Impetigo (See Color Plate)

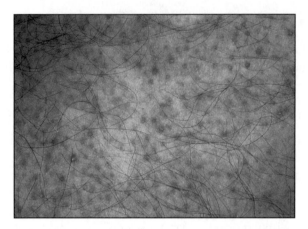

Figure 5-15 Folliculitis

FOLLICULITIS is a superficial infection of the hair follicle caused by infection, trauma, or possibly irritation (**Figure 5-15**). It is primarily caused by *S. aureus* and is characterized by pruritus, localized swelling, and the formation of tiny dome-shaped pustules and red papules at follicular openings. This condition is often observed in the axillary and/or genital area secondary to shaving.

A *CARBUNCLE* is a coalescence of several inflamed follicles into a single inflammatory mass with purulent drainage from multiple follicles (**Figure 5-16**) (Goldstein, 2009).

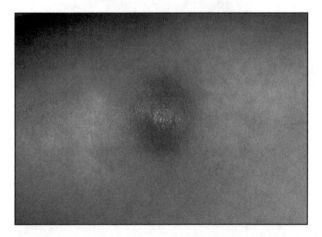

Figure 5-16 Carbuncle

Fungal Infections

CANDIDIASIS, caused by *Candida albicans*, is commonly seen in the diaper area and presents with well-defined erythema, often with maceration in inguinal creases and with satellite lesions (**Figure 5-17**). It may also present as thrush, creamy-white plaques on the buccal mucosa and the tongue.

TINEA INFECTIONS, also called dermatophytes, are defined by the anatomic site of infection: tinea capitis (head), tinea corporis (body), tinea pedis (athlete's foot), tinea cruris (jock itch), and tinea unguium or onychomycosis (nail fungus).

- ➤ *TINEA CAPITIS* is found on the scalp with or without alopecia (Figure 5-18). It is defined by well-demarcated, round, scaly lesions, often with broken hairs, crusting, pustules, and surrounding moist, boggy areas. Lymphadenopathy can be palpated in the occipital nodes.
- ➤ *TINEA CORPORIS* produces an annular, sharply defined papulovesicular border, with central clearing (**Figure 5-19**). It is located on the trunk, face, and extremities.
- ➤ *TINEA VERSICOLOR* is shown in **Figure 5-20**. Presents with fine scaling in hypopigmented, hyperpigmented, and/or erythmatous macules on the trunk and upper extremities.
- ➤ *TINEA PEDIS* causes small, scaly, pruritic, erythematous vesicles and fissures between and under the toes (**Figure 5-21**). It is found in chronically warm, moist feet.

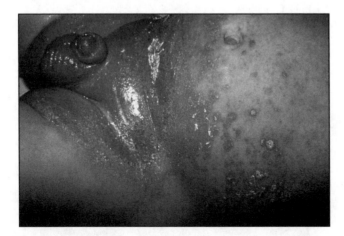

Figure 5-17   Candida Albicans

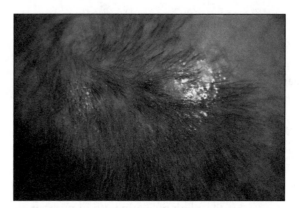

Figure 5-18   Tinea Capitis

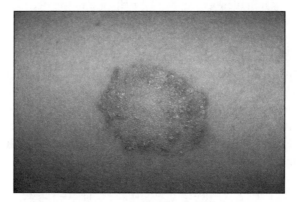

Figure 5-19   Tinea Corporis

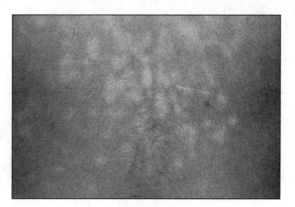

Figure 5-20   Tinea Versicolor (See Color Plate)

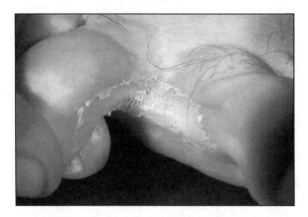

Figure 5-21   Tinea Pedis

> ➤ *TINEA CRURIS* causes well-marginated, erythematous, scaly plaques in the inguinal folds and between the thighs. It is most often seen in adolescent males due to moisture, warmth, friction, obesity, and tight-fitting garments.
> ➤ *TINEA UNGUIUM* is rare in children, although it may be associated with tinea pedis. It presents with distal thickening and yellowing of the nail plate.

Viral Infections

VERRUCAE is a human papillomavirus (HPV) infection that typically presents as warts. These warts are classified according to their clinical presentation: common warts (Verrucae vulgaris), plantar warts (Verrucae plantaris) and flat warts (Verrucae plana).

> ➤ *COMMON WARTS* are the most common and occur on the dorsal surface of the hands, nails, and feet (**Figure 5-22**). They are round, flesh-colored papules with well-defined borders, rough, hard nodules, and an irregular surface.
> ➤ *PLANTAR WARTS* present on the plantar surface of the feet. They are characterized by thick, painful endophytic plaques (**Figure 5-23**). The lesion is often covered by a thick callous, with punctate blood vessels revealed underneath. This type of wart most commonly affects adolescents and young adults.
> ➤ *FLAT WARTS* are the least common. They are flat, flesh-colored papules and present most commonly on the face and dorsal surface of the hands.

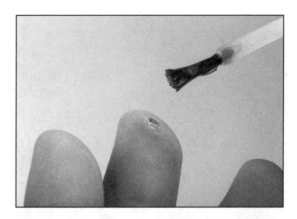

Figure 5-22   Common Wart

MOLLLUSCUM CONTAGIOSUM is a poxvirus that presents as pearly colored, dome-shaped papules with central umbilication. These papules frequently present in groups on the face, upper body, and axillae, although they may appear anywhere on the body. See **Figure 5-24**.

HERPES SIMPLEX TYPE I occurs in children as orolabial lesions, or "cold sores." The lesions present as small vesicles on an erythematous background. A major complication is self-inoculation secondary to scratching the infected area. See **Figure 5-25**.

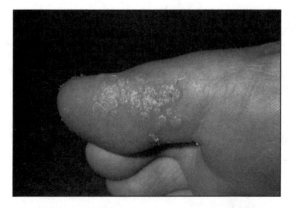

Figure 5-23   Plantar Warts

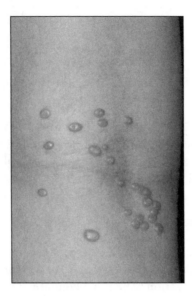

Figure 5-24 Molluscum Contagiosum

HERPES SIMPLEX TYPE II, or herpes genitalis, produces soft, fleshy papules that occur in the anogenital area. The papules are also known as genital warts and are usually asymptomatic.

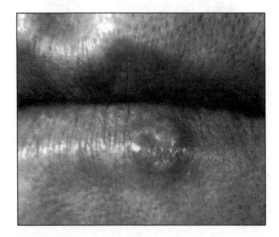

Figure 5-25 Herpes Simplex Type I/Herpes Labialis

Infestations

PEDICULOSIS IS AN INFESTATION OF PEDICULOSIS CAPITIS, or head lice. Lice present with pruritus specifically located in the occipital and postauricular areas. Their effects become more intense at night. They are oval in shape and firmly attached to the hair shaft.

SCABIES, OR SARCOPTES SCABIEI, is caused by mites, which are transmitted by close person-to-person contact. The condition presents with pruritus, which increases at night, and an erythematous, papular rash. Distribution is generally in intertriginous sites such as interdigital, axillary, cubital, popliteal, and inguinal areas. See **Figure 5-26** and **Figure 5-27**.

Inflammatory Disorders

ATOPIC DERMATITIS is characterized by persistent pruritus and scratching that eventually leads to papules, erythema, excoriation, serous discharge, crusting, and lichenification. The most common example is eczema. The areas most commonly affected are the flexor surfaces such as the antecubital and popliteral fossae, wrist angles, and neck. Lichenification is a term used to describe thickening of the skin or epidermal thickening secondary to constant scratching.

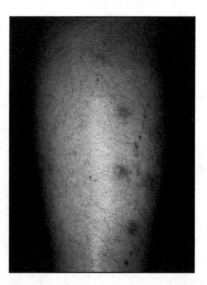

Figure 5-26 Scabies

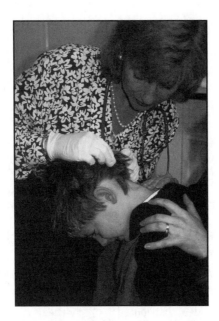

Figure 5-27 Head Lice

DIAPER DERMATITIS is the most common irritant contact dermatitis of childhood. Etiology of skin breakdown is based on urine pH, urine frequency, stool consistency, digestive enzymes in the stool, and type of diaper used, as well as detergent and cleaning agents used. Presentation is erythematous vesicles, papules, and scaling on skin that comes in direct contact with the diaper. Skin folds are generally spared.

SEBORRHEIC DERMATITIS is also called cradle cap. It generally presents within the first 3–4 months of life. Presentation is thick, whitish–yellowish scaly, oily plaques on the scalp. It may also present on the face and trunk and in skin folds.

CONTACT DERMATITIS presents as a localized area of erythema and/or pruritus. It is the result of direct contact with an irritant or allergen that causes a localized reaction. Lesions can be characterized by erythema, scaling, and vesicles.

ACNE VULGARIS is predominately seen in adolescence and presents with inflammation of the sebaceous follicle in which excess sebum, keratinous debris, and bacteria accumulate, producing microcomedones.

Write-Up of Skin Findings

When describing skin lesions, note characteristics, exudates, location, pattern of arrangement, and distribution. In your overall assessment, the following information should be summarized:

1. Identification of the primary lesion
2. Distribution of the lesion
3. Identification of associated findings
4. Age of the patient

Terms used in describing skin lesions include the following:

Lesion	Characteristic	Example
Annular	Ring shaped	Ringworm
Linear	Arranged in lines	Poison ivy
Grouped	Clustered together	Impetigo
Diffuse	Widely distributed	Rubeola
Discrete	Distinct and separate	Varicella
Confluent	Lesions run together	Viral exanthems
Eczematoid	Vesicles with oozing crust	Eczema
Multiform	More than one shape	Erythema multiform
Reticulated	Lacelike	Fifth disease
Telangiectatic	Dilated superficial blood vessels	Stork bite
Zosteriform	Linear along a nerve distribution	Herpes zoster

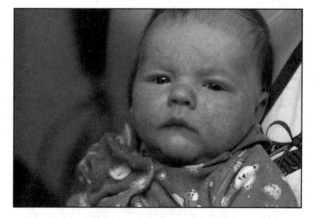

Figure 5-28   Eczema

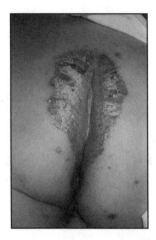

Figure 5-29 Diaper Dermatitis

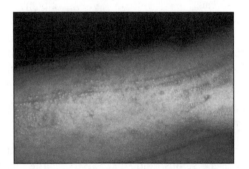

Figure 5-30 Poison Ivy

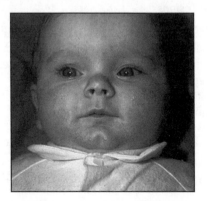

Figure 5-31 Infant Acne

Primary Skin Lesions

Skin lesions are classified into two categories: primary and secondary. *Primary skin lesions* are variations in color or texture that may be present at birth, such as moles or birthmarks. They arise from normal skin as the result of anatomic changes in the epidermis, dermis, or subcutaneous tissue. Primary skin lesions are listed in the following tables.

Flat Nonpalpable Lesions

Lesion	Characteristic	Example
Macule	< 1 cm	Freckle, mole
Patch	> 1 cm	Café au lait spot

Solid Mass, Palpable Lesions

Lesion	Characteristic	Example
Papule	< 1 cm	Nevus, wart
Nodule	1–2 cm	Lipoma
Plaque	> 1 cm	Raised/thickened skin, psoriasis, seborrhea
Wheal	Superficial cutaneous edema	Hives, insect bite
Tumor	> 2 cm	Neoplasma

Fluid-Filled Palpable Lesions

Lesion	Characteristic	Example
Vesicle	< 1 cm, serous fluid	Blister, herpes simplex
Bulla	> 1 cm, serous fluid	Large blister
Pustule	< 1 cm, filled with pus	Impetigo, pimple

Special Primary Skin Lesions

Lesion	Characteristic	Example
Comedo	Plugged sebaceous gland	Blackhead
Burrow	Slightly raised tunnel in epidermis	Scabies
Cyst	Encapsulated, filled with semisolid liquid	Sebaceous gland
Abscess	Pus-filled lesion	Localized infection/larger than furuncle
Furuncle	Inflammation of hair follicle	Infection on back of neck
Milia	Tiny white papules	Noted on infant's face

NONPALPABLE

A. Macule: Localized changes in skin color of loss than 1 cm in diameter
Example: Freckle

B. Patch: Localized changes in skin color of greater than 1 cm in diameter
Example: Vitiligo, stage 1 pressure ulcer

PALPABLE

C. Papule: Localized changes in skin color of loss than 1 cm in diameter
Example: Warts, elevated nevi

D. Plaque: Solid, elevated lesion greater than 0.5 cm in diameter
Example: Psoriasis

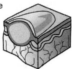

E. Nodules: Solid and elevated; however, they extend deeper than papules into the dermis or subcutaneous tissues, 0.5-2.0 cm
Example: Lipoma, erythema nodosum, cyst

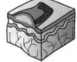

F. Tumor: The same as a nodule only greater than 2 cm
Example: Carcinoma (such as advanced breast carcinoma); **not** basal cell or squamous cell of the skin

G. Wheal: Localized edema in the epidermis causing irregular elevation that may be red or pale
Example: Insect bite or a hive

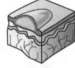

FLUID-FILLED CAVITIES WITHIN THE SKIN

H. Vesicle: Accumulation of fluid between the upper layers of the skin; elevated mass containing serous fluid; less than 0.5 cm
Example: Herpes, simplex, herpes zoster, chickenpox

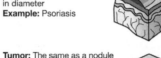

I. Bullae: Same as a vesicle only greater than 0.5 cm
Example: Contact dermatitis, large second-degree burns, bulbous impetigo, pemphigus

J. Pustule: Vesicles or bullae that become filled with pus, usually described as less than 0.5
Example: Acne, impetigo, furuncles, carbuncles, folliculitis

K. Cyst: Encapsulated fluid-filled or a semi-solid mass in the subcutaneous tissue or dermis
Example: Sebaceous cyst, epidermoid cyst

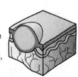

Figure 5-32 Morphology of Primary Lesions

Source: Adapted from Jarvis, *Physical Examination & Health Assessment*, Saunders; Bickley, *Bates' Guide to Physical Examination and History Taking*, Lippincott; Seidel, Ball, Dains, & Benedict, 2006.

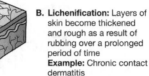

ABOVE THE SKIN SURFACE

A. Scales: Flaking of the skin's surface
Example: Dandruff or psoriasis, xerosis

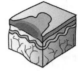

B. Lichenification: Layers of skin become thickened and rough as a result of rubbing over a prolonged period of time
Example: Chronic contact dermatitis

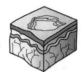

C. Crust: Dried serum, blood, or pus on the surface of the skin
Example: Impetigo

D. Atrophy: Thinning of the skin surface and loss of markings
Example: Striae, aged skin

BELOW THE SKIN SURFACE

E. Erosion: Loss of epidermis
Example: Ruptured chicken-pox vesicle

F. Fissure: Layers of skin become thickened and rough as a result of rubbing over a prolonged period of time
Example: Chapped hands or lips, athlete's foot

G. Ulcer: A depressed lesion of the epidermis and upper papillary layer of the dermis
Example: Stage 2 pressure ulcer

H. Atrophy: Fibrous tissue that replaces dermal; tissue after injury
Example: Surgical incision

I. Keloid: Enlarging of a scar past wound edges due to excess collagen formation (more prevalent in dark-skinned persons)
Example: Burn scar

J. Excoriation: Loss of epidermal layers exposing the dermis
Example: Abrasion

Figure 5-33 Morphology of Primary Lesions

Source: Adapted from Jarvis, *Physical Examination & Health Assessment*, Saunders; Bickley, *Bates' Guide to Physical Examination and History Taking*, Lippincott; Seidel, Ball, Dains, & Benedict, 2006.

Secondary Skin Lesions

A *secondary skin lesion* results from changes in the skin caused by primary skin lesions, either as a natural progression or due to scratching or irritation to the skin. Secondary skin lesions are listed in the following table.

Lesion	Characteristic	Example
Erosion	Loss of epidermis, leaving a shallow depression	Due to rubbing/ picking
Fissure	Linear crack in the dermis	Athlete's foot
Excoriation	Loss of epidermis, dermis exposed	Abrasion
Atrophy	Thinning of skin surface	Stria
Scaling	Keratinized cells, flaking	Psoriasis
Crusting	Dried serum, blood, exudates	Scab
Petechia	Red pinpoint spots/hemorrhage	Infection
Purpura	Purple discoloration due to bleeding	Infection
Ecchymosis	Discoloration of skin due to injury	Bruise healing
Scar	Fibrous tissue replacing dermis	Healed wound
Keloid	Increased collagen formation	Burn scar
Lichenification	Rough, thickened epidermis	Chronic dermatitis

> **Red Flags**

Concerning skin rashes are those that present with associated systemic symptoms such as fever. Rashes that do not blanch require further investigation. Rashes with increased erythema, warmth, and/or drainage need to be assessed further. Alopecia, or loss of hair, needs further workup. An abnormal hairline in an infant that extends to mid-forehead may indicate chromosomal abnormalities.

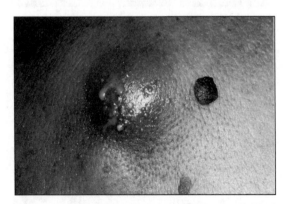

Figure 5-34   Carbuncle (See Color Plate)

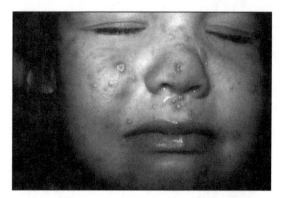

Figure 5-35 Typical Varicella Lesions

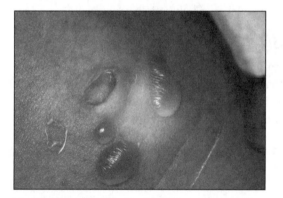

Figure 5-36 Bullous Impetigo (See Color Plate)

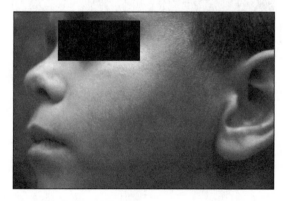

Figure 5-37 Fifth's Disease (See Color Plate)

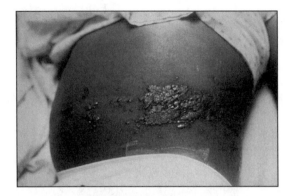

Figure 5-38   Herpes Zoster

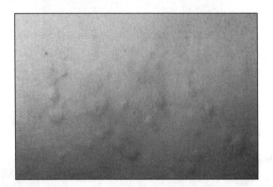

Figure 5-39   Hives

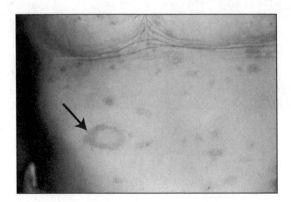

Figure 5-40   Pityriasis Rosea: Herald Patch

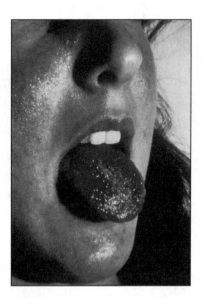

Figure 5-41 Strawberry Tongue

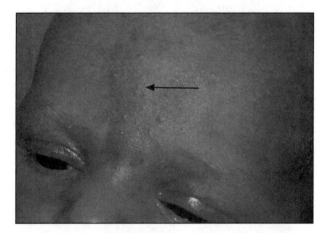

Figure 5-42 Stork Bite (See Color Plate)

TABLE 5-2   CLINICAL MANIFESTATIONS INSECT BITES AND STINGS

Type	Clinical Manifestation	Clinical Therapy
Mosquitoes and Fleas Local inflammation results from injected foreign protein or chemicals.	**Local reactions:** ■ Discrete, red papules and edema at the bite site with itching, burning, pain, and hives; minimal discomfort ■ Pruritic wheals and bullae tend to develop with repeat exposure **Systemic reactions:** ■ Wheezing, urticaria ■ Laryngeal edema ■ Shock	■ Cold compresses or ice applied to the site ■ Antihistamine medication ■ Systemic reactions need emergency medical treatment
Bee or Wasp Sting Hymenoptera Venoms contain enzymes that affect vascular tone and permeability.	**Local reactions:** ■ Mild, local pain ■ Erythema and edema **Systemic reactions:** ■ Generalized urticaria, flushing, angioedema, pruritis ■ Wheezing ■ Anaphylaxis is rare	■ Remove stinger as soon as possible ■ Use ice or cold compresses and elevate extremity ■ Massage a dash of meat tenderizer (papain powder) and a drop of water into the skin for 5 minutes to relieve the pain ■ Antihistamine medication ■ Treat systemic reactions with glucocorticoids and antihistamines or epinephrine ■ Desensitization for severe reactions
Fire Ants Venom is hemolytic and neurotoxic, causing a histaminelike response.	**Local reactions:** ■ A black center at the point of the bite, or trail of lesions across skin ■ Initial wheal becomes a vesicle in a few hours; in 24 hours, the fluid is cloudy, and the vesicle has a red halo ■ Pruritis, erythema, edema, induration ■ Systemic and anaphylactic reactions can occur	■ Ice or cold compresses ■ Antihistamine medication ■ Elevate extremity ■ Systemic reactions— same as bees and wasps

TABLE 5-2 CLINICAL MANIFESTATIONS INSECT BITES AND STINGS		
Type	**Clinical Manifestation**	**Clinical Therapy**
Black Widow Spider Venom is neurotoxic.	■ Stinging sensation at time of bite ■ Localized edema and erythema, two fang marks, petechiae branching from site ■ Systemic reaction in 1–3 hours, symptoms peak in 3–12 hours, diminish in 72 hours ■ Muscle rigidity of torso and abdomen, priapism, muscle cramps near the bite ■ Malaise, sweating, nausea, vomiting, dizziness, restlessness, insomnia ■ Hypertension and arrhythmias ■ Oliguria	■ Ice ■ Diazepam for muscle spasms ■ Opioids for pain management ■ Antihistamine medication ■ Hydrocortisone may decrease the inflammatory response ■ Antivenom IV is used in severe reactions after negative skin test for hypersensitivity to horse serum
Brown Recluse Spider Venom contains proteolytic enzymes and sphingomyelinase D, a cytotoxic factor.	■ Itching, pain, and erythema at bite site in first 6 to 12 hours, evolves to purple bull's eye lesion that signals beginning of necrosis; reddish blisters; a white ring is surrounded by an irregular erythematous ring (Zeglin, 2005) ■ Severe progressive reactions may occur in 12–72 hours, including fever, chills, restlessness, malaise, joint pain, and nausea and vomiting	■ Ice or cold compresses ■ Cleanse the wound and provide good wound care ■ Analgesics ■ Oral anti-inflammatory agent ■ Antibiotics for secondary infection ■ Excision and skin grafting in cases of severe necrosis

Write-up of the Skin

EXAMPLE FOR INFANTS: Skin: brown, warm to touch, turgor within normal limits (WNL). Skin is without erythema, papules, vesicles, or scaling. Mongolian spot 3 × 5 cm noted over lumbar sacral area. Full head of dark brown hair. Scalp without crusting or lesions.

EXAMPLES FOR SCHOOL-AGE CHILDREN AND ADOLESCENTS:

➤ *SKIN*: warm to touch, clear without lesion, without rashes, bruising, or pallor.
➤ *SKIN*: cluster of three small lesions with erythematous base and honey-colored crust on left upper lip. Skin otherwise clear.

Case Study: Skin Assessment— Changes in Skin Lesions

Billy, a 4-year-old boy, presents to your office with lesions grouped together on his right lower leg. His mother initially thought they were insect bites because they were pruritic. They have since progressed from papules to vesicopustules and now present with an erythematous base with honey-colored crust.

Physical examination is noncontributory. Vital signs are normal, patient is afebrile.

Questions

1. What organisms are most likely responsible for these lesions?
2. What is the difference between the two dermatologic manifestations that may present?
3. What is your recommended treatment plan?

Answers

1. The most likely organisms are *Staphylococcus aureus* and group A hemolytic streptococci.
2. Nonbullous impetigo is the most common form of impetigo. Lesions begin as papules that progress to vesicles surrounded by erythema. Subsequently, they become pustules that enlarge and break down to form thick, adherent crusts with a characteristic golden appearance, usually involving the face and extremities; this evolution usually occurs over about a week. Multiple lesions may develop but tend to remain well localized. Regional lymphadenitis may occur, although systemic symptoms are usually absent.

Bullous impetigo is a form of impetigo seen in young children in which the vesicles enlarge to form flaccid bullae with clear yellow fluid that later becomes darker and more turbid; ruptured bullae leave a thin brown crust. Usually there are fewer lesions than in nonbullous impetigo, and the trunk is more frequently affected.

3. The topical drug of choice is mupirocin, which is applied three times daily. The treatment of choice for oral antibiotic therapy, which should be used for bullous impetigo if wide spread, is cephalexin, clindamycin, or dicloxacillin (Baddour, 2009).

References

Baddour, L. (2009). Impetigo. *Uptodate.com*. Retrieved from http://www.uptodate.com/patients/content/topic.do?topicKey=~HHLSIGqvYqv1h5

Goldstein, B., & Goldstein, A. (2009). General principles of dermatologic therapy and topical corticosteroid use. Retrieved from http://www.uptodate.com

Seidel, H., Ball, J., Dains, J., Benedict, G. (2006). *Mosby's guide to physical examination* (6th ed.). Boston: Mosby.

Zeglin, D. (2005). Brown recluse spider bites. *American Journal of Nursing, 105*(2), 64–68.

Resources

Colyar, M. (2003). *Well-child assessment for primary care providers*. Philadelphia: F.A. Davis, Company.

Estes, M. (1998). *Health assessment and physical examination*. Albany, NY: Delmar Publishers.

Habif, T. (2004). *Clinical dermatology* (4th ed.). New York: Mosby.

Marieb, E. (1995). *Human anatomy and physiology* (3rd ed.). Redwood City, CA: Benjamin/Cummings Publishing Company.

Potts, N., & Mandleco, B. (2007) *Pediatraic nursing* (2nd ed.). Victoria, Australia: Thomson, Delmar Learning.

Wolff, K., Johnson, R. A., & Suurmond, D. (2005). *Fitzpatrick's color atlas and synopsis of clinical dermatology* (5th ed.). New York: McGraw Hill.

Zitelli, B., & Davis, H. (2002). *Atlas of pediatric physical diagnosis* (4th ed.). St. Louis, MO: Mosby.

Examination of the Eye

Anatomy and Physiology of the Eye

The visual system consists of the eyeballs, protective orbital bones, lids and lashes, lacrimal apparatus, extraocular muscles, the intraocular fluid system, and the neural pathways that mediate vision.

External Anatomy

The eye itself is protected by the bony orbital cavity. The external structures of the eye include the eyelids, conjunctiva, lacrimal glands, and extraocular muscles. The eyelids consist of smooth muscle covered with a very thin layer of skin that protects and maintains lubrication of the eye, as well as protects the eye from injury. The eyelashes are in double and triple rows that curve outward from the lid margins and filter out dust. The interior surface of the lid is lined with a pink mucous membrane called the palpebral conjunctiva; the palpebral fissure is the elliptical open space between the eyelids.

Within the upper lid are the tarsal plates, which are strips of connective tissue containing the meibomian glands. These sebaceous glands secrete a lubricating substance onto the lids that helps to decrease evaporation. The lacrimal glands lie within the bony orbit above and lateral to the eyeball. Fluid (or tears) that protects the conjunctiva and cornea from drying and also inhibits microbial growth comes from three sources: meibomian glands, conjunctival glands, and lacrimal glands. These tears then pass into the nasolacrimal duct, which drains into the nose through the lacrimal puncta.

The *conjunctiva* is a thin vascular mucous membrane that lines the lids and anterior portion of the globe. Because it is very vascular, when the blood vessels are dilated either due to irritation or infection, the eye has a pink appearance (hence "pink eye"), a condition known as conjunctivitis.

Eye movements are controlled by six *extraocular muscles* that work in a conjugate parallel manner. For example, when a child turns his or her head to look left, the left lateral rectus and the right medial rectus muscles contract to turn the eyes to the left. This movement involves the oculomotor nerve (cranial nerve III) and the abducens nerve (cranial nerve VI). When a child turns his or her head and looks down and to the right, the right inferior rectus muscle (cranial nerve III) is principally responsible for moving the right eye, while the left superior oblique muscle (cranial nerve IV) is principally responsible for moving the left eye when looking downward (Bickley, 2003, p. 122). The lateral rectus muscle, which is innervated by the abducens nerve (cranial nerve VI), turns the eye laterally. Overall, the movement of the extraocular muscles is controlled by three cranial nerves: the abducens (cranial nerve VI), which innervates the lateral rectus muscle, thus abducting the eye away from the nose; the trochlear (cranial nerve IV), which innervates the superior oblique muscles; and the oculomotor (cranial nerve III), which innervates the superior, inferior, and medial rectus and the inferior oblique muscles.

Internal Anatomy

The internal anatomy is comprised of three separate tunics, or layers. The outer tunic is composed of the sclera and the cornea, the middle tunic consists of the choroids and ciliary body and iris, and the inner tunic is composed of the retina.

The *sclera* is an opaque covering that appears white and covers the structures inside the eye. The extraocular muscles insert into the sclera and physically support the internal structure of the eye. The cornea is a nonvascular transparent surface that covers the iris and the pupil and is continuous with the conjunctival epithelium. The cornea is very sensitive to touch, as noted when a speck of dirt gets into the eye. It is the trigeminal nerve (cranial nerve V) that is stimulated when assessing the corneal reflex. The cornea separates the anterior chamber (aqueous humor) from the exterior environment. The anterior chamber is the space between the cornea and the iris. The aqueous humor is produced by the ciliary body in the posterior chamber. It circulates through the pupil into the anterior chamber and is removed through the canal of Schlemm.

The iris contains pigment cells that produce the color of the eye. The central aperture of the iris is the pupil, which constricts and dilates, allowing light to travel to the retina. The pupil is controlled by the parasympathetic and sympathetic system (the fight-or-flight mechanism). Stimulation of the sympathetic system dilates the pupil, whereas stimulation of the parasympathetic system constricts the pupil.

The middle layer, or tunic, is composed of the choroid, which prevents light from reflecting internally and is vascularized to deliver blood to the retina. This layer also contains the ciliary bodies. These bodies control the thickness of the lens, which is a biconvex disc located posterior to the pupil. The lens refracts light, focusing an object on the retina of the eye. Behind the lens and in front of the retina is the vitreous humor, which helps maintain the shape of the eye.

The inner layer of the eyeball is composed of the retina, which is the innermost structure of the eye. Within the retina is the optic disc, retinal vessels, the physiologic cup, macula and fovea centralis, and cones and rods. It is this part of the eye that is seen through an ophthalmoscope.

When looking through the ophthalmoscope, the first observation is the red reflex, which is the reflection of light off the retina. The retina lines the innermost layer of the eyeball and is an extension of the optic nerve. It receives light impulses that are transformed into electrical impulses and transmitted to the occipital lobe of the brain.

In the fundus of the eye, paired retinal vessels branch out from the optic disc toward the periphery, growing smaller as they extend outward. Retinal arteries are smaller and lighter red than veins and often have a reflection of a silvery light. Normal arterial to venous width is a ratio of 2:3 or 4:5.

Farther back in the eye is the optic disc, located on the nasal side of the retina. It is oval or round, and its margins are distinct, flat, and sharply demarcated. The color varies from creamy yellow-orange to a pinkish tone. The physiologic cup is the smaller circular area inside the disc where the retinal blood vessels enter and exit. The macula is a small, round area approximately the size of the disc; it is located approximately 3.5 mm temporal to the disc. It is easily seen because it is devoid of retinal vessels. In the center of the macula is the fovea centralis, the area of sharpest vision. The cones are located at the fovea and are responsible for color perception. The rods are located on other portions of the retina and provide dark and light discrimination, as well as peripheral vision. **Figures 6-1** through **6-5** showcase different areas of the eye.

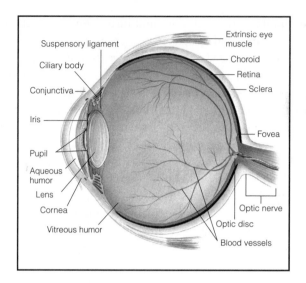

Figure 6-1 Eye Ball (See Color Plate)

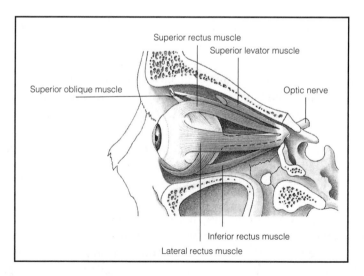

Figure 6-2 The Extraocular Muscles

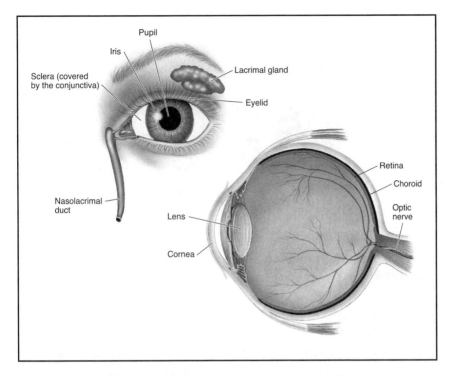

Figure 6-3   Glands and Ducts of the Eye

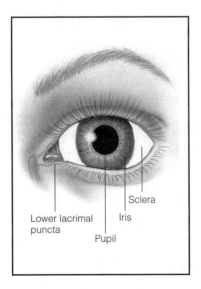

Figure 6-4   External View of the Eye

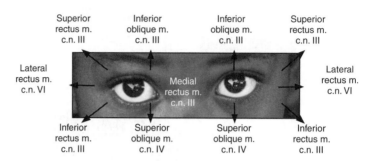

Figure 6-5 Direction of Movement
Source: Pat Thomas, 2006.

Visual Pathways

Through the visual pathways, objects in the field of vision reflect light that is received by sensory neurons in the retina. The images are received upside down and reversed. From there, they pass along nerve fibers through the optic disc and the optic nerve. Fibers from the left half of each eye pass through the optic chiasm to the right side of the brain, and fibers from the right side of each eye pass to the left side of the visual cortex of the occipital lobe of the brain. At the optic chiasm, nasal fibers cross over; thus, the left optic tract has fibers from the left half of each retina, and the right optic tract has fibers *only from the right.*

An example of a common defect found on visual field testing is left homonymous hemianopsia, which results from damage to the optic tract and the occipital lobe. This condition is characterized by loss of vision of the left half of the fields of both eyes. A patient with a left upper homonymous quadrantanopsia has a visual field defect/cut in one quadrant, limiting vision on the upper left side of both eyes. An example of a defect in both temporal fields is bitemporal hemianopsia, which is characterized by loss of peripheral vision in the temporal fields or on both right and left sides. This is assessed through the confrontation test.

Development of the Eye

The eye forms during the first 8 weeks of gestation, although development of the eye is not complete at birth. Continued development of vision is

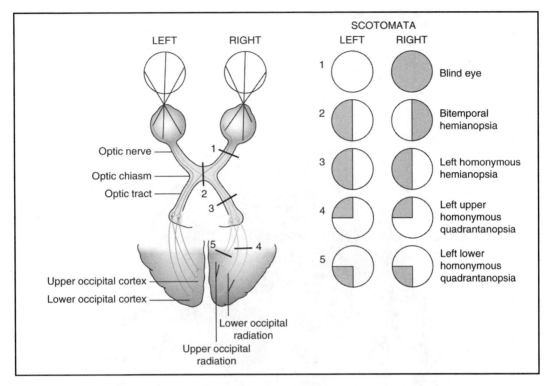

Figure 6-6 Visual Field Defects

Source: This article was published in Textbook of Physical Diagnosis: History and Examination, 5th edition, Swartz. Visual field defects. Copyright Saunders (2005).

dependent upon maturation of the nervous system. In newborns the sclera appears blue-white because it is very thin, allowing the coloration of the choroid to show through. At birth there is only a small amount of pigment in the iris, which explains why all babies are born with blue eyes. Pigmentation is completed by 6 months of age. The infant develops a blink reflex within the first 2 months of life. At birth the nasolacrimal duct is often blocked, which presents with chronic tearing or watery discharge referred to dacryostenosis or nasolacrimal duct obstruction. In most infants, this blockage resolves spontaneously within the first year, although for some babies, surgical intervention is necessary. Tears generally present at around 2 months of age. Newborns' eyes should move together, although eye movements often appear disconjugate until the third month of life due to weak eye muscles. Visual acuity cannot be measured in the newborn, although you can assess visual reflexes and direct and consensual pupillary constriction in response to light.

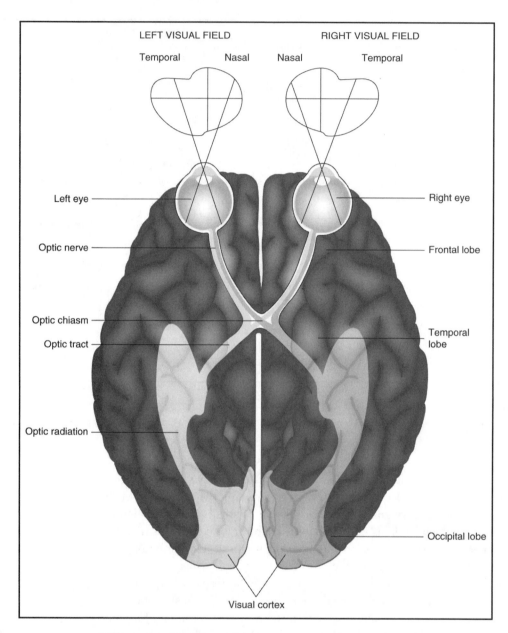

Figure 6-7 Visual Pathway

Source: This article was published in Textbook of Physical Diagnosis: History and Examination, 5th edition, Swartz. Visual pathway, page 289. Copyright Saunders (2005).

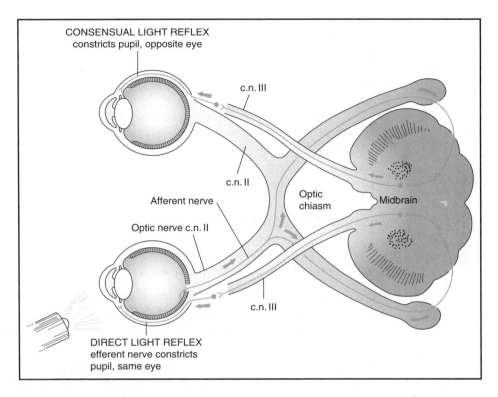

Figure 6-8   Consensual/Direct Light Reflex

Source: This article was published in Textbook of Physical Diagnosis: History and Examination, 5th edition, Swartz. Visual pathway, page 289. Copyright Saunders (2005).

During the internal, or ophthalmoscopic, examination, the red reflex of the newborn can be observed; it is often lighter in color than the normal red or orange color noted in older children. It is difficult to examine the optic disc in infants; however, the concern of *papilledema* associated with trauma such as shaken baby syndrome, subarachnoid hemorrhage, or meningitis is reduced because the fontanelles and open sutures allow for increased intra-cranial pressure. In young children, the shape of the eyeball is less spherical than that of the adult, although the lens is more spherical at birth.

Most infants are born hyperopic, or farsighted; as the child grows, hyperopia gradually decreases. In early childhood, as the child's head and brain develop, the globe of the eye becomes rounder. Visual acuity develops over the first year of life and is achieved at approximately 6 years of age. (Bickley, 2003, p. 674).

Visual development is described as follows:

- *BIRTH*: The baby blinks and regards faces.
- *1 MONTH*: The baby fixes on objects.
- *1.5–2 MONTHS*: Eye movements become coordinated, and horizontal following to midline.
- *3 MONTHS*: Eyes converge, the baby starts to reach for toys, and good horizontal and vertical following is seen.
- *12 MONTHS*: Visual acuity is approximately 20/50.

Assessment Considerations: Subjective Information

Infants

Eye considerations pertinent to the infant include:

- Did the mother have a vaginal infection at the time of delivery? Gonorrhea and genital herpes both have ocular sequelae for the newborn that may present as conjunctival irritation, exudates, redness, or granular development.
- Was the newborn preterm or low birth weight? If so, there are concerns of retinopathy of prematurity (ROP). ROP may result in retinal scarring and/or retinal detachment.
- Does the infant gaze at the mother's face or at bright objects?
- Does the infant blink when bright lights or threatening movements are directed at the face?
- Are there concerns regarding cataracts, which may present as a white area in the pupil rather than "red eye" (or as the red reflex) in photographs? This finding may be an indication that one eye is not able to reflect light properly, which can indicate a lesion in front of the retina such as a retinoblastoma.
- Is there excessive tearing over the lower eyelid in one or both eyes? If so, it may indicate a blocked nasolacrimal duct, a condition called dacryostenosis.
- Is strabismus noted some or all of the time? Intermittent convergent strabismus (esotropia) or intermittent divergent strabismus (exotropia) is within normal limits in the newborn period due to ocular motor weakness. If the condition persists beyond 3 months, it needs to be referred to an ophthalmologist (Bickley, 2003).
- Is there concern regarding redness or bleeding into the sclera? Subconjunctival hemorrhage is common in newborns due to rupture of small

vessels during the pressure of delivery. The red area may be large or small, but it is always confined to the limits of the sclera. It is asymptomatic and does not affect vision.

- Is there nystagmus, wandering or shaking eye movements, persisting several days after delivery? Persistent nystagmus may indicate a CNS disorder and should be referred to a neurologist.
- Is there swelling or redness in the conjunctiva? Chemical conjunctivitis often occurs after application of silver nitrate at birth as prophylaxis against gonorrheal conjunctivitis or ophthalmia neonatorum. Some nurseries have changed to erythromycin eye ointment following delivery because it causes less irritation.
- In babies or toddlers, is the child unable to reach for and pick up small objects, or does he bring objects close to examine them?

School-Age Children and Adolescents

Eye considerations pertinent to school-age children and adolescents include:

- Are there concerns regarding diplopia?
- Are there concerns regarding redness, swelling, itching, or discharge?
- Does the child wear glasses or contact lenses, and when was the child's last eye examination?
- Does the child under- or overreach for objects? Ask the parent if he or she notices the child squinting, stumbling, or walking into things?
- In school-age children, does the child need to sit close to the front of the classroom to see the board? Does the child have a history of poor progress in school that is not explained by intellectual ability?
- Does the child have a relevant medical or surgical history? Consider the history of medications and allergies, and the immunization status.

Family History

During the subjective assessment, also consider the child's family history of visual disorders, such as glaucoma, blindness, nystagmus, retinoblastoma, congenital cataracts, strabismus, and photophobia. Also ask about a family history of diabetes, thyroid disease, sickle cell hemoglobinopathies, neurologic disorders, connective tissue disorders, congenital heart disease, and rheumatoid arthritis.

It is important to keep in mind that the eye is composed of various types of tissue, which makes it susceptible to a variety of diseases. Because of its transparency, the eye is the only organ in the body in which the provider can directly see and assess the health of both the veins and the arteries, thus gaining important clues to the diagnosis of systemic diseases.

Review of Systems

Review all bodily systems with special emphasis on the skin; eye; nose; neck; and respiratory, musculoskeletal, neurologic, and endocrine systems. Pay particular attention to the following:

EYE: Consider the child's history of eye infections, photophobia, excessive tearing, pruritus, discharge, strabismus, and cataracts. Does the child wear glasses or contact lenses, and when was the last eye exam? In younger children, has the child experienced problems with fixing, tracking, squinting, head tilting, eye–hand coordination, or balance, or has the child exhibited changes in the ability to maintain eye contact? For older children, has the child experienced visual loss or blurring, diplopia, spots, and/or halos?

SKIN: Consider allergic disorders that may have ocular manifestations such as atopic dermatitis.

NOSE: Consider nasal polyps, allergic rhinitis, history of sinusitis, and environmental allergies.

Assessment Considerations: Objective Information

Examination of the External Eye

When examining the eyes of an infant or toddler, it is best if the child is held by the parent or is sitting in the parent's lap. The child should be held upright so you can observe the whole face. When examining a child who is school age or older, he or she can sit alone facing you.

Before actually picking up the ophthalmoscope or touching the child, it is important to note the position and spacing of the eyes. Start by inspecting placement of the eyes, noting whether they are wide set (hypertelorism) or close set (hypotelorism). If you are unsure, measure the distance between the inner canthi. The average distance between inner canthi is 2.5 cm, or 1 inch. Hypertelorism is noted in children with Down syndrome. Continue by inspecting the vertical folds that partially or completely cover the inner canthi. These epicanthal folds are normally found in Asian children. Epicanthal folds can also be an indication of Down syndrome, glycogen storage disease, and renal agenesis. Inspect the slant of the eye by drawing an imaginary line across the inner canthi. The palpebral fissures lie horizontally along this imaginary line. In the newborn, the upper eyelids often show epicanthal folds running medially downward and obscuring the inner canthus. This observation in conjunction with a wide, flat bridge of the nose may create the illusion of crossed eyes, or pseudostrabismus, which can be dispelled by noting a symmetrical light reflex on the pupils. Note that Asian children have an upward slant of the palpebral fissure, as do children with Down syndrome. See **Figure 6-9**, **Figure 6-10**, and **Figure 6-11**.

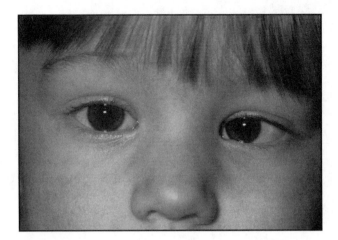

Figure 6-9   Pseudostrabismus

Inspect the eyelids for placement, noting that the eyelid falls between the upper border of the iris and the upper border of the pupil. Drooping eyelid, or ptosis, may be associated with damage or paralysis of the oculomotor nerve (cranial nerve III), or it may be due to neuromuscular immaturity. Incomplete eye closure due to lid lag may be associated with hyperthyroidism. In addition, the "sunset sign" may occur when the iris deviates downward and increased sclera is noted between the upper lid and the iris. The sunset appearance is associated with increased intracranial pressure.

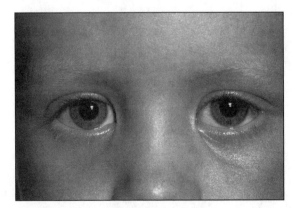

Figure 6-10   Epicanthal Folds

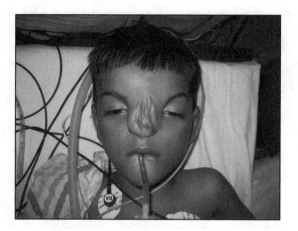

Figure 6-11 Hypertelorism

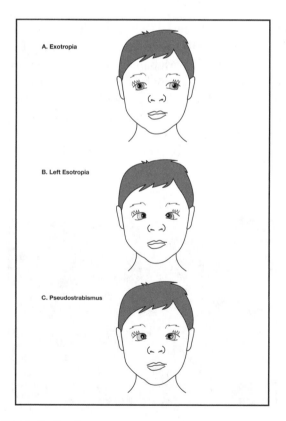

Figure 6-12 Muscle Dysfunction

Inspection of the conjunctivae involves pulling down the lower lid as the child looks up. Inspect the upper lid by rolling the eyelid over a cotton-tipped applicator. The conjunctivae should be pink and glossy. Inspect the bulbar conjunctiva for color. It should be clear and transparent, allowing the white of the sclera to be clearly visible.

Next inspect the sclera, which is white and clear. In the newborn, the sclera may appear to have a bluish tint due to its relative thinness. Dark-skinned children may present with small black marks in the sclera; this is a normal variant. A yellow appearance of the sclera indicates jaundice; this is not a normal finding.

On further inspection of the eyes, assess the irises for color, shape, and inflammation. The irises should be round and clear, but occasionally you may note different colors. Typically the iris color at birth is grayish-blue in light-skinned infants and grayish-brown in dark-skinned infants. The infant's eye color becomes permanent as the result of increased production of pigment at around 6–12 months of age. If there is an absence of color and pinkish tint to the iris, consider the possibility of albinism. In conjunction with Down syndrome, you may observe Brushfield spots, a ring of white or light speckling of the iris.

Next inspect the pupils for size, equality, and response to light. Pupils are normally round and of equal size, although unequal pupils (anisocoria) may be a normal finding if other findings are all normal. Pupils should respond briskly to light, and consensual response is expected when light is shown in the contralateral eye. To assess pupillary response, darken the room slightly and place the side of your hand down the midline of the nose to observe the response of each pupil when light is shone directly into the eye. A normal response is written as PERRLA (pupils equal, round, reactive to light, and accommodation).

When examining the eyelids, note the color and whether there are erythematous lesions such as hemangiomas or vascular malformations. Observe small linear creases on the lower eyelid, which are associated with allergies. Overall, inspect for edematous eyelids, which may be associated with congestive heart failure, hypoproteinemia, or nephritic syndrome. A less concerning cause of edematous eyelids may be associated with itching due to an allergic reaction to environmental allergens.

Use of the Ophthalmoscope

Before examining the fundus, or the interior, of the eye, dim the light in the room to allow for better visualization. There are two dials on the ophthalmoscope: One adjusts the light apertures and filters; the other changes the lenses to correct for the refractive errors of both the examiner and the patient.

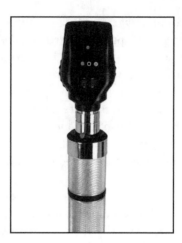

Figure 6-13 Ophthalmoscope

When examining the right eye of the patient, hold the ophthalmoscope in your right hand and up to your right eye. Ask the patient to look straight ahead and to focus on a distant target. Start with the small aperture and the lens diopter dial set to 0. The myopic examiner should start with minus lenses, which are the red numbers; the hyperopic examiner should start with plus lenses, which are the black or green numbers. Keep your index finger on the dial to move it up or down for focusing. Place the ophthalmoscope against your forehead over the eye you are going to use. Place your other hand on the patient's head to give you a frame of reference. While looking through the ophthalmoscope, approach the patient at eye level, approximately 15 inches away, and angle the light at the outer canthus of the patient's eye. Slowly come around with the light until you are directly in front of the patient's eye. Coming in from an angle will decrease papillary constriction and allow for better visualization. The light should be directly shining on the pupil, and a red glow, the red reflex, can be seen.

This part of the examination is relatively easy and can be performed on an infant as well as a toddler. You can accomplish this procedure by holding the light 20 to 30 inches away as well, thereby avoiding fear and crying in a young child. In an older child, you will be able to move further in beyond the red reflex and begin to observe the blood vessels in the periphery. To inspect the other eye, repeat the same procedure by placing the ophthalmoscope in your left hand and near your left eye; then focus the light on the patient's left eye.

A brief overview of the dials on the ophthalmoscope follows:

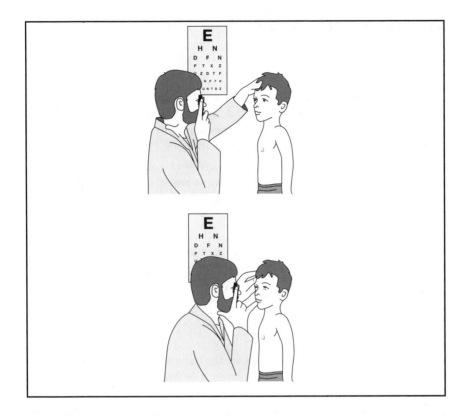

Figure 6-14   Eye Exam

The *SMALL APERTURE* provides easier view of the fundus through an undilated pupil. It is recommended to start your examination with this aperture and proceed to the large aperture to illuminate a larger portion of the fundus.

The *LARGE APERTURE* is the standard aperture for dilated pupils and for general examination of the eye.

The *FIXATION APERTURE* is the aperture with the pattern of an open center and thin lines. It permits easy observation of eccentric fixation without masking the macula. The graduated crosshairs can be used to estimate either the amount of eccentric fixation relative to the macula or the size or location of a lesion on the retina.

The *SLIT LAMP* is helpful in determining various levels of lesions, particularly tumors.

The *COBALT FILTER*, or the purple light, is helpful in eliciting fluorescence when the dye fluorescein is used. It allows for visualization of corneal lesions and abrasions (Welch Allyn Medical Diagnostic Equipment Manufacturer, 1996).

Assessment of the optic fundus is important because it can provide details about the vasculature of other systemic diseases in the pediatric patient such as diabetes, AIDS, endocarditis, and hypertension. It is also an important assessment in the examination of a child with shaken baby syndrome and/or head trauma. Because the eye is an extension of the nervous system, examination of the optic fundus can reveal important information on many neurologic disorders in children.

Examination of the Internal Eye

Internal inspection of the eye requires the ophthalmoscope. In babies and young children, it may be possible only to illicit the red reflex. In an older child who can cooperate, you may be able to visualize the retina, optic disc, macula, fovea centralis, and the veins and arteries noted in the eye grounds. It is helpful to darken the room before beginning so the child's pupil will dilate and make visualization easier. If the infant has his or her eyes closed, do not try to pry them open. Instead, sit the baby up or have the parent hold the baby; you will find that the infant will then open his or her eyes. This is a good opportunity to assess for the red reflex, which will appear very light in color, almost white. The peripheral vessels will not be well developed. At the same time, you may make fleeting eye contact with the infant and may even get the infant to follow your face in a horizontal pattern.

With the school-age child or adolescent ask him or her to sit on the table and focus on something straight ahead, such as a picture on the wall. Use your right eye to examine the child's right eye and your left eye to examine

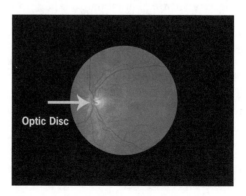

Figure 6-15 Optic Disc (See Color Plate)

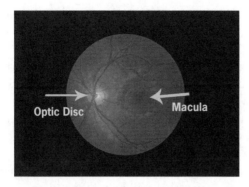

Figure 6-16   Macula (See Color Plate)

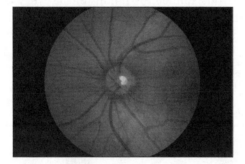

Figure 6-17   Optic Disc (See Color Plate)

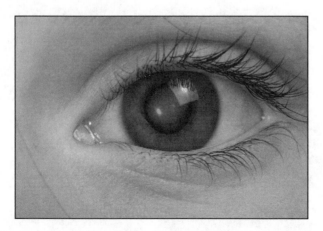

Figure 6-18   Corneal Light Reflex (See Color Plate)

the child's left eye. In children and adolescents, the red reflex will present as a red or orange glow. Looking further into the back, or fundus, of the eye, you will note the retinal vessels. By following the vessels from the periphery, you will note that they become larger as they lead you to the physiologic cup. At this point, you are looking at the optic disc and noting its size, color, and margins. To the left of the optic disc, approximately two disc widths removed, is the macula. It is lateral to the cup and appears isolated, as it is devoid of retinal vessels. In the center of the macula is the fovea, a depressed area where the cones are located.

It is often difficult to exam the back of the eye in toddlers or young school-age children because they will have difficulty focusing while you are shining the bright light into their eyes. Ask the late school-age or adolescent child to remain seated on the examination table and to focus on a picture on the far wall as you examine the fundus of the eye, which is detailed in the previous section. A helpful hint when examining the back of the eye is to angle the light of the ophthalmoscope on the side of the face near the eye so that when you come in from the side, the bright light will not cause pupillary constriction. Angle the light at the outer canthus of the eye and gradually come around so you are looking directly into the eye. To observe

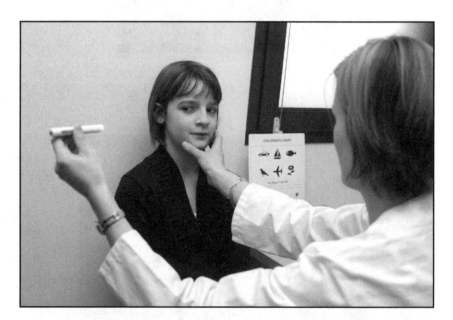

Figure 6-19 Eye Exam Extraocular Movements

the optic disc, it is helpful to direct the light downward on the nasal side of the retina.

Visual Examination Techniques

Extraocular Movements

The next part of the eye exam is inspection of *extraocular movements (EOMs),* which tests for weakness in the extraocular muscle groups. In the assessment of EOMs, you are examining the six cardinal fields of gaze, which coordinate with the six muscles that control eye movement. Children younger than 4 years of age may not be able to cooperate for this test, although using a finger puppet is a helpful way to get a child's attention as you move your finger through the six cardinal gazes. Making a game out of this procedure is both helpful to you and fun for your patient. It is often necessary to stabilize the child's head by holding a finger under his or her chin. Ask the child to follow your other finger (possibly using the finger puppet to hold the child's attention) as you move it **slowly** in a large circle. For a child who knows letters, explain that you want him or her to follow your finger as you draw an imaginary *H.* Start by placing a finger puppet on your index finger and hold your finger approximately 10 inches from the patient's nose. From the midline, first move your finger approximately a foot to the patient's right and stop, then move it up about 8 inches and stop, then move it down about 16 inches and stop, and, lastly, slowly move your finger back to the midline.

Deviations from normal are noted when eye movements are not coordinated or parallel, or when one or both eyes fail to follow your finger in any given direction. In addition, when looking to the extreme side, you may observe a quick rhythmic movement of the eyeball in the direction of gaze, called end-gaze nystagmus or far lateral gaze nystagmus. Nystagmus is defined as a rhythmic oscillation of the eyes. There are many causes, such as impairment of vision during early childhood development, disorders of the labyrinth of the ear and the cerebellar system, and drug toxicity (Bickley, 2003, p. 610). End-gaze nystagmus is considered within normal limits. Other presentations of nystagmus require referral to a neurologist.

Cover/Uncover Test

This test is performed to determine eye muscle weakness or strabismus. While examining a young child, have the child sit on a parent's lap. Ask them to look at a picture on the wall behind you. At the same time, cover one of their eyes with a 3- × 5-inch card. Observe the uncovered eye as it focuses on the picture. The uncovered eye should remain in place without movement. As the card is removed from the covered eye, observe that eye for movement. If the eyes are in alignment, there will be *no* movement of either eye. If the uncovered eye shifts position as the other eye is covered, a misalignment of the eye exists. The test demonstrates a weakness in one of the eyes—either *esotropia*, which is when the eyeball moves inward or toward the nasal side, or *exotropia*, which is when the eyeball moves toward the temporal side or outward. If your patient continues to look at you rather than at the picture behind you, ask the parent to stand a few feet behind you and call the child's name to get his or her attention. This approach will help to demonstrate the same findings.

Corneal Light Reflex

This test can be performed in the infant as well as in the young child. Using a pen light, shine the light directly into the eyes from a distance of approximately 16–20 inches, and observe the reflection of the light in each pupil. A normal response is reflection of the light as it appears symmetrically located in both pupils. Deviation from normal is when the light reflection appears at different spots in each eye. In a child younger than 6 months of age, you may notice an asymmetric response, which can be within normal limits. If the child is older than 6 months, referral is required. If the room is bright enough, you may just need to inspect both eyes for reflection of the light reflex off the cornea without using a pen light.

Visual Fields

Visual fields, or confrontation, can be assessed at 3–4 years of age. The overall evaluation is dependent on the cooperation of the child, and your ability to engage the child. A visual field is the entire area seen by an eye when it looks at a central point (Bickley, 2003, p. 119). This test is a gross assessment of peripheral vision; it compares the child's peripheral vision with your own, assuming that yours is normal. Have the child sit on a parent's lap, and sit in front of the child at eye level. Again, using a finger puppet is a helpful way to gain the child's attention and cooperation. Next, ask the child to look at your nose, and with both of your arms extended in opposite directions, ask the child to tell you which puppet is wiggling. The child may not tell you but may look at the puppet instead, which tells you that the child saw the movement in his or her peripheral vision. You can make a game out of this as well by repeating this test three or four times, moving your fingers in different positions in accordance with the six cardinal fields of gaze. In an older child, you can play a game by holding up several fingers and asking the child to tell you how many fingers are up, while making sure the child is looking at you or focusing on your nose. It may take several attempts before the child understands.

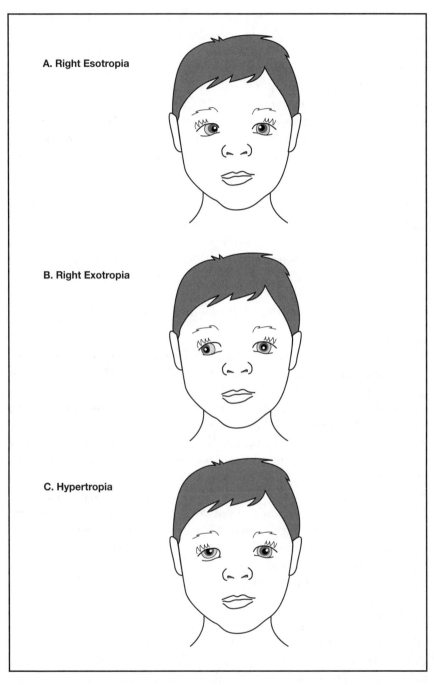

A. Right Esotropia

B. Right Exotropia

C. Hypertropia

Figure 6-20 Muscle Dysfunction

In older children, this test is performed by asking the child to sit on the exam table and you as the examiner stand at eye level, approximately two to three feet away. Ask the child to look into your eyes while you return the gaze. Place your hands about two feet apart lateral to the child's ears, and while wiggling fingers of both hands move them along a line of an imaginary bowl and toward the line of gaze until the child can identify them. Repeat this pattern in both the upper and lower temporal quadrants. This is comparing the child's peripheral vision with your own assuming that your peripheral vision is normal. If the child cannot see your wiggling fingers when you see them, this suggests that there may be a peripheral field loss and referral to an ophthalmologist is recommended.

Assessing for field defects is important in a child, particularly after head trauma, when a child is increasingly losing his or her balance, or when there is concern of seizures. Also, neurologic disorders associated with tumors often present with visual field defects. Although this test may be difficult to perform in a young child, it can detect gross hemianopsia, or blindness, in one-half of the visual fields in one or both eyes. For more precise evaluation, referral to a pediatric ophthalmologist is recommended.

Color Vision

Color vision is assessed by using the Ishihara test for color deficiency. This test was named after its creator, Dr. Shinobu Ishihara (1879–1963). Color blindness is an inherited condition in which certain colors cannot be distinguished. Red and green are the colors most commonly affected. The test consists of a number of colored plates that each contain a circle of dots appearing in randomized color and size. Commonly, the dots appear in shades of green and light blues with a number differentiated in shades of brown, or the dots appear in shades of red, orange, and yellow with a number in shades of green. For those with impaired color vision, the numbers are not discernible. The full test consists of 38 plates, although the presence of a deficiency is apparent after displaying just a few plates. This test can initially be performed on children between 4 and 5 years of age if they can both cooperate and recognize numbers. There is no treatment for color blindness. Color blindness plates are shown in **Figure 6-21**.

Accommodation

In accommodation, the pupils constrict when viewing nearby objects and dilate when focusing on distant objects. In a well-lit room, and with the child sitting on the parent's lap, ask the child to look into your eyes, or hold a finger puppet in front of the child and ask him or her to look at it. Then instruct the child to look at a picture on the wall or in the distance. A normal response is initial constriction of the pupils when looking at the near object and dilation when looking at the far object.

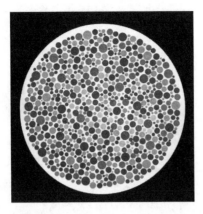

Figure 6-21 Color Blindness Plates (See Color Plate)

Accommodation is a reflection of the sympathetic and parasympathetic nervous system, or the fight-or-flight response. Deviation from normal is abnormal pupillary size or anisocoria, which is defined by unequal pupil size, although both react to light and accommodation. Inequality may be congenital or may be due to inflammation of neurophthalmic pathways. Other examples of pupil abnormality are associated with drug ingestion (such as small, fixed pupils observed in opiate ingestion) or severe head trauma (a fixed dilated pupil).

Visual Acuity

To assess acuity in the infant, observe for blinking in response to a bright light. Also, when the child is 2–3 months of age, observe for brief eye contact; when 4 months of age, observe fixating on a brightly colored object, such as a red ball, and move the ball in a horizontal plane. If you can make eye contact, move your head in a horizontal plane, continuing to maintain eye contact with the child and noting whether the baby follows you by moving his or her head and maintaining eye contact. By 6 months of age, the child should be able to follow in both a horizontal and vertical plane. If the child does not follow or fixate, referral is necessary. See **Figure 6-22** for an example of following.

In young children, several tests can be performed to assess visual acuity. While a test of visual acuity is the most frequently recommended vision screening test for preschool children, most guidelines also recommend a test of stereopsis, or binocular depth perception. In choosing an appropriate test of stereopsis for preschool children, several features are important to consider. The first is that the test should be a test of stereopsis in which monocular cues are minimized or absent. The Random Dot E (RDE) stereo-test meets this requirement and has been recommended for use in preschool

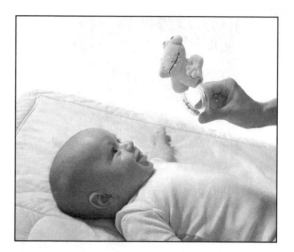

Figure 6-22   Following

vision screening by the American Academy of Pediatrics (2003). **Figure 6-23** is an example of the RDE stereotest.

An older child's vision can be tested using Allen cards or E cards. The Allen cards show pictures of familiar objects in graduated sizes. The E cards show the letter *E* in different orientations and in graduated sizes. The child is asked to point to the direction in which the feet of the *E* are turned: up, down, left, or right. Start by using the E cards, and have the child indicate the direction of the *E*'s legs with his or her fingers, or use

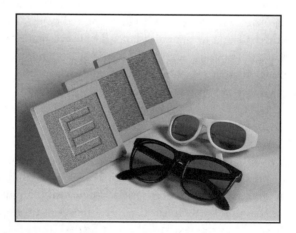

Figure 6-23   Random Dot E (RDE) Stereotest

a large cardboard *E* for the child to move in the appropriate direction (American Academy of Pediatrics, 2003).

Common Eye Infections in Children

The following is a description of opthalmic disorders you may encounter when assessing a child's eyes.

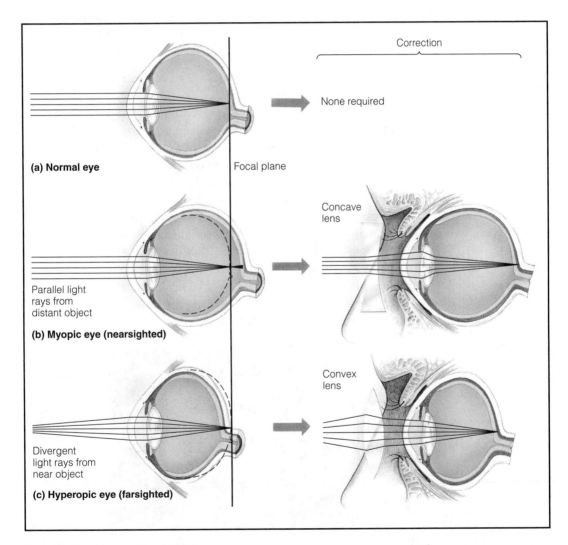

Figure 6-24   Common Visual Problems

BLEPHARITIS is a chronic inflammatory condition at the eyelid margins that causes itching and crusting at the lash line. There are varying degrees of erythema at the lid margins. This condition is often seen in conjunction with seborrhea dermatitis.

CHALAZION is an inflammation of the meibomian glands. It produces a nontender, localized nodule over the tarsus of the upper or lower eyelid. It is not on the lid margin as is a sty, but is on the actual eyelid and is easily palpable. See **Figure 6-25**.

HORDEOLUM, also called a sty, is a localized staphylococcal infection of the gland of Zeis. It presents superficially at the margin of the eyelid as a red, swollen, tender pustule. See **Figure 6-26**.

CONJUNCTIVITIS, or pink eye, is a very common disease of the eye. There are three types: bacterial, viral, and allergic.

> *BACTERIAL CONJUNCTIVITIS* presents unilaterally with diffuse hyperemia of the bulbar and tarsal conjunctiva, purulent discharge, and matting of the eyelashes upon awakening. See **Figure 6-27**. It spreads to the other eye within 48 hours (Graham & Uphold, 2003).

> *VIRAL CONJUNCTIVITIS* is the leading cause of conjunctivitis in children and is highly contagious. It presents bilaterally, with conjunctival hyperemia, edema, and watery discharge. There is risk of bacterial conjunctivitis with viral conjunctivitis, which may require antibiotic therapy.

> *ALLERGIC CONJUNCTIVITIS* presents with the hallmark signs of itching and watery eyes. There may be mild lid edema, fine papillary hypertrophy, bulbar conjunctival hyperemia, mucoid discharge, and nasal congestion. See **Figure 6-28**.

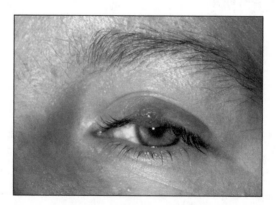

Figure 6-25 Chalazion

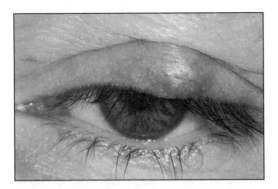

Figure 6-26   Hordeolum

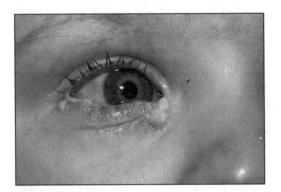

Figure 6-27   Bacterial Conjunctivitis

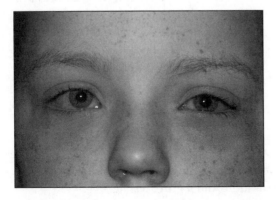

Figure 6-28   Allergic Conjunctivitis

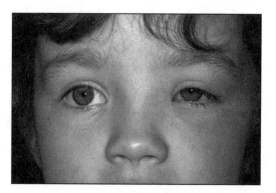

Figure 6-29   Orbital Cellulitis

NEONATAL CONJUNCTIVITIS, also called ophthalmia neonatorum, presents during the first 12 to 24 hours of life and is most frequently caused by silver nitrate drops instilled at birth to prevent gonococcal infection. It presents as a mild conjunctivitis. Actual *Neisseria gonorrhoeae* presents within the first two to five days of life, causes acute conjunctival inflammation with erythema, and copious amounts of purulent discharge.

TRACHOMA is the most common cause of blindness worldwide, although it is rarely seen in the United States. It is prevalent in third-world countries and is characterized by conjunctivitis with small lymphoid follicles in the conjunctiva.

PERIORBITAL CELLULITIS is an infection of structures around the eye. It presents with erythema, induration, and tenderness of the periorbital tissues, usually without signs of systemic infection. Periorbital cellulitis often requires inpatient treatment with antibiotics.

ORBITAL CELLULITIS is infection of the orbit with restricted and painful eye movement, proptosis, edema of the conjunctiva, and decreased visual acuity. It is much more concerning than periorbital cellulitis and requires immediate referral. See **Figure 6-29**.

CORNEAL ABRASION results from scratching or abrading the cornea, often caused by a foreign object. Injuries present with pain, tearing, photophobia, foreign body sensation, and a gritty feeling.

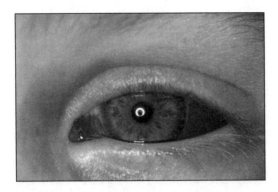

Figure 6-30 Conjunctival Hemorrhage

CONGENITAL CATARACT presents with a white pupillary reflex. Identification of the red reflex in newborns and infants is necessary to avoid missing a congenital cataract. Refer to an ophthalmologist as soon as possible to avoid visual impairment.

> **Red Flags**

- Among the signs to worry about when examining an infant is the absence of a blink reflex. During an ophthalmic exam, partial or white reflex instead of a red reflex warrants immediate referral, as does retinal hemorrhage associated with head injury, which often results from shaken baby syndrome.

- Concerns in the toddler and older child include constriction of the pupils (*miosis*), which occurs with the use of certain drugs (e.g., morphine). Dilatation of the pupils (*mydriasis*) can be related to specific drugs, trauma, and circulatory arrest. Fixed unilateral dilation of one or both pupils indicates local eye trauma or severe head injury. Limitation of or pain resulting from eye movement in conjunction with bulbar erythema and edema may be associated with orbital cellulitis. A child who does not make eye contact when interacting may be showing signs of autistic like behavior. Newly observed vertical nystagmus or lateral nystagmus, other than end-gaze nystagmus, requires immediate referral.

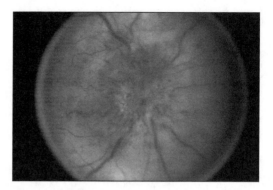

Figure 6-31 Papilledema (See Color Plate)

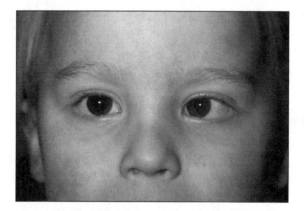

Figure 6-32 Esotropia

- Papilledema presents with swelling of the optic nerve as it enters the back of the eye. It is present in both eyes and is caused by increased intracranial pressure. See **Figure 6-31**. It requires immediate referral. Papilledema is relatively uncommon in infants because the bones of the skull are not fully fused. It may be present in the older child secondary to trauma, infection, or CNS lesions.

Write-Up of the Eye

EXAMPLE FOR INFANTS: Brows, lids, and lashes intact, eyes appropriately placed, pupils, equal, round, react to light, accommodation (PERRLA); makes fleeting eye contact; blinks to bright light; without lid lag, ptosis, discharge, or crusting. Corneal light reflex symmetric, no strabismus, conjunctiva clear, sclera white, no lesions. Bilateral red reflex.

EXAMPLE FOR SCHOOL-AGE CHILDREN AND ADOLESCENTS: Brows, lids, and lashes intact; no tearing; conjunctiva clear; sclera white without lesions or redness; pupils reactive equally to light and accommodation. Cornea clear without lesions. Extraocular movements intact, no nystagmus, visual fields full to confrontation. Cover/uncover test without evidence of deviation. Corneal light reflex symmetric without strabismus. Fundi: red reflex present bilaterally, discs with well-defined borders bilaterally, AV ratio of vessels 2:5, no crossing changes noted. Background has even color, no hemorrhage or exudates, macula present. Acuity by Snellen chart: O.D. 20/20, O.S. 20/20 without glasses.

Case Study: Eye Assessment for Drainage

Alex, an 18-month-old boy, is brought to your office with a 24-hour history of drainage from his left eye, rhinorrhea, and cough. He is afebrile but has been fussy for the past 2 days. His history is significant for two previous episodes of otitis media. He is in day care 4 days a week.

On examination:

- *Eyes*: PERRLA. In the left eye, the conjunctiva is injected with palpebral and bulbar edema. The right eye is within normal limits. There is minimal evidence of purulent drainage.
- *Ears*: The right tympanic membrane is gray with mobility. The left tympanic membrane is dark gray and dull with decreased mobility.
- *Oropharynx*: Moist without erythema
- *Nose*: Dried mucopurulent drainage in both nares
- *Neck*: Supple without lymphadenopathy
- *Lungs*: Clear without adventitious sounds

Questions

1. What is the difference between viral, bacterial, and allergic conjunctivitis in children?
2. What is the association between conjunctivitis and otitis media?
3. What is your treatment plan for Alex?

Answers

1. *Bacterial conjunctivitis* is characterized by conjunctival injection, purulent drainage, edema of the palpebral and bulbar conjunctiva, photophobia, and crusting on the eyelashes. It generally presents in one eye with eventual infection of the other eye. *Viral conjunctivitis* is characterized by redness, itching, and serous drainage that affects both eyes. It is associated with adenovirus. *Allergic conjunctivitis* presents with the hallmark signs of ocular itching and watery drainage. It is often accompanied by a history of atopic disease.

2. The association between conjunctivitis and otitis media is based on the communicating anatomic location of the conjunctival sac, the middle ear, and the nasopharynx, which leads to conjunctivitis-otitis syndrome.

3. The treatment plan for Alex includes erythromycin ophthalmic ointment, sulfa ophthalmic drops, or polymyxin/trimethoprim drops. The dose is one-half inch (1.25 cm) of ointment deposited inside the lower lid or 1 to 2 drops instilled four times daily for 5–7 days. Ointment is preferred over drops for children because it stays on the lids and has a therapeutic effect even if a minimal amount is applied directly to the conjunctiva (Jacobs, 2008).

References

American Academy of Pediatrics: Eye Examination in Infants, Children, and Young Adults by Pediatricians, Committee on Practice and Ambulatory Medicine, Section on Ophthalmology. (2003). *Pediatrics. 111*(4), 902-907.

Bickley, L. (2003). *Bates' guide to physical examination and history taking* (8th ed.). New York: Lippincott Williams & Wilkins.

Graham, M.V. & Uphold, C. R. (2003). *Clinical guidelines in child health*, (3rd ed.). Barmarrae Books.

Jacobs, D. (2008). Conjunctivitis. *Uptodate.com.*

Welch Allyn Medical Diagnostic Equipment Manufacturer, 1996. Skaneateles Falls, NY.

Resources

Burns, C., Dunn, A., Brady, M., Starr, N., & Blosser, C. (2000). *Pediatric primary care: A handbook for nurse practitioners* (3rd ed.). St. Louis, MO: Saunders.

Estes, M. (1998). *Health assessment and physical examination*. Albany, NY: Delmar Publishers.

Jarvis, C. (2004). *Physical examination and health assessment* (5th ed.). St. Louis, MO: Elsevier.

Marieb, E. (1995). *Human anatomy and physiology* (3rd ed.). Redwood City, CA: Benjamin/Cummings Publishing Company.

Potts, N., & Mandleco, B. (2007) *Pediatraic nursing* (2nd ed.). Victoria, Australia: Thomson, Delmar Learning.

Swartz, M. H. (2009). *Textbook of physical diagnosis* (3rd ed.). St. Louis, MO: Saunders.

Tortora, G. J, Grabvowski, S. R. (2003). *Principles of anatomy and physiology* (10th ed.). New York: Wiley.

Examination of the Head, Neck, and Lymphatic System

Anatomy and Physiology

The Cranium

The skull is composed of two sets of bones, the *cranial bones*, or cranium (**Figure 7-1**), which enclose and protect the brain, and the facial bones, which form the framework of the face. The cranium is made up of eight bones: the frontal bone, two parietal bones, two temporal bone, the occipital bone, the sphenoid bone, and the ethmoid bone. The bones of the skull are not firmly joined at birth and are separated by sutures and by two fontanelles. This allows for the change and mobility of the head as it proceeds through the birth canal. The sutures that intersect with the cranium bones are the coronal suture, which crowns the head from ear to ear at the union of the frontal and parietal bones. The sagittal suture separates the head lengthwise and is where the two parietal bones meet at the cranial midline. The lambdoid suture separates the parietal bones crosswise and is where the parietal bones meet the

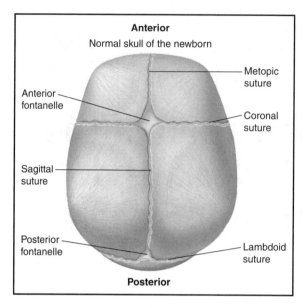

Figure 7-1 Cranium

occipital bone posterior. These sutures gradually ossify during early childhood.

The *FRONTAL BONE* forms the anterior portion of the cranium, which includes the forehead, and roof of the orbits. The smooth portion of the forehead between the orbits is called the glabella. The frontal sinuses are located at the areas lateral to the glabella.

The *PARIETAL BONES* are large, curved bones that form most of the superior and lateral aspects of the skull.

The *OCCIPITAL BONE* forms most of the posterior wall and base of the skull. Importantly, the occipital bone internally supports the cerebellum of the brain, and in the base of the occipital bone is the foramen magnum. It is through this opening that the inferior part of the brain, the medulla oblongata, connects with the spinal cord.

The *TEMPORAL BONES* have a complicated shape. Part of the temporal bone forms the zygomatic arch, which is the projection of the cheekbone. Another part of the bone on the inferior surface of the zygomatic process forms the movable temporomandibular joint (TMJ). Another part of the temporal bone is the mastoid process, which can be palpated posterior to the ear. The mastoid region is adjacent to the middle ear cavity and is a

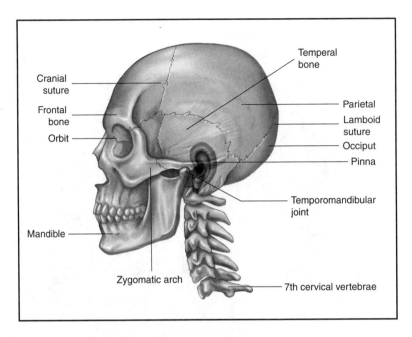

Figure 7-2 Structure of the Head

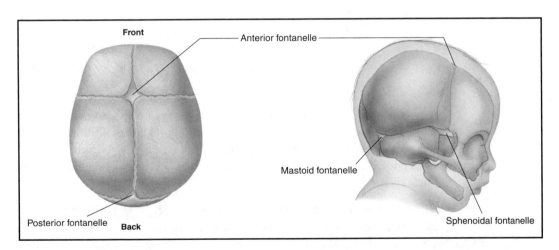

Figure 7-3 Fontanels and Bones of the Newborn Skull Viewed from Above and Lateral View of Newborn Skull Showing Fontanels and Bones

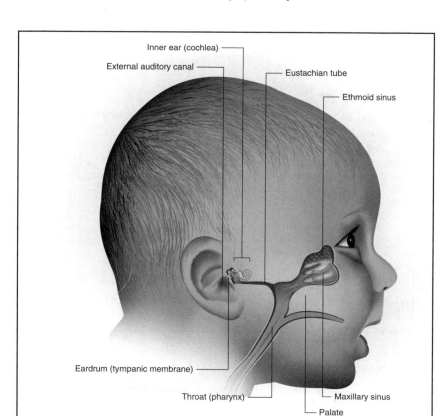

Figure 7-4 Eustachian Tube and Posterior Pharynx

high-risk area for infection emitting from the throat and is a difficult infection to treat because it may easily spread to the brain.

The *SPHENOID BONE* is considered the keystone of the cranium because it articulates as a central wedge with the other cranial bones. Within the body of the sphenoid bone are the sphenoid sinuses. Further within the sphenoid bone is the sella turcica, or Turk's saddle, a saddlelike depression that encloses the pituitary gland.

The *ETHMOID BONE* also has a complicated shape. It lies between the sphenoid and the nasal bones of the face and forms the bony area between the nasal cavity and the orbit. The ethmoid sinuses are located in this area. Extending medially are the turbinates, which protrude into the nasal cavity. The parts of the brain underlying the various parts of the skull will be discussed in Chapter 13.

The Facial Bones

The major facial bones include the mandible, maxilla, zygomatic, nasal, concha, lacrimal, palatine, and vomer bones, as well as the inferior nasal conchae. The major landmarks of the face are the palpebral fissures and the nasolabial folds. The facial muscles are innervated by the trigeminal nerve (cranial nerve V) and the facial nerve (cranial nerve VII).

The *MANDIBLE* is the largest and strongest bone of the face and forms the chin and lower jaw, extending up to the TMJ. This bone anchors the lower teeth.

The *MAXILLARY BONES* form the upper jaw, and all facial bones except the mandible articulate with the maxillae; these bones are therefore considered the keystone bones of the face. Incorporated in the maxillary bones are the maxillary sinuses that flank the nasal cavity laterally. These sinuses are the largest of the paranasal sinuses, extending from the orbits to the upper teeth. Figure 7-5 illustrates the sinuses. When infected, the maxillary sinuses produce dark shadows under the eyes referred to as "raccoon eyes."

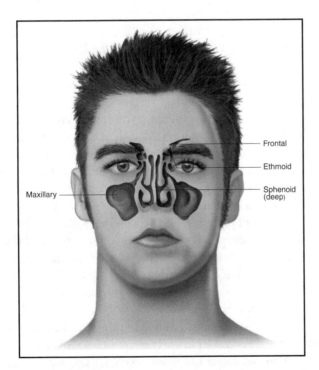

Figure 7-5 Diagram of Sinuses

The *ZYGOMTIC BONES*, called the cheekbones, articulate with the zygomatic processes of the temporal bones.

The *NASAL BONES* form most of the skeleton of the external nose.

The *LACRIMAL BONES* are small, delicate bones that form the medial walls of each orbit. They house the lacrimal sac, which allows tears to drain from the eye into the nasal cavity.

The *PALATINE BONES* complete the posterior portion of the hard palate, or the roof, of the mouth.

The *VOMER BONE* is a slender, plow-shaped bone located within the nasal cavity. It forms part of the nasal septum.

The *INFERIOR NASAL CONCHAE* are the thin, curved bones in the nasal cavity that form the lateral walls of the nasal cavity.

The Neck

The structure of the neck is formed by the seven cervical vertebrae that support the head and allow mobility. The major neck muscles are the sternocleidomastoid and the trapezius muscles, which are innervated by cranial nerve XI, the spinal accessory. Together, the skull and neck provide protective covering and housing for the brain and the complex matrix of the nervous system. The first cervical vertebra, C1 or the atlas, is different from the rest and is so named from the mythological character, Atlas, who supported the world on his shoulders. The second vertebra, C2 or the axis, acts as a pivot on which the head rotates, allowing it to turn from side to side. The seventh cervical vertebra, C7, is called the vertebra prominens. It has a single large spinous process that serves as a useful landmark when performing physical assessment of the neck, back, and thorax.

The major muscles of the neck divide each side of the neck into two triangles, the anterior and posterior, by the *sternocleidomastoid* and the *trapezius* muscles. The sternocleidomastoid muscles extend from the upper portion of the sternum and the clavicle to the mastoid process, allowing the head to bend laterally, rotate, flex, and extend. The trapezius muscles extend from the occipital bone down the neck and insert at the outer third of the clavicles at the acromion process of the scapula along the spinal column at the level of the thoracic spinal nerve 12 (T12). These muscles allow the shoulders and scapula to move up and down and rotate medially. The neck muscles are further divided into two triangles that lie above and below the hyoid bone. The anterior triangle is formed by the mandible, the trachea, and sternocleidomastoid muscles; it contains the anterior cervical lymph nodes, the trachea, and the thyroid gland. The posterior triangle is the area between the sterno-cleidomastoid and the trapezius muscles with the clavicle at the base; it contains the posterior cervical lymph nodes. See **Figure 7-6.**

The *thyroid gland* is the largest endocrine gland in the body. It secretes thyroxine (T4) and triiodothyronine (T3), which regulate the rate of cellular metabolism. It is composed of two lobes, butterfly shaped, each curving posteriorly between the trachea and the sternomastoid muscle. The lobes are connected in the middle by a thin isthmus lying over the second and third tracheal rings and below the cricoid cartilage. See **Figure 7-7.** The cricoid cartilage is the landmark for making an emergency airway, or tracheostomy.

The thyroid cartilage, or Adam's apple, consists of two fused plates of hyaline cartilage that form the anterior wall of the larynx. It is usually larger in males than in females and is used as a landmark in examining the neck. Thyroid disease occurs less frequently in children than in adults, although hypothyroidism is screened for in the newborn period.

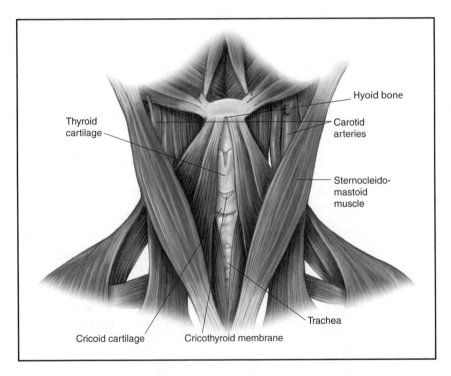

Figure 7-6 Midline Neck Structure

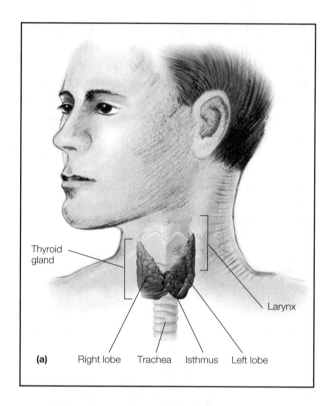

(a) Right lobe   Trachea   Isthmus   Left lobe

Figure 7-7 Thyroid Gland

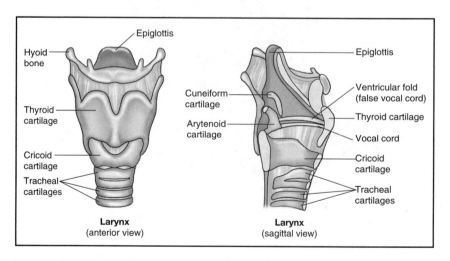

Larynx
(anterior view)

Larynx
(sagittal view)

Figure 7-8 Larynx

The Lymphatic System

The lymphatic system consists of two parts, the lymphatic vessels and the lymphoid tissue. The lymphatic vessels transport fluids from the tissue space and return it to the bloodstream. Excess fluid in the tissue space would build up in the interstitial space and produce edema if not retrieved by the lymphatic system and returned to the bloodstream. The lymphatic vessels drain into the two main trunks, which empty into the venous system at the subclavian veins. The right lymphatic duct empties into the right subclavian vein. It drains the right side of the head and neck, right arm, right side of the thorax, right lung and pleura, right side of the heart, and right upper section of the liver. The thoracic duct drains the rest of the body and empties into the left subclavian vein.

The lymphatic system has three main functions: (1) conserve fluid and plasma proteins that leak out of the capillaries, (2) contribute to the immune system in defending the body against disease, and (3) absorb lipids from the intestinal tract. Lymph nodes are small oval clumps of lymphatic tissue arranged in groups located at intervals along the vessels. The nodes filter the lymphatic fluid and filter out pathogens before the fluid is returned to the bloodstream. These pathogens are then exposed to lymphocytes in the lymph nodes, and an antigen-specific response is mounted to eliminate the pathogens.

Four superficial groups of nodes are accessible to inspection and palpation:

1. The cervical nodes, which drain the head and neck
2. The axillary nodes, which drain the breast and upper arm
3. The epitrochlear nodes, which are in the antecubital fossa and drains the hand and lower arm
4. The inguinal nodes, which are in the groin and drain most of the lymph of the lower extremities, the external genitalia, and the anterior abdominal wall

Development of the Lymphatic System

In children, the lymphatic system is still developing and is less effective at creating antibodies, leaving young children more vulnerable to infection. The lymphatic system matures and reaches peak development at around 10–12 years of age. Lymph tissue then gradually decreases in size during adolescence. In children, the lymph nodes are relatively large, particularly the superficial ones, and can be easily palpated without signs of infection. During an infectious process, such as pharyngitis, excessive swelling and hyperplasia of the lymph tissue occurs and is noted in enlarged tonsils. Children often have palpable lymph nodes as their immune system responds to environmental pathogens to which they are exposed. An example is slightly enlarged movable, non-tender nodes that are palpated along the anterior cervical chain. These are referred to as shotty nodes associated with otitis media and other upper respiratory infections.

In children with enlarged or tender cervical lymph nodes, it is important to determine their acuity and whether they have developed over the past few days or have been there for several weeks. Also note whether they are unilateral or bilateral. The anterior cervical lymph nodes are enlarged in a variety of infections of the head and neck, such as pharyngitis or Epstein-Barr virus. Infections may be bacterial, such as streptococcal and staphylo-coccal, or viral. Most children with enlarged anterior cervical adenopathy have acute self-limiting infections. A common infection in children with lymphadenopathy is cat-scratch disease. The infection may result from a cat scratch or from a cat licking a child's broken skin. Often, cervical ade-nitis develops, and lymphadenopathy is generally present.

The most common ages noted for lymphadenopathy are between 3 and 5 years (Swanson, 2009). Cervical and inguinal nodes are more common after 2 years of age than in the first six months. Small occipital and postauricular nodes are common in infants, but less common in older children. Occipital nodes can be palpable in conjunction with scaling infected lesions on the scalp such as tinea capitis. Postauricular and postcervical node enlargement is commonly noted with acute mononucleosis. Epitrochlear and supracla-vicular adenopathy are uncommon at any age. Lymphadenopathy in these areas is a red flag and is associated with malignancy and cancer such as lymphoma and leukemia (Swanson, 2009). Generalized lymphadenopathy is usually associated with systemic diseases such as HIV.

Assessment Considerations: Subjective Information

Infants

Considerations pertinent to the infant in the assessment of the head and neck include:

- What is the prenatal history? Include in this history the mother's use of alcohol or drugs, or specific treatment for abuse. Alcohol abuse during pregnancy places the fetus at risk for fetal alcohol syndrome, which produces distinct facial features such as smooth philtrum, thin upper lip, and small palpebral fissures.
- What is the birth history? Was the delivery vaginal or by cesarean section? Also consider the presentation and difficulty of the delivery and whether forceps were used. Use of forceps increases the risk for caput succedaneum (localized edematous swelling of the soft tissue of

the scalp resulting from the birthing process) and cephalhematoma (subperiosteal hemorrhage resulting from the birthing process).

- Are there abnormalities in the shape and size of the head? Molding of the skull bones is a common cause of temporary asymmetry that occurs during the birthing process. Unusual head shape may be due to a congenital anomaly or positioning in utero. Congenital anomalies include meningomyelocele, encephalocele, upslanting palpebral fissures (associated with Down syndrome), and downslanting palpebral fissures (associated with Noonan syndrome).
- Did the results of the neonatal screen indicate any concerns, such as hypothyroidism?
- Are the concerns regarding the patterning, quality, and texture of hair or the location of the hairline? Low anterior and posterior hairlines and hypopigmentation may be associated with genetic disorders.
- Are there concerns about bulging or depressed fontanelles?
- Is there facial asymmetry or paralysis, such as Bell's palsy, due to birth injury?
- Are there concerns about dysmorphogenesis? If so, examine the parents and siblings, noting growth and development, head circumference, height, and weight.

School-Age Children and Adolescents

Considerations pertinent to the school-age child or adolescent in the assessment of the head and neck include:

- Is the child experiencing headaches? If so, determine the frequency, quality, duration, location, character, pattern, and associated symptoms. Headaches will be reviewed in greater detail in Chapter 13.
- Does the child have a history of neck injury, including limitation of movement, pain with movement, swelling of the neck, and radiation pattern?
- Does the child have a history of temperature intolerance? Change in hair, skin, or nail texture? Change in emotional stability, energy level, weight, and/or bowel habits? All of these findings are associated with thyroid disease.
- Does the child have a history of head injury, with associated loss of consciousness?
- Does the child have a history of changes in the menstrual cycle (increased or decreased flow)?

Family History

During the subjective assessment, also consider the child's family history in regard to head, neck, and lymphatic conditions:

- History of congenital anomalies such as dysmorphic disorders
- History of cognitive delay or mental retardation
- History of seizures
- History of thyroid disease
- History of diabetes (which may predispose the child to acquired hypothyroidism) (Ball, 2010, p. 1269)

Review of Systems

The review of systems should include the following:

- *WEIGHT*: Gain or loss
- *SKIN*: Changes in color or texture
- *HAIR*: Changes in quality, texture, or distribution
- *NAILS*: Changes in appearance or texture
- *HEAD*: Head injury, dizziness, headaches
- *NECK*: Swelling, stiffness, pain, masses, node enlargement, limitation of movement, hoarseness
- *HEART*: History of fatigue, bradycardia
- *GASTROINTESTINAL SYSTEM*: History of constipation or change in bowel habits
- *GENITALIA*: Delayed puberty
- *NEUROLOGIC SYSTEM*: Delayed developmental milestones, change in deep tendon reflexes due to muscle weakness
- *ENDOCRINE SYSTEM*: Changes in weight, heat/cold intolerance, change in energy level

Assessment Considerations: Objective Information

Examination of the Head of the Infant

Inspection

Start by measuring the infant's head circumference, and compare the results with the expected size for age on a growth chart. Also inspect the skull for symmetry. Molding, or overlapping, may be noted in the newborn secondary to the birthing process. Overlapping of the cranial bones may occur, causing the head to appear asymmetric. The head usually regains normal shape in approximately 1–2 weeks. Inspect for normal spacing of the facial features, noting excessive hair or an unusually low hairline, anterior or posterior. Note symmetry and/or paralysis of facial features, skin color, and skin texture. Observe the infant's head control, position, and movement, noting any inability to move the head in one direction, jerking, or tremorlike movements. Inspect the scalp veins for dilatation, which can be associated with increased intracranial pressure.

In the older infant, asymmetry of the head, or *plagiocephaly*, may be noted. See **Figure 7-9**. This condition is defined by flattening of one side of the head, primarily the occipitoparietal region, due to positioning. With today's guidelines suggesting that infants lie on their back to prevent SIDS, there have been more reported cases of *plagiocephaly*. In addition, frontal bossing, or abnormal skull contour in which the forehead becomes prominent, may be observed in the premature infant or in the infant with hydrocephalus. An infant's skull may present with swelling over the occipitoparietal region, a condition called *caput succedaneum* that is due to subcutaneous edema, which crosses over the suture line and resolves in several days. See **Figure 7-10**. Edematous areas with margins that are limited to suture line margins and that often require weeks to recede are subperiosteal hemorrhages, or *cephalohematomas*. An important difference between caput succedaneum and cephalohematoma is that swelling never extends across the suture lines in cephalohematoma, although more than one cranial bone may show evidence of edema.

Palpation

When palpating the infant's head, place the infant in a sitting position while you are assessing the sutures and fontanelles. With your finger pads,

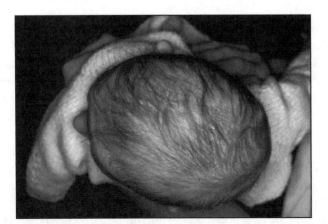

Figure 7-9   Plagiocephaly

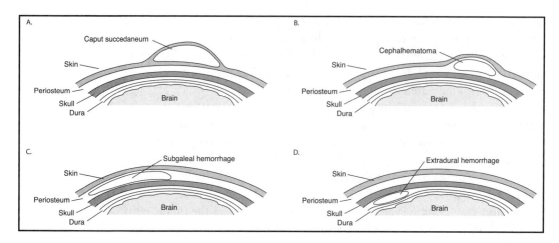

Figure 7-10 Caput Succedaneum

palpate the *sagittal* suture line, the *coronal* suture line, and the *lambdoidal* suture, assessing for suture lines that are open or overlapping. Premature closure of the cranial sutures gives the head an unusual shape referred to as *craniosynostosis*, which can be palpated as a bony ridge over the suture line. Molding is a temporary or transient overlapping due to the birthing process, whereas craniosynostosis can cause severe brain compression. The shape of the newborn's head gradually rounds out, although there are certain metabolic disorders where there is premature ossification of the sutures, such as microcephaly, which results in a narrow, conelike shape to the head.

On further examination of the infant's head, palpate the anterior fontanelle at the junction of the sagittal, coronal, and frontal sutures. Palpate the posterior fontanelle at the junction of the sagittal and lambdoidal sutures. Assess for bulging, fullness, pulsations, and size. The anterior fontanelle is typically 4–6 cm at birth and gradually closes between 9 and 18 months of age. Many times when an infant is 6 months to 1 year of age, the anterior fontanelle is not palpable, although the cranial bones have not actually fused yet. The posterior fontanelle is much smaller, 0.5–1.5 cm, and gradually closes between 1 and 3 months of age. An exceptionally large anterior fontanelle (greater then 3 cm) may be associated with hydrocephaly, hypothyroidism, osteogenesis imperfecta, and vitamin D deficiency or rickets (see **Figure 7-13**). A depressed anterior fontanelle associated with dehydration is a late sign when assessing an infant's hydration status. A posterior fontanelle larger then 1.5 cm may also be associated with congenital hypothyroidism.

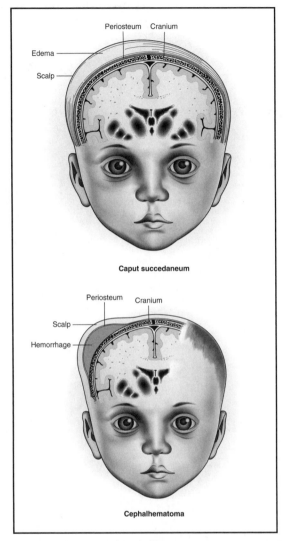

Figure 7-11 Caput Succedeneum and Cephalhematoma

Source: This article was published in Physical Examination and Health Assessment, 5th edition, Jarvis. Caput succedaneum and Cephalhematoma, page . Copyright Saunders (2007).

Further palpation of the scalp above and behind the ears detects *craniotabes*, which is a soft depressable area of the skull bone (usually parietal bones). It is most commonly found in premature infants associated with syphilis and/or rickets (Thureen, Deacon, O'Neill, & Hernandez, 2004, p. 123). Transillumination of the skull is performed in infants in whom there is increasing head circumference and suspicion of CNS disease. In a

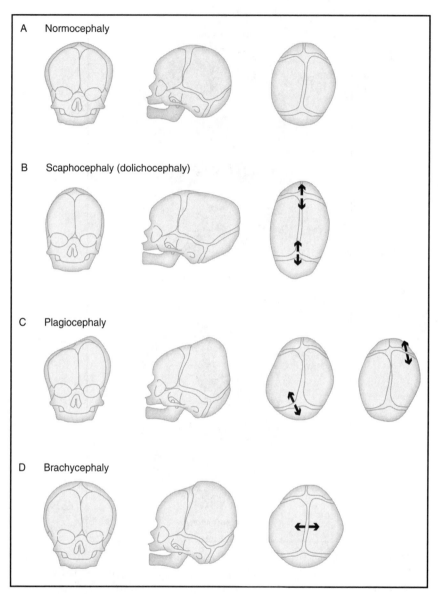

Figure 7-12 Craniosynostosis

Source: Potts/Mandleco. Pediatric Nursing, (2nd ed). © 2007 Delmar Learning, a part of Cengage Learning, Inc. Reproduced by permission. www.cengage.com/permissions

completely darkened room, a transilluminator, or flashlight fitted with a soft rubber collar, is placed firmly against the infant's scalp. In a normal infant, you would expect to see a 2-cm ring of light beyond the rim of the

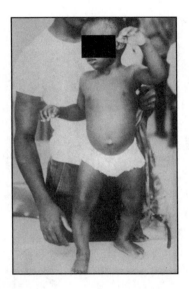

Figure 7-13 Child with Rickets

flashlight. If the rim of light is well beyond 2 cm or the entire head lights up, suspect *hydranencephaly*, which is reduced size of the cerebral cortex (**Figure 7-15**). Hydranencephaly is a rare condition in which the brain's cerebral hemispheres are absent and replaced by sacs filled with cerebrospinal fluid. This condition should not be confused with hydrocephaly, in which there is an excessive buildup of cerebral spinal fluid. This accumulation of cerebral spinal fluid is due to an imbalance between production and absorption (Boon, 2009).

Percussion
There is minimal percussion of the infant's head, although *Macewen sign*, or "cracked pot" sound, is elicited in older infants after fontanelle closure in conjunction with increased intracranial pressure.

Auscultation of the infant's skull is generally not performed.

Examination of the Head and Face of the School-Age Child and Adolescent

Inspection
Inspection of the head starts by assessing size, shape and symmetry, and head position. Note if the head is normocephalic, which is a round symmetric skull that is appropriate to body size. Inspect the scalp by parting the hair, noting any lesions, scaling, scabs, nits, or parasites. Specifically, inspect behind the ears, noting scaling or skin breakdown associated with atopic dermatitis.

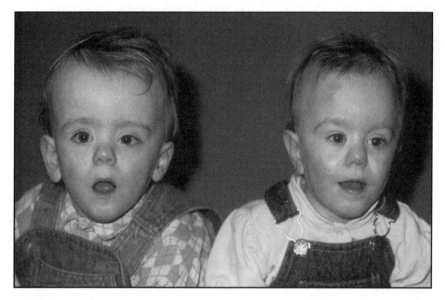

Figure 7-14 Hydrocephaly

Assess for abnormal facies, including the shape of the eyes as well as the placement of, symmetry of, and distance between the inner canthi.

Inspect the face for absence of eyelashes or eyebrows, eyebrows extending to midline (or synophrys), fusion of the eyebrows in the midline (a rare disorder associated with Cornelia de Lange syndrome), ptosis of the eyelid, shape of the nose (noting a depressed, wide, or prominent nasal bridge), hypoplastic nares, large nares, or beaklike nose. Assess the definition of the nasolabial fold, size of the philtrum, size of the mandible, fullness of the cheeks, protrusion of the forehead (also referred to as frontal bossing), shape of the head, and distribution of hair and hairline. Keep in mind, unusual facies may not be readily apparent until later in childhood.

Look for familial similarities between the child and the parents and siblings. If you have concerns about a child, inspect the parents' and siblings' facies, obtaining additional head circumferences when necessary.

Palpation

When palpating the child's head, use the pads of your fingers and position the child's head so it is slightly flexed and cradled in your hands. Palpate all areas of the cranium for tenderness or masses, assessing for contour and for the presence of lymph nodes. Palpate the child's hair, noting its color, distribution, and texture. While palpating, locate the TMJs with your fingertips.

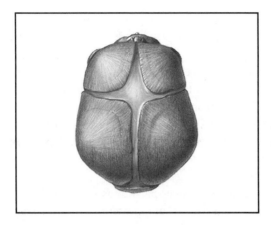

Figure 7-15   Anterior Fontanel
Source: © Adam.com

They are located anterior to the tragus of the ear. Place your fingertips into the joint space and ask the child to gently open and close his or her mouth. Assessment of crepitus, locking, or popping can indicate dysfunction of the TMJ.

Examination of the Neck of the Infant

During *inspection* of the infant's neck, it is helpful to support the infant's shoulders and tilt the head back slightly. Note symmetry, size, and shape of the neck, and the presence of edema, distended neck veins, pulsations, masses, and webbing (which may be associated with Down or Turner syndrome). Assess head control and head position as well as symmetry of accessory neck muscles.

During *palpation* of the infant's neck, it is important to check for mobility. You can assess muscle development and passive range of movement by cradling the infant's head in your hand and gently turning it from side to side. Also test flexion, extension, and rotation in this manner. Palpation of the infant's neck generally does not reveal palpable lymph nodes.

Examination of the Neck of the Child and Adolescent

Lymphadenopathy, although unusual during infancy, is common during childhood. The most common cause of a neck mass in a child is benign lymphadenopathy, and the majority of findings are non-neoplastic.

Lesions, or masses, are primarily of an inflammatory nature, such as viral or bacterial. The child's lymph nodes reach their maximum size around 10–12 years of age (Ball, 2010, p. 217.) During minor viral and bacterial illnesses, the child's lymph nodes, including the anterior and posterior cervical chain, are likely to be enlarged and/or tender. Once treated, you may still be able to palpate small, nontender nodes, referred to as shotty nodes, which may persist for 3–6 weeks following the inflammatory process. These benign nodes are a normal finding in toddlers and preschool-age children. They are related to environmental antigen exposure or residual effects of a prior illness such as pharyngitis. Enlargement of the occipital nodes can occur with tinea capitis secondary to infected scaling lesions on the scalp. Palpable occipital and posterior cervical nodes may also be noted in conjunction with acute mononucleosis.

When palpating, use the finger pads to assess the submental, submandibular, tonsillar, anterior cervical chain, posterior cervical chain, supraclavicular preauricular, posterior auricular, and occipital lymph nodes. Note the location, size, shape, tenderness, mobility, and associated skin inflammation of any enlarged nodes. Enlarged lymph nodes of greater concern are those that are hard or fixed to underlying tissue. Lymph nodes palpated in the *supraclavicular area* are always abnormal and raise the concern of malignancy.

In the assessment of mobility of the neck, the presence of *nuchal rigidity* (inability to touch the chin to the chest when the head is flexed forward), particularly in a child with a fever, is a reliable indicator of meningeal irritation. Other tests used to assess nuchal rigidity are the Brudzinski sign and the Kernig sign. See **Figure 7-16** and **Figure 7-17**. The Brudzinski sign is elicited when the child is lying supine with the head flexed forward. In this position, the child will automatically flex the hips and knees. The Kernig sign is evoked when the child is lying supine with the hips flexed. If meningeal irritation is present, the child will resist your attempt to extend the leg. (Meningitis is discussed in greater detail in Chapter 13.)

Further palpation of the neck includes assessment of the thyroid gland. Familiarity with the midline neck structures is important in examining the thyroid gland. Structures in the midline of the neck, from uppermost to lowermost, are as follows:

- The hyoid bone, which lies just below the mandible at the angle of the floor of the mouth
- The thyroid cartilage, which is shaped like a shield
- The cricoid cartilage, which is the uppermost ring of the trachea and is palpable just below the thyroid cartilage
- The tracheal rings
- The isthmus of the thyroid, which lies across the trachea below the cricoid cartilage

In the infant, the thyroid usually cannot be palpated. If you can palpate it, then it is enlarged and should be referred. In assessing the infant's thyroid,

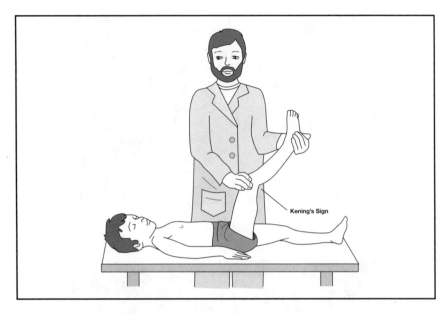

Figure 7-16   Kernig's Sign

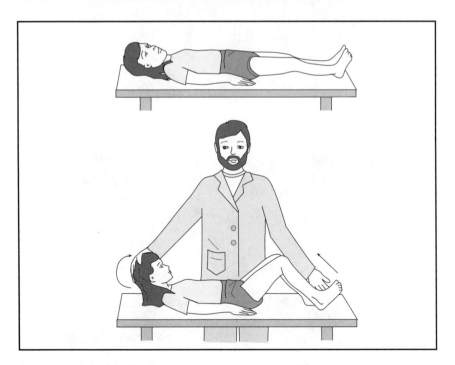

Figure 7-17   Brudzinski's Sign

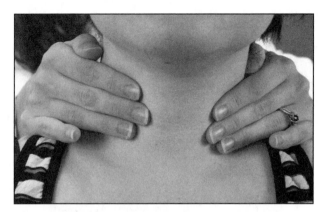

Figure 7-18 Posterior Approach for Palpation of the Thyroid Gland

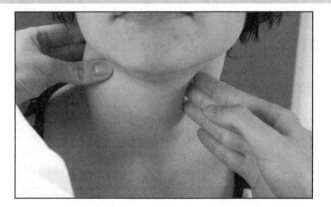

Figure 7-19 Anterior Approach for Palpation of the Thyroid Gland

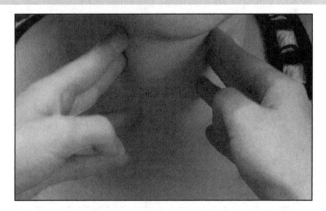

Figure 7-20 Palpation of the Thyroid Gland

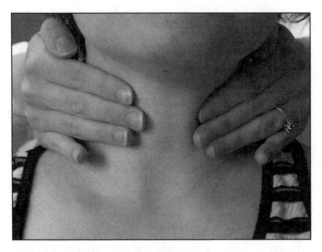

Figure 7-21 Posterior Approach to Thyroid Exam

place your hand under the scapula and raise the child's shoulders. Allow the child's head to fall back gently, and observe the thyroid gland for enlargement. Palpate with one finger on either side of the gland (Colyar, 2003, p. 64). In toddlers and preschool children, place your fingers on the front of the trachea by the cricoid and palpate for lumps.

For school-age children and adolescents, palpate with your finger pads. Ask the child to sit up straight and bend his or her head slightly forward and to the right, which will relax the neck muscles. The thyroid gland can then be examined by either standing facing the child or standing behind the child. If standing in front of the child, use your finger pads to displace the trachea slightly to the right, palpating the left lobe of the thyroid. To encourage swallowing, give the child a cup of water and ask him or her to swallow when you displace the trachea to either the right or the left side. If standing behind the child, repeat the same procedure, displacing the trachea to the left and palpating the right lobe of the thyroid.

During this procedure, you are assessing for size, tenderness, consistency, and presence of nodules. The gland's normal consistency is soft, and its contours can barely be seen or palpated. The thyroid gland in a school-age child is approximately the size of the thumb from the interphalangeal joint to the tip (Goldbloom, 2003, p. 337). An enlarged thyroid gland can be associated with thyroiditis. An enlarged and tender thyroid with nodules can be associated with nodular goiter, subacute thyroiditis, or thyroglossal duct cyst (Colyar, 2003, p. 64).

Common Disorders of the Neck

Common congenital neck lesions include thyroglossal duct cysts, branchial cleft cysts, cystic hygromas, and hemangiomas. Descriptions of these as well as other conditions follow.

THYROGLOSSAL DUCT CYSTS are generally located midline in the neck and inferior to the hyoid bone. They are usually noted after 2 years of age as an inflamed tender mass. When not inflamed, they may be palpated as firm, mobile, and nontender lumps that move upward with the tongue.

BRANCHIAL CLEFT CYSTS present anterior to the middle of the sterno-cleidomastoid muscle as small dimples or openings. They are associated with a sinus tract infection. See **Figure 7-22**.

HYGROMAS are lymphatic malformations that present as painless transilluminated soft masses in the supraclavicular fossa. The majority are present at birth.

TORTICOLLIS, also called wry neck, may present in the neonate following trauma to the sternocleidomastoid muscle due to birth injury or intrauterine malposition. See **Figure 7-23**.

PREAURICULAR CYSTS AND SINUSES are generally benign congenital malformations of the preauricular soft tissue. They are pin-sized openings located anterior to the helix of the ear and are lined with squamous epithe-

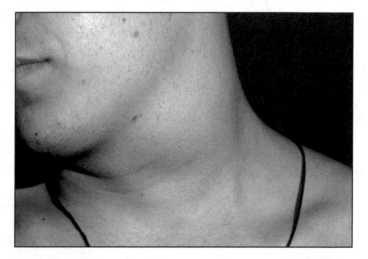

Figure 7-22 Branchial Cyst

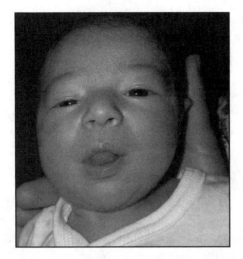

Figure 7-23 Torticollis

lium that may become infected. They may be bilateral or unilateral and are referred for further investigation and their relation to hearing deficits.

LYMPHADENOPATHY is lymph node enlargement. It is secondary to localized infection or antigenic stimulation proximal to the involved node. In children, cervical lymphadenopathy is a common finding associated with frequent viral infections of the upper respiratory tract. *Lymphadenitis* is inflammation or infection of the lymph node that is erythematous, warm, tender to palpation, and often fluctuant. It is usually associated with a proximal bacterial infection.

EXCESS SKIN may be noted in the neck and may be a feature of genetic syndromes. Examples include Turner syndrome, in which the neck appears webbed because of redundant skin along the posterolateral line, and Down syndrome, in which there may be excess skin at the base of the neck posteriorly (McKee-Garrett, 2009).

THYROID DISORDERS of the thyroid gland present with either inadequate or excessive production of thyroid hormone.

CONGENITAL HYPOTHYROIDISM is decreased production of thyroid hormone that can be either congenital or acquired. Congenital hypothyroidism is due to inadequate production of thyroid hormone, most often due to partial failure of the thyroid gland to adequately develop. This disorder is screened for through the state-established newborn screening program.

Lack of attention to this disorder can result in jaundice, hypotonia, and mental retardation, to name a few of the symptoms.

ACQUIRED HYPOTHYROIDISM, also called *Hashimoto thyroiditis*, is an autoimmune disease. It is the most common cause of acquired hypothyroidism in children. Due to pituitary or hypothalamic dysfunction, there is a deficiency of thyroid-stimulating hormone (TSH). Symptomatology in children includes weight gain, decreased height velocity, delayed bone and dental age, muscle weakness, and delayed puberty.

 Red Flags

- Concerns in the infant are premature closure of the cranial sutures or a large anterior fontanelle (greater than 3 cm). Significant head lag after 6 months requires further evaluation. An irregular or misshapen head requires referral.

- Concerns about the infant's face regarding unusual or irregular facies, without confirmation of familial tendencies, require further evaluation.

- Concerns about the neck of the infant include limited or painful movement and resistance to flexion associated with meningeal irritation. Lateral resistance to motion can be associated with torticollis. Webbing and extra or excess skin folds are a concern for chromosomal abnormalities.

- In the toddler and older child, an enlarged thyroid gland needs further investigation.

Write-Up of the Head and Neck

EXAMPLE FOR INFANTS:
- ➤ *HEAD*: normocephalic, anterior fontanelle palpable, scalp without lesions or tenderness, well-spaced facial features
- ➤ *NECK*: supple with full range of motion, symmetric, no masses, without palpable lymph nodes, trachea midline

EXAMPLE FOR SCHOOL-AGE CHILDREN AND ADOLESCENTS:
- ➤ *HEAD*: normocephalic, scalp without lesions or tenderness, well-spaced facial features
- ➤ *NECK*: trachea midline and freely moveable, thyroid lateral and borders palpable, no enlargement or nodules noted, no palpable lymph nodes, full range of motion, good strength

Case Study: Head and Neck

A 10-year-old boy presents to your office with a runny nose and congestion for the past 10 days. He complains of a mild sore throat and cough that gets worse at bedtime. He also complains of a frontal headache.

Physical Examination

- Low grade fever
- Skin: clear without rash
- Nose: inflamed nasal mucosa
- Pharynx: postnasal mucopurulent discharge and malodorous breath
- Neck: supple without lymphadenopathy
- Lungs: clear to auscultation

Questions

1. What sinuses are commonly implicated in sinusitis in a child of this age?
2. What are the signs and symptoms of acute sinusitis?
3. What is the plan of care for this patient?

Answers

1. The sinuses commonly implicated are the maxillary and ethmoid sinuses.
2. Signs and symptoms include:
   - More severe or prolonged URI
   - Coughing during the day, but often worse at night
   - Low-grade fever
   - Clear or mucopurulent rhinorrhea and post nasal drip
   - Facial pain
   - Sore throat
   - Headache
   - Halitosis
3. Plan of care includes:
   - Antibiotic therapy for 10 days
   - Decongestants/antihistamines
   - Topical steroid nasal spray
   - Comfort measures such as analgesics, increased humidity, and increased oral fluids

References

Ball, J., Bindler, R., Cowen, K. (2010). *Child health nursing* (2nd ed.). Pearson.

Bickley, L. (2003). *Bates' guide to physical examination and history taking* (8th ed.). New York: Lippincott Williams & Wilkins.

Boon, J. (2009). Etiology and evaluation of macrocephaly of infants and children. *UpToDate.*

Colyar, M. (2003). *Well-child assessment for primary care providers*. Philadelphia: EA Davis Company.

Goldbloom, R. (2003). *Pediatric clinical skills*. New York: Churchill Livingston.

McKee-Garrett, T. M. (2009). Assessment of the newborn infant. *Uptodate.com.* Retrieved June 23, 2010, from http://www.uptodate.com/patients/content/topic.do?topicKey=~f.3PJ4DC/TiCXif

Swanson, D. (2009). Diagnostic approach to and initial treatment of cervical lymphadenitis in children. *Uptodate.com.* Retrieved June 23, 2010, from http://www.uptodate.com/patients/content/topic.do?topicKey=~tSbLIRvYvRVw5

Thureen, P., Deacon, J., O'Neill, P., & Hernandez, J. (2004). *Assessment and care of the well newborn* (2nd ed.). Philadelphia: Saunders.

Resources

Berkowitz, C. (2008). *Pediatrics: A primary care approach* (3rd ed.). Philadelphia: Saunders.

Burns, C., Dunn, A., Brady, M., Starr, N., & Blosser, C. (2000). *Pediatric primary care: A handbook for nurse practitioners* (3rd ed.). St. Louis, MO: Saunders.

Friedman, S., Nelson, N., Weitzman, M., & Seidel, H. (2001). *Hoekelman's Primary Pediatric Care* (4th ed.). St. Louis, MO: Mosby.

Jarvis, C. (2004). *Physical examination and health assessment* (5th ed.). St. Louis, MO: Elsevier.

Marieb, E. (1995). *Human anatomy and physiology* (3rd ed.). Redwood City, CA: Benjamin/Cummings Publishing Company.

Potts, N., & Mandleco, B. (2007). *Pediatric nursing* (2nd ed.). Victoria, Australia: Thomson Delmar Learning.

Seidel, H., Ball, J., Dains, J., Benedict, G. (2006). *Mosby's guide to physical examination* (6th ed.). Boston: Mosby.

Examination of the Ear, Nose, and Throat

Anatomy and Physiology

The Ear

The ear is a paired sensory organ comprised of the auditory system, which is focused on sound, and the vestibular system, which is focused on maintaining balance and equilibrium. The ear can be divided into three distinct parts both functionally and anatomically: the external ear, the middle ear, and the inner ear. The external ear is also called the auricle and is made up of six parts: the helix, antihelix, external auditory meatus, tragus, antitragus, and lobule. These parts are also anatomic landmarks that are useful when you are documenting findings.

The auricle, also called the pinna, is a shell-shaped projection that functions to collect and direct sound waves through the ear canal to the tympanic membrane. The external auditory canal is approximately 1.25 inches (2.5 cm) long and contains modified sweat glands that secret cerumen, or earwax. The earwax is a sticky substance that functions as a method to trap foreign bodies and repel insects. In many people, the cerumen dries and falls out by itself; in others, it builds up and becomes compacted, which can lead to hearing impairment. The color of cerumen ranges from a deep dark honey color to a light cream color and is reflective of its composition.

The middle ear is separated from the external ear by the tympanic membrane, which is a thin translucent membrane more commonly referred to as the eardrum. Sound waves cause the eardrum to vibrate, in turn transmitting sound waves to the tiny bones of the middle ear and putting them into vibration. The middle ear connects to the throat and nasopharynx via the eustachian tube. This tube runs downward, linking the middle ear cavity with the nasopharynx, which is continuous with the same mucosa as the middle ear. The eustachian tube equalizes air pressure on both sides of the eardrum. Swallowing or yawning can open the eustachian tube, which equalizes the pressure in the middle ear cavity with the external air pressure. In order for the eardrum to vibrate, there must be equal pressure on both sides. When there is unequal pressure, one has the sensation of ear popping, experienced particularly while flying in an airplane or driving up or down a steep hill. This popping occurs until equal pressure is obtained.

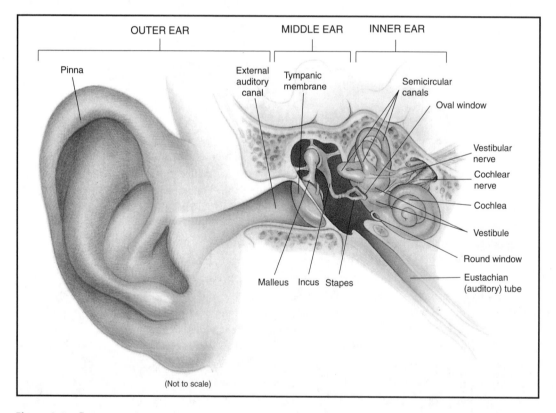

(Not to scale)

Figure 8-1   Ear

The tympanic cavity is composed of three tiny bones, the ossicles, which are the smallest bones in the body. These bones are named for their shape—the malleus, which is shaped like a hammer; the incus, which is similar to an anvil; and the stapes, which looks like a stirrup. The incus articulates with the malleus laterally and the stapes medially. Sound is conducted from the tympanic membrane to the inner ear by vibrations. The short process and handle of the malleus attach directly to the tympanic membrane. The head of the malleus articulates directly with the incus, which then articulates with the head of the stapes, also referred to as the footplate, which attaches to the oval window of the inner ear. The middle ear has three main functions: (1) It conducts sound vibrations from the external ear to the hearing receptors in the inner ear, (2) it protects the inner ear by reducing the amplitude of loud noise, and (3) the eustachian tube provides equalization of air pressure on each side of the tympanic membrane, protecting it from rupture. The tympanic membrane is pearly gray in color and composed of two parts, the pars flaccida, which is the superior small, slack section of the drum, and the pars tensa, the lower and more taut portion of the drum. The mallelus, the largest of the three bones, includes the handle, or

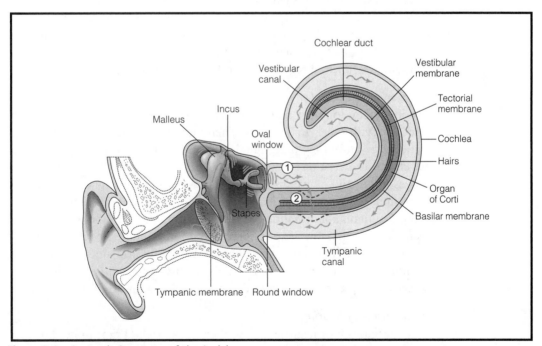

Figure 8-2   Anatomic Structures of the Auricle

umbo, which extends downward onto the tympanic membrane. It is often visible if the drum is translucent.

The inner ear, also referred to as the bony labyrinth, is a second series of interconnecting membranous sacs within the bony labyrinth which is filled with fluid called perilymph. Within this labyrinth is the vestibule that houses receptors that react to equilibrium and changes in head position. The semicircular canals project from the posterior aspect of the vestibule, and their function is to help maintain balance. Extending from the anterior portion of the vestibule is the cochlea, which contains the hair cells of the organ of Corti, where the receptor cells for hearing are located. Nerve impulses are generated in the inner ear and travel along the vestibulocochlear nerve (cranial nerve VIII), which leads to the brain, or cerebral cortex, where they are interpreted.

Interestingly, alterations in this area can affect control of the eyes, leading to nystagmus. When electrical impulses are transmitted to the vestibular portion of the eighth cranial nerve, synapses occur in the vestibular and oculomotor nuclei producing nystagmus, or rapid compensatory movements of the eyes. Nystagmus is an involuntary rhythmic movement of the eyeballs that may be pendular oscillations or jerky drifts of one or both eyes. These movements can be horizontal, vertical, rotary, or a combination. They can be caused by disease of the inner ear or the retina of the eye, or by disease or lesions in the central nervous system (Burns, Dunn, & Brady, 2000, p. 721). New onset of nystagmus without relation to testing oculomotor function requires referral to a neurologist.

Development of the Ear

Auditory development and the three divisions of the ear develop in conjunction with other vital organs. Therefore, deformities of the ear are significant because they may signal malformations of other organ systems or chromosomal alterations. External ear development begins at week 5 of gestation, and by week 6, middle ear development occurs. By week 9 of gestation, the ears are particularly vulnerable to developmental malformation. Common abnormalities include abnormal folds in the pinna, prominence of the ears, low-set positioning, abnormal rotation of the pinna, and even absence of the pinna. When these types of abnormalities are observed, it should alert the provider that other systemic abnormalities, such as renal agenesis, may also have occurred in conjunction with ear development.

Mechanisms of Hearing

The mechanism of hearing is described by Marieb (1995) in her book on anatomy and human physiology:

> Sounds set up vibrations in air that beat against the eardrum that pushes a pair of tiny bones that press fluid in the inner ear against membranes that set up shearing forces that pull on the tiny hair cells that stimulate nearby neurons that give rise to impulses that travel to the brain which interprets them—and you hear (p. 530).

In understanding the mechanism of hearing, the auditory system is divided into three levels: peripheral, brainstem, and cerebral cortex. The ear transmits sound and converts its vibrations into electrical impulses that are interpreted by the brain at the peripheral level. An example is the sound of a foghorn. The sound waves cause vibrations of the tympanic membrane, which are carried by the middle ear occicles (three small bones) to the oval window of the inner ear. These sound waves then travel through the cochlea, and the frequency of the sound bends the hair cells of the organ of Corti. They mediate the vibrations into electric impulses that are then transmitted by the cranial nerve VIII (vestibulocochlear) to the brainstem. From the brainstem, these messages are conducted to the cerebral cortex where they are interpreted (Jarvis, 2008).

There are three types of hearing loss: conductive, sensorineural, and mixed.

CONDUCTIVE HEARING LOSS is caused by mechanical dysfunction of the external or middle ear. It can occur from anything that interferes with the transmission of sound from the outer to the inner ear. Some of the causes for conductive hearing loss in children are middle ear infections (otitis media and otitis media with effusion), the most commonly encountered problem in children. Conductive hearing loss may also be caused by cerumen impaction; perforation of the tympanic membrane, which can be caused by infection; and trauma such as a head injury, a blow to the ear, or an object poked into the ear such as a pencil or stick.

SENSORINEURAL HEARING LOSS indicates pathology of the inner ear, cranial nerve VIII (vestibulocochlear), or parts of the cerebral cortex that process auditory information. In children, certain viral or bacterial infections such as mumps or meningitis can lead to the loss of hair cells in the choclea in the inner ear. Use of certain otoxic drugs that affect the hair cells in the chochlea such as aminoglycosides, gentamicin, tobramycin, and neomycin, particularly in the premature newborn, can cause permanent hearing loss.

MIXED HEARING LOSS is a combination of both conductive and sensorineural.

The Nose and Paranasal Sinuses

The nasal cavity is formed by the ethmoid and sphenoid bones of the skull, and the nose is the only externally visible part of the respiratory system. It serves several functions: It humidifies and moistens air entering the lungs, it filters and cleanses the inspired air, and it houses the olfactory, or smell, receptors. In addition, it is the primary organ that serves as a first-line immunologic defense. As inspired air comes in contact with the nose, the mucous membranes that line the nose contain immunoglobulin A (IgA) that acts as an immunologic defense against bacteria entering the body.

The nose is divided into an external and internal portion. The external nose consists of paired nasal bones and upper and lower cartilage. This part of the nose is composed of pliable hyaline cartilage that makes the external nose flexible. The upper third of the external nose is made up of bone. Under the surface of the external nose are the nares, or nostrils. Each naris broadens into the anterior part of the nose, or the vestibule, which is lined with numerous coarse nasal hairs, or vibrissae, that filter coarse material from the air. The remainder of the nasal cavity is lined with ciliated columnar epithelium that filter out dust and bacteria as well as move mucus from the nasal cavity and paranasal sinuses toward the nasopharynx where it is swallowed. An interesting point is that the nasal mucosa has a dark pink or reddish color, which is due to the rich blood supply necessary to warm inhaled air. Consequently, the lining of the nose often appears redder in color than the oral mucosa. The amount of mucus produced can more than double when the nose and/or sinuses are inflamed.

The nasal cavity is divided by the septum into a right and left side. Along the anterior part of the septum is a rich supply of blood vessels called the Kiesselbach plexus. This is the most common site for nosebleeds. Along the lateral nasal wall of each nasal cavity are the superior, middle, and inferior turbinates (see **Figure 8-3**). They increase the surface area so that the mucous membranes with a rich supply of blood vessels can warm, humidify, and filter the inhaled air. The opening of the sinuses is located under the middle turbinate, and tears from the nasolacrimal duct drain into the anterior aspect of the inferior turbinate, which explains why when you cry your nose also runs.

General innervation to the nose is controlled by the parasympathetic nervous system, which controls secretions. The olfactory receptors (cranial nerve I) are found on the superior portion, or roof, of the septum and cribriform region. They originate in the olfactory bulb, which is located under the frontal lobe, pass directly through the cribriform plate, and enter into the nasal cavity. These smell receptors then transmit information to the temporal lobe in the brain where it is interpreted.

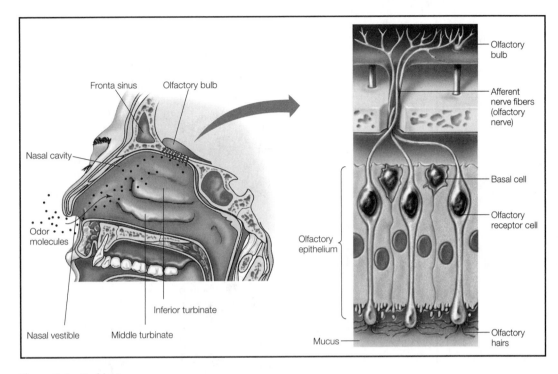

Fronta sinus

Olfactory bulb

Nasal cavity

Odor molecules

Nasal vestible

Middle turbinate

Inferior turbinate

Olfactory epithelium

Mucus

Olfactory bulb

Afferent nerve fibers (olfactory nerve)

Basal cell

Olfactory receptor cell

Olfactory hairs

Figure 8-3 Turbinates

The paranasal sinuses develop during gestation as four paired para-nasal invaginations of the nasal cavity. The first sinuses to develop are the maxillary sinuses, which are present at birth and become pneumatized by 4 years of age. The ethmoid sinuses are present at birth, although they do not become pneumatized until 6–8 years of age. The sphenoid sinuses become pneumatized by 5 years of age and attain adult size by 12 years. The frontal sinuses are the last to develop at age 12 years, reaching adult size by 20 years. Radiographically, the maxillary and ethmoid sinuses are evident in early infancy, the frontal sinuses by 6 years, and the sphenoid sinuses by 8 years. By the end of adolescence, all the sinuses have enlarged to reach adult size.

The development of the nose and paranasal sinuses is directly linked with the development of the facial part of the skull and dentition. These air-filled openings located in the frontal, sphenoid, ethmoid, and maxillary bones are hollow openings in the skull that help to lighten the weight of the skull bones. The sinuses are lined with the same ciliated mucous membrane

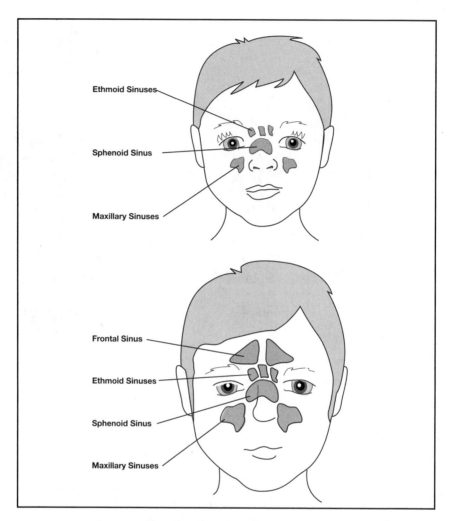

Ethmoid Sinuses

Sphenoid Sinus

Maxillary Sinuses

Frontal Sinus

Ethmoid Sinuses

Sphenoid Sinus

Maxillary Sinuses

Figure 8-4 Anterior View of the Cranial Sinuses—Child and Adult

as the nasal cavity. They communicate by draining into the nasal cavity beneath the middle and superior turbinates via small openings called ostia. This flow is unidirectional toward the ostia, which ultimately prevents the flow of bacteria from the nose back into the sinuses. Often, with the stasis of secretions, this opening becomes occluded, leading to inflammation and ultimately a sinus infection. A partial vacuum can also develop in the sinuses, which is characterized by a sinus headache localized over the inflamed areas (Marieb, 2000).

The Mouth and Pharynx

The floor of the nasal cavity is the hard palate, which is also the roof of the mouth (**Figure 8-5**). The unsupported posterior portion of the nasal cavity is the soft palate, or posterior portion of the palate. The nasopharynx lies above the mouth and serves as a passageway for air. During swallowing, the soft palate and the uvula move forward, which closes off the nasopharynx and thereby prevents food from entering the nasal cavity. This sealing action does not occur when children are laughing while eating and swallowing, and consequently liquid enters the nasal cavity and squirts out of the nose.

The oral cavity is bounded anteriorly by the lips, laterally by the cheeks, superiorly by the hard palate, and inferiorly by the mucosa covering the superior surface of the tongue. Included in this cavity are the upper and

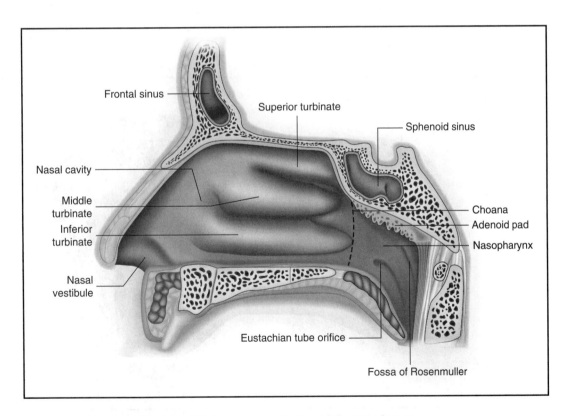

Figure 8-5   Anatomy of the Lateral Wall of the Nasal Cavity and the Nasopharynx

lower dentition, the tongue, salivary glands, mucosal glands, and the mucosal tissue, which are rugae covering the hard palate.

In examination of the mouth and throat, bear in mind that there are proportional differences between the infant and the child. The oral cavity in the newborn is small and is occupied by the tongue, which is broad and flat and appears to be large due to a small and slightly retracted lower jaw. The tongue is posteriorly connected to the hyoid bone and anteriorly connected to the floor of the mouth by the frenulum. In addition, the newborn has buccal fat pads, also called sucking pads. These pads are deposits of adipose tissue located in the space between the buccinators and masseter muscles that provide stability for the infant during sucking. At the back of the oral cavity, the soft palate and the epiglottis are in contact, which provides an additional safety mechanism to prevent aspiration. The infant also has additional protection of the airway by the larynx and hyoid cartilage, which are higher in the neck and closer to the base of the epiglottis. The infant's eustachian tube is also different than the older child's. It runs horizontally from the middle ear into the nasopharynx, and as the child grows, the eustachian tube changes and gradually assumes a more vertical angle; it

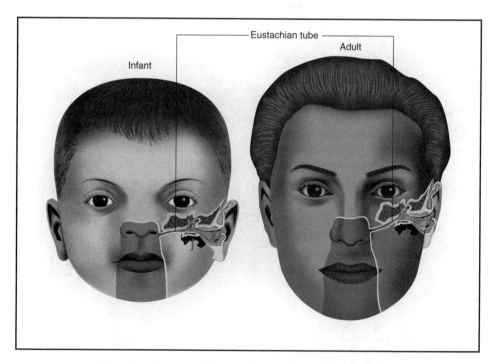

Figure 8-6 Comparison of Eustachian Tube in Child and Adult

lengthens and its pharyngeal orifice moves inferiorly. This change is important because when an older child or adolescent develops an upper respiratory infection with nasal congestion, fluid that backs up into the eustachian tube is better able to drain, thereby decreasing the frequency of inflammation and middle ear infections. In the young child, fluid from the nose backs up into the eustachian tube, eventually pushing against the tympanic membrane and leading to otitis media with effusion.

The palate, which forms the roof of the mouth, is composed of the hard palate anteriorly and the soft, muscular, flexible palate posteriorly. Projecting downward from the soft palate is the uvula. During swallowing, the soft palate and uvula are drawn upward, or superiorly, closing off the nasopharynx and, therefore, preventing food from entering the nasal cavity. In children with cleft palate, the embryonic facial processes do not properly fuse, which results in a fissure of the palate. This fissure may occur in the soft palate or may extend into the hard palate as well. Because the palate forms the roof of the oral cavity and the floor of the nose, a cleft in any

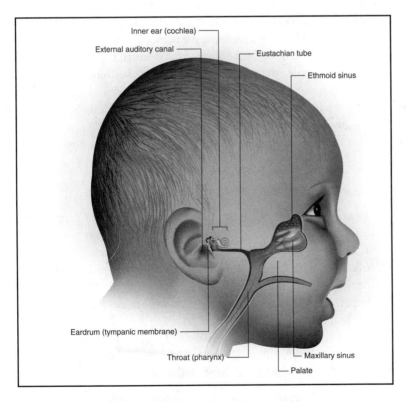

Figure 8-7 Eustachian Tube and Posterior Pharynx

part of the palate provides open communication between these two cavities. This ultimately results in complex problems regarding feeding, speech, and middle ear infections.

An extension of the soft palate is the uvula, which consists of an epithelial layer that surrounds a core of smooth muscle. The epithelium contains mast cells and macrophages that form a protective barrier against microbial invasion. Along the lateral sides of the soft palate are the palatine arches or pillars where the tonsils are located. There are three sets of tonsils. The palatine tonsils, composed of lymphoid tissue, are located on either side at the posterior end of the oral cavity. These are the largest of the tonsils and are the ones that most often become infected. The lingual tonsils lie at the base of the tongue, and the pharyngeal tonsils (or adenoids) are located in the posterior wall of the nasopharynx. See **Figure 8-8**.

The salivary glands, of which there are three, lie mainly outside of the oral cavity (**Figure 8-9**). They include the parotid, the largest gland, which lies anterior to the ear and opens into the oral cavity next to the second molar in the upper jaw. It is inflammation of the parotid glands with myxovirus that causes the childhood disease mumps. The virus is spread from person to person in saliva. Today, with mumps, measles, and rubella vaccine, mumps is rarely seen. The submandibular gland runs beneath the mucosa of the oral cavity and opens under the tongue at the base of the frenulum. The sublingual gland lies anterior to the submandibular gland and opens via many ducts under the tongue. The purpose of the salivary glands is to cleanse the mouth, dissolve and moisten food so it can be tasted, and start the digestive process through enzymes that initiate the chemical breakdown of starchy foods.

Developmental Milestones of Hearing

Newborns are screened in the hospital for hearing using brainstem auditory-evoked response (BAER), and parents are given a written report confirming the status of the infant's hearing test. If they did not pass, the pediatrician should follow up with further evaluation. Auditory-evoked response reflects activity of the cochlea, the auditory nerve (cranial nerve VIII), and auditory brainstem pathways. It is conducted through surface electrodes applied to the scalp (Ball, Bindler, & Cowen, 2010, p. 818).

Visual cues to observe for confirmation of a baby's hearing can be noted by observing developmental milestones at various ages.

During the first 3 months, the baby will:

- React to loud sounds with a startle, or Moro, reflex
- Be soothed and quieted by music or soft sounds

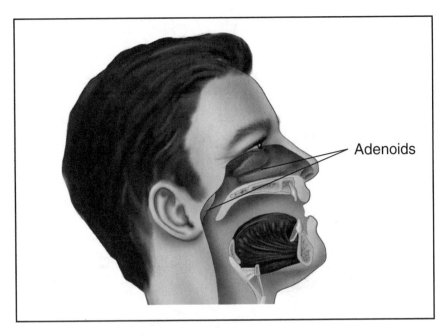

Figure 8-8 Adenoids

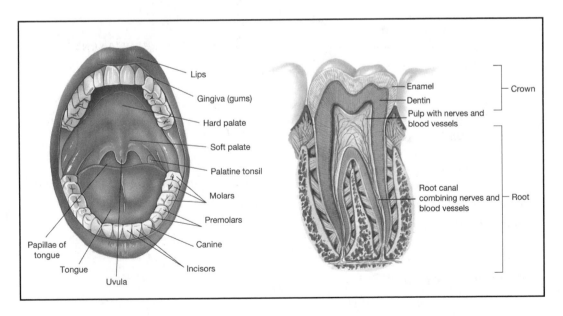

Figure 8-9 Mouth (Oral Cavity)

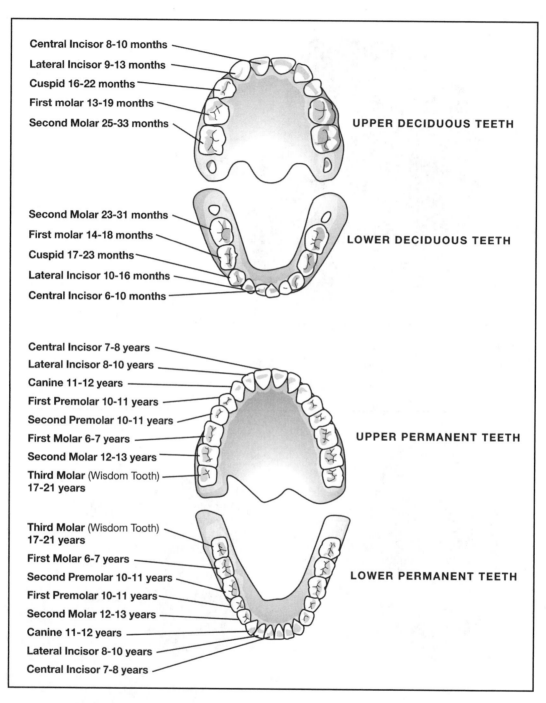

Central Incisor 8-10 months
Lateral Incisor 9-13 months
Cuspid 16-22 months
First molar 13-19 months
Second Molar 25-33 months

UPPER DECIDUOUS TEETH

Second Molar 23-31 months
First molar 14-18 months
Cuspid 17-23 months
Lateral Incisor 10-16 months
Central Incisor 6-10 months

LOWER DECIDUOUS TEETH

Central Incisor 7-8 years
Lateral Incisor 8-10 years
Canine 11-12 years
First Premolar 10-11 years
Second Premolar 10-11 years
First Molar 6-7 years
Second Molar 12-13 years
Third Molar (Wisdom Tooth) 17-21 years

UPPER PERMANENT TEETH

Third Molar (Wisdom Tooth) 17-21 years
First Molar 6-7 years
Second Premolar 10-11 years
First Premolar 10-11 years
Second Molar 12-13 years
Canine 11-12 years
Lateral Incisor 8-10 years
Central Incisor 7-8 years

LOWER PERMANENT TEETH

Figure 8-10 Upper and Lower Deciduous Teeth

- Turn his or her head toward you when you speak
- Be awakened by loud noise
- Recognize your voice and stop crying and/or smile upon hearing your voice
- Look or turn toward a new sound

By 3 to 6 months, the baby will:

- Respond to "no" and changes in your tone of voice
- Imitate his or her own voice by babbling
- Enjoy and reach out to rattles and other toys that make sounds
- Begin to repeat sounds (such as *ooh*, *aah*, and *ba-ba*)
- Be scared by a loud voice or noise and begin to cry

By 6 to 12 months, the child will:

- Responds to his or her own name
- React to the telephone ringing by becoming quiet and looking toward it
- Understand and respond to expressions, such as waving to the words "bye-bye"
- Make babbling sounds with increasing intonations when playing alone

By 12 to 18 months, the child will:

- Point to or look at familiar objects or people when asked to do so
- Imitate simple words and sounds, and possibly use a few single words meaningfully
- Enjoy games like peekaboo and pat-a-cake

By 18 months to 2 years, the child will:

- Follow simple directions, such as, "Give me the ball."
- Use single words such as "cookie" and "ball"
- Start to put two to three words together
- Know 10 to 20 words
- Point to some body parts when asked

A good way to remember the development of expressive language skills is with the phrase "2 years, 2 words." By two years of age children are generally putting two to three words together.

Assessment Considerations: Subjective Information

The following sections provide questions to consider when assessing a child's ear, nose, and mouth.

The Ear

Infants

- Consider the infant's response to sound: Does the infant turn his or her head? Blink? Cry? Startle?
- Does the infant babble, using different pitches or intonations?
- Is the infant breast- or bottle-fed? There is an increased occurrence of otitis media secondary to bottle-feeding and bottle-propping.
- Does the infant have a history of frequent ear infections?
- Is the infant in day care?
- Does the infant have a history of ear injury or hearing problems related to trauma?
- Was the baby premature? Certain drugs are ototoxic, such as strepto-mycin, kanamycin, and neomycin.
- Does the infant have a history of illness such as meningitis or encephalitis?
- As a baby, were BAERs done in the nursery? If so, what were the results?

School-Age Children

- How does the parent clean the child's ears? With Q-tips? Encourage parents not to use Q-tips.
- Has the child ever had his or her ears tested? If so, when and by whom?
- Are the ears abnormally shaped? Malformed ears may be associated with renal or chromosomal abnormalities or craniofacial malformations.
- Do the child's ears appear to be low or obliquely set?
- Does the child turn the television up loudly?
- When spoken to, does the child not respond or ask the person to repeat what was said?
- Is the child progressing poorly in school despite having no intellectual deficits?
- Is the child's language acquisition delayed, or is the child losing language milestones? Loss of language milestones requires prompt referral.
- Does the child have a history of environmental allergies?

Adolescents

- Does the adolescent have a history of frequent ear infections associated with swimming?
- Does the adolescent have a history of ear trauma secondary to sports?
- How does the adolescent clean his or her ears?
- Is there concern of hearing loss due to constant loud noise such as playing in a rock band?
- Does the adolescent have a history of environmental allergies?

The Nose

Infants

- Does the infant have a history of nasal discharge? If so, serous or purulent?
- Is the infant in day care?
- Does the infant have a history of frequent upper respiratory infections?
- Does the infant have a history of environmental allergies?

School-Age Children

- Does the child have a history of epistaxes (nosebleeds)?
- Does the child have a history of nasal discharge? If so, serous or purulent?
- Does the child have a history of frequent upper respiratory infections?
- Does the child have a history of sleep apnea or noisy breathing?

Adolescents

- Does the adolescent have a history of intranasal use of cocaine?
- Does the adolescent have a history of frequent use of nasal spray?
- Does the adolescent have a history of environmental allergies? Postnasal drip?

The Mouth

Infants

- Does the infant have a history of congenital defects such as cleft palate or craniofacial abnormality?
- Does the infant use a pacifier?
- Does the infant suck his or her thumb?
- Does the infant go to sleep with a bottle of milk?
- Does the infant have a history of dental decay (bottle mouth)?

School-Age Children

- What is the child's history of dental care? Consider factors such as last dental appointment, braces, exposure to fluoridated water or fluoride supplementation, and frequency of brushing?
- Does the child have a history of frequent sore throats?
- Does the child have a history of excessive sugar intake, including sugared cereals and candy?

Adolescents

- Does the adolescent smoke cigarettes or chew tobacco? If so, frequency and number of years?

- What is the adolescent's history of dental care? Consider factors such as last dental appointment, flossing, braces, crowns, and frequency of brushing?
- Does the adolescent wear a mouth guard during sports?
- Does the adolescent have a history of frequent sore throats?

Family History

During the subjective assessment, also consider the child's family history, including such considerations as the following:

- Is there a family history of hereditary renal disease?
- Is there a family history of abnormally shaped ears?
- Is there a family history of hearing problems or hearing loss?
- Is there a family history of mental retardation, renal disorders, or chromosomal abnormalities?
- Is there a family history of maternal gestational diabetes?

Review of Systems

EARS: Consider concerns about hearing, both expressive and receptive speech, pulling at ears, discharge from ears and odor, frequency of ear infections and treatment, cerumen presentation, and the method of ear cleaning.

NOSE: Consider concerns about sense of smell, discharge, epistaxis history, difficulty or noisy breathing, mouth breathing, frequent colds, sneezing, allergies, nasal salute, and nose picking.

SINUSES: Assess for dark circles under the eyes, thick nasal discharge lasting more than 10–14 days, frontal headaches, facial pain, halitosis, and a cough that increases at night.

MOUTH AND THROAT: Consider sores on the tongue or mucous membranes; drooling; problems chewing and swallowing; hoarseness; history relating to dental care/hygiene, dental visits, and teeth brushing; need for orthodontia; use of pacifier; thumb sucking; and frequency of sore throats.

NECK: Check for swelling and masses or node enlargement.

LUNGS: Consider difficulty breathing, flaring nostrils, cough, and allergies.

Assessment Considerations: Objective Information

Examination of the External Ear

Examination of the child's ear is similar for all age groups.

Inspection

(Inspection of the ears of the newborn is covered in Chapter 4.)

Inspect the external ears by assessing their shape and symmetry. Assess the placement of the ears, observing from the front. You can draw an imaginary line from the outer canthus of the eye to the top of the ear. The top of the ear, or the top of the pinna, should be even with the outer canthus of the eye. Low-set ears are associated with mental retardation, renal agenesis, and chromosomal disorders. At the same time, note the size of the pinna, inspecting for any pits, tags, or fistulae around the ears, which may indicate hearing deficits and should be further investigated. Inspect the shape, noting if the external ear is oval. Small, rounded external ears may be a normal deviation but are also associated with Down syndrome (Roizen, 2010).

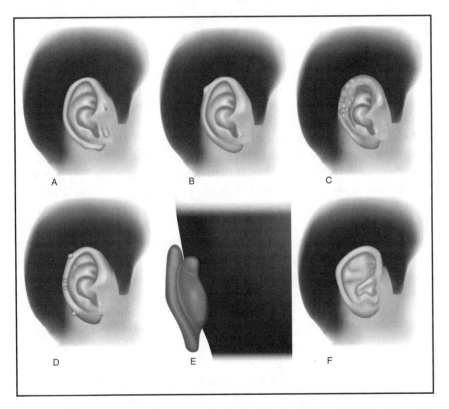

Figure 8-11   Ear Malformations—A: Preauricular Skin Tag, B: Darwin's Turbercle, C: Cauliflower Ear, D: Tophi, E. Malformation of the Auricle, F: Sebaceous Cyst

Based on inherited familial characteristics, there are numerous variations observed in the size, shape, and attachment of the ears. Malformations of the external ear or deviations from normal may represent variations or more obvious abnormalities that may be signs of teratogenicity. Position of the ear is characteristic of many syndromes and chromosomal abnormalities that may also signify aberrations of internal organs, particularly the kidneys.

One of the more common malformations is the posteriorly rotated ear, which gives the false impression of being low set. Children with trisomy 17 and trisomy 18 may present with malformation of the pinna and/or abnormal ear attachment.

A number of normal variations, such as overly prominent or protruding ears, are due to defects in the amount and position of the antihelix. If this alteration is bilateral, it is considered an inherited familial characteristic. If unilateral, this variation may be associated with other congenital ear abnormalities and requires further investigation. Darwin's tubercle is a normal variant that is characterized by a small thickening or nodule along the posterior segment of the helix. It was first described by Charles Darwin in 1871 and is considered to represent the top of formerly erect and pointed mammalian ears (see **Figure 8-12**). Incomplete scapha helix development is commonly observed in premature infants. It is considered a normal variant in the full-term infant. The scaphae develop and gradually take on normal presentation as the infant matures.

Preauricular skin tags are another alteration that may be an inherited family trait with no associated abnormalities. Other times skin tags can be associated with renal anomalies. If the child has dysmorphic features and/or other major anomalies, he or she should be referred for a genetic workup. Overall, preauricular skin tags are a common minor congenital abnormality. They may be single or multiple, pedunculated or sessile (meaning without a stalk and attached directly at the base). They may be associated with hearing loss in approximately 5% of cases, and, therefore, a routine hearing evaluation is recommended. In addition, because of the risk of an associated renal anomaly, an abdominal scan is also recommended (Ipp, n.d.).

Preauricular cysts, pits, fissures, and sinuses are benign congenital malformations of the preauricular soft tissues. Preauricular pits or fissures are located near the front of the ear and mark the entrance to a sinus tract that may travel under the skin near the ear cartilage. These tracts are lined with squamous epithelium and may isolate bacteria that eventually lead to infection. Preauricular tags are epithelial mounds or pedunculated skin that arise near the front of the ear around the tragus. They have no bony, cartilaginous, or cystic components and do not communicate to the ear canal or middle ear.

(a)   (b)

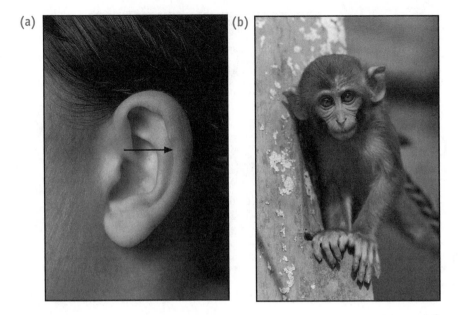

Figure 8-12   Darwin's Tubercle: (a) Human Ear; (b) Monkey

Simple preauricular cysts should not be confused with first branchial cleft cysts. Branchial cleft anomalies are closely associated with the external auditory canal, the tympanic membrane, the angle of the mandible, and/or the facial nerve. Children identified with preauricular pits or cysts should be examined for other congenital anomalies (eMedicine, n.d.).

Palpation
Palpate the external ear for tenderness, including the mastoid process. Pull gently on the pinna and tragus, noting if there is any pain. In children with external otitis (or swimmer's ear), there will be severe pain due to inflammation in the ear canal. Remember, the tissue making up the pinna and external ear is continuous with the external ear canal.

Pain on palpation of the mastoid process may be associated with a middle ear infection or more commonly is associated with mastoiditis. Mastoiditis is uncommon today due to vigilant use of antibiotics associated with otitis media, but it can be potentially life threatening. It is inflammation of the mucoperiosteal lining of the mastoid air cells with subsequent swelling and obstruction of drainage from the mastoid.

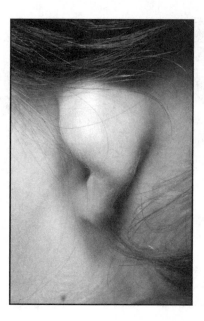

Figure 8-13   Microtia

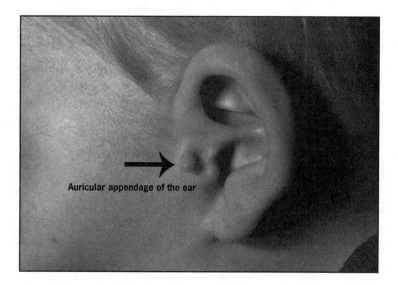

Auricular appendage of the ear

Figure 8-14   Preauricular Appendages

Examination of the Middle Ear

Otoscopic Assessment
Otoscopic assessment varies by age group.

Infants

Otoscopic assessment of the middle ear of the infant can be performed on the examination table with the child in a supine position. Gently insert the speculum into the ear canal. Assessment of the middle ear in the neonate is generally obscured by vernix caseosa, particularly during the first few days of life. In the infant, the tympanic membrane will be visible, although the light reflex is diffuse due to the thicker, grayer, and more vascular tympanic membrane. The drum of the infant is also more horizontal, making it more difficult to observe and easy to confuse with the canal wall. By 1 month of age, the drum is in a vertical or oblique position, making inspection easier; by 4 months of age, the drum becomes more cone shaped.

Toddlers

In toddlers and early school-age children, save the otoscopic examination for last. The ear canal is sensitive and therefore may be painful for the child. In addition, the young child is often fearful and not able to remain still for this intrusive examination.

Because ear infections are very common during early childhood, it is important to develop skill in examining the ears and in using the insufflator to correctly diagnose middle ear problems.

Adequate restraint is usually necessary to examine the external canal and the tympanic membrane. There are several positions that you can try in examining the child's ears. If the child is on the parent's lap, place the child's legs between the parent's legs, and ask the parent to gently restrain the child by placing one arm around the child's body, holding the arms in place, and using the other arm to help steady the child's head against the parent's chest. If this approach does not work and the child is difficult to hold, another option is to place the child on the examination table in a supine position. Extend the arms overhead alongside the ears, and have the parent secure them. You can then hold the child's head to one side while you hold the otoscope with the other hand. For school-age children who are somewhat apprehensive, they can sit upright on the table and you can play a game about peeking into their ear and looking for Mickey Mouse or any character that works. Often, letting them hold the otoscope and shine the light helps to alleviate some of their fear.

Once you have the child in position, hold the otoscope and insufflator in one hand. With the handle of the otoscope facing down toward the child's

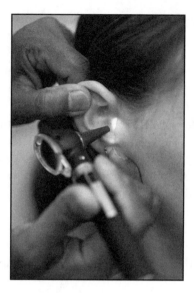

Figure 8-15 Otoscopy Examination

feet, pull up on the pinna and gently place the speculum into the ear canal. Because of the curvature of the canal in the infant, you need to grasp the lower portion of the pinna and retract the ear downward and backward to straighten the canal. By the time the child is 3 to 4 years of age, the canal has changed somewhat and, therefore, the pinna should be pulled up and back. Doing so helps to straighten the ear canal and improve visualization of the drum.

School-Age Children

Methods for assessing the middle ear of a school-age child are the same as those used for an adult. Keep in mind, if the child is there for assessment of otitis media, remember to inspect the normal ear first, thus giving you a frame of reference before viewing the ear with the inflammation. If the child has been crying, the tympanic membrane may appear red to pink on visualization.

To begin, ask the child to sit on the table. Tilt the child's head slightly away from the ear being examined. Hold the otoscope in your dominant hand and place the largest speculum on the otoscope that will fit comfortably in the child's ear canal. You can hold the otoscope with the handle pointing upward and the back of your hand resting against the child's head, which gives you a little leverage. You can also hold the otoscope with the handle pointing down. Either way is acceptable depending upon which position is more comfortable for you and provides you with the best visualization. Slowly insert the speculum into the external canal, assessing for inflammation, cerumen, exudates, lesions, and foreign bodies. In young children, it is not unusual to observe a small toy lodged in the ear canal.

It is important to note, do not flush the foreign object out of the ear until you have properly identified it. Small beans, or peas may swell in size when water is added to the ear, further obstructing the canal. Also when inspecting the ear canal, you may note a small colored tube (e.g., blue, yellow, green) that resembles a push tack. It is a myringotomy tube, which is placed in the tympanic membrane to provide for better drainage in children with chronic otitis media with effusion.

Continue to insert the speculum into the external canal until the tympanic membrane is visualized. Remember to gently pull the ear up and back in children 3–4 years of age and older in order to straighten the canal. In some patients, the ear drum is directly at the end of your speculum; in others, you must pull a little more to straighten the canal to see the drum. When the drum is visualized, identify the color, the light reflex, and other landmarks such as the umbo, the short process, and the long handle of the malleus. Inspect for perforations, lesions, bulging, or retraction of the drum, noting if there are blood vessels, bubbles, or a fluid line on the drum. A fluid line means that the lower part of the drum will look darker in color than the upper portion due to the collection of fluid behind the tympanic membrane. The line is the point of differentiation between the lower and upper portions of the drum.

Repeat the same process on the other ear. The canal should appear pink and may have tiny hairs. You may also observe cerumen. In some children, the cerumen will be thick and dark and occlude visualization of the drum. In this case, ear irrigation is necessary for further visualization. Doing so is particularly important if the child is febrile and the source of the fever needs to be determined. The normal tympanic membrane is pearly gray or very light pink in color; it is often translucent, allowing you to visualize the bony landmarks. Again, if the child has been crying, the drum may appear red in color. When inspecting for the light reflex, it generally appears between 4 and 6 o'clock on the drum on the right ear, and between 6 and 8 o'clock on the drum on the left ear. When the tympanic membrane appears dark gray in color without a light reflex, think otitis media with effusion. If the tympanic membrane is pink or red in color, you are visualizing inflammation of the middle ear. You may observe a light reflex on the drum even though there is inflammation. This finding means there is infection of the drum, but no fluid behind the tympanic membrane.

Adolescents

Methods for assessing the adolescent's middle ear are the same as those used for an adult. With the adolescent in an upright position, slowly insert the speculum into the ear canal, approximately 1.0 to 1.5 cm. As you are inserting the speculum, inspect the canal for discharge, cerumen, erythema, foreign bodies, and scaling. The ear canal should have a minimal amount of cerumen, the color of the tissue should be uniformly pink, and you may observe small hairs on the outer end of the canal.

With the speculum firmly in place, inspect the tympanic membrane, noting the color, contour, and perforations. Inspect for the bony landmarks and the light reflex. The color should be pearly gray and translucent, and the membrane is conical in shape. No perforations should be present. In an adolescent with a history of chronic ear infections as a young child, you may note silver scarring or dense white plaques on the drum. These findings indicate previous perforations. In addition, a bulging tympanic membrane with a distorted light reflex may be observed, indicating effusion, with pus or fluid behind the drum. A retracted tympanic membrane with decreased mobility is associated with obstruction of the eustachian tube, which causes a vacuum in the middle ear. On further inspection of the drum, you may note a color other than pearly gray (such as amber), fluid, or air bubbles that are caused by serous fluid in the middle ear.

Pneumatic Otoscopy

One of the major differences in the examination of the child's ear versus the adult's ear is use of pneumatic otoscopy. Pneumatic otoscopy refers to the use of an insufflator, a rubber bulb attached to the otoscope, to instill air into the middle ear. This method allows you to assess the mobility of the tympanic membrane for a more accurate diagnosis. Tympanic membrane mobility helps to determine the amount of middle ear effusion, the degree of negative or positive pressure, and other changes on the tympanic membrane.

To use pneumatic otoscopy correctly, the examiner must obtain a tight fit between the speculum and the ear canal. To obtain a proper fit, you must select the correct speculum size. If you choose a speculum that is too small, you will not obtain a tight seal in the canal and will produce a false-positive or lack of movement of the tympanic membrane. (If the speculum is too small and a seal is not obtained, air will leak out around it.)

Once the speculum is placed in the ear canal and air is introduced, you will see an inward movement of the drum indicating positive pressure and absence of effusion. When you release the pressure on the bulb, air is removed from the cavity and the tympanic membrane will move outward toward you due to the negative pressure that is created. You can repeat this process several times, noting the to-and-fro movement of the tympanic membrane. If there is no movement of the drum as you introduce negative and positive pressure, there is most likely fluid behind the tympanic membrane (otitis media with effusion), which will decrease mobility of the drum. Remember, after treatment of acute otitis media with effusion, fluid may remain behind the tympanic membrane for several weeks. In this case, when you examine the child, you will note decreased mobility of the drum. This finding does not require further antibiotic treatment but does require follow-up to ensure adequate hearing.

The concern with a history of chronic otitis media with effusion is decreased hearing and eventually speech delay. For a child with chronic ear infections, referral to otolaryngology is necessary to evaluate for further treatment with a myringotomy (a surgical incision of the tympanic membrane). *Tympanostomy tubes are* small plastic tubes that are surgically inserted into the middle ear to prevent the accumulation of fluid and to maintain ventilation of the middle ear. These ventilating tubes remain in place for 6 months to several years. Eventually, they will move out of the eardrum (extrude) and remain in the ear canal or fall out on their own. The insertion of tympanostomy tubes is one of the most common surgical procedures performed on children (Vaile, Williamson, Waddell, & Taylor, 2006). (For more information on tympanostomy tubes, refer to a text on otolaryngology.)

Tests for Inspecting the Middle Ear

Tympanometry is a test used to quantify information about the presence of fluid in the middle ear, mobility of the middle ear system, and ear canal volume. It is particularly helpful in determining the persistence of otitis media with effusion when a question remains following pneumatic otoscopy. The test is performed by placing a probe in the ear canal, forming a pressurized seal. This device changes the air pressure in the canal, which causes the tympanic membrane to move back and forth. This movement is then recorded on a graph and, based on configuration, may indicate effusion.

An *audiogram* or *pure-tone audiometry* measures the ability to hear pure tones of various frequencies as a function of intensity measured in decibels. This test measures the quietest sounds a child can hear. It does not measure how well a child can understand connected speech. The threshold for each tone is determined by finding the intensity level at which the child can detect the tone 50% of the time. The test is conducted in a sound-treated room, using pure tones directed through headphones or a sound field via speakers. It gives a basic understanding of what a child can or cannot hear (Sanford, 2010).

The *Rinne test* and the *Weber test* are used to assess bone and air conduction. To perform the Rinne, place a vibrating tuning fork on the child's mastoid process behind the ear and ask the child to tell you when he or she no longer hears the vibrations. Then move the tuning fork next to the ear and ask the child again to tell you when he or she no longer hears the vibrations. Normally, air conduction is twice as long as bone conduction. Repeat this test on the other ear. A child who hears sound longer by bone conduction than air conduction may be experiencing a conductive hearing loss; a child who hears the vibrations longer by air conduction than bone conduction may be experiencing sensorineural hearing loss in that ear.

The Weber is performed by placing the vibrating tuning fork midline on top of the child's head and asking the child to tell you where the sound is heard best. It may be in both ears equally or in one ear. The sound should be heard equally in both ears. If it is heard better in one ear, a conductive hearing loss lateralizes to the deaf ear. Both the Rinne and the Weber tests are gross assessments of hearing; if there is any concern regarding hearing loss, more definitive testing, such as an audiogram, should be performed.

Inspection and Palpation of the Nose

Inspection and palpation of the nose vary by age group.

Infants

General inspection of all facial features is important to assure that the child has normal facies. Abnormalities of the face may be an indication of genetic and/or chromosomal abnormalities. On generalized inspection, the nose should be symmetrical and centrally placed. Children of African or Asian descent may have a flattened bridge, which is a normal variation.

In infancy, assessment for patency is the most important component of the nasal exam. Because most infants are obligate nose breathers, you can gently occlude each nostril alternately while holding the infant's mouth closed, or you can observe for quiet and comfortable respirations. The concern is to be sure there is not choanal atresia, which is a membranous or bony blockage of the nasal passage. If there is any question, an appropriate-sized catheter can be passed through the nares to ensure there is no blockage. There are several indications of respiratory distress, although when referring to the nose and the upper airways, the primary indication is nasal flaring. There may also be increased respiratory rate, color change, and possible grunting if there is upper airway blockage.

Next, inspect the nose to be sure the septum is midline by gently shining the light from the otoscope into the nose. If necessary, use a large speculum and gently insert it into the vestibule of the nose.

School-Age Children

In toddlers or early school-age children who are apprehensive, have them sit on the parent's lap. Older children can sit on the examination table. Use a large speculum on the end of your otoscope, and tilt the child's head backward and push the tip of the nose upward. Gently place the speculum in the vestibule of the nose, inspecting the mucous membrane, which should be moist and pink in color. Assess for nasal septal deviation and the presence of polyps. Also inspect the turbinates, noting their color. Diffuse redness and swelling is associated with inflammation such as new onset of an upper respiratory infection. Pale, boggy, or bluish turbinates are associated with allergies. The presence of polyps may also be associated with allergies and/or asthma. Unilateral discharge that is malodorous and purulent may be indicative of a foreign object.

Adolescents

Inspection of an adolescent's nose is the same as that of an adult. With the adolescent in an upright position, start by inspecting for deviation in shape and size. In an adolescent, there may be swelling across the bridge of the nose secondary to chronic trauma to the nose. Inspect the nares, noting any discharge, flaring, or extreme narrowing. They should be oval in shape and symmetrically placed. Flaring of the nostrils is associated with respiratory distress. If there is discharge present, the character and color should be noted. The character of the discharge is associated with various disorders: Clear rhinorrhea is associated with allergies, whereas mucoid discharge is more typical of upper respiratory infections.

Inspect the nose for a transverse crease between the junction of the cartilage and the bony structure of the nose. This finding is often associated with chronic nasal allergies and itching. On palpation of the nose, assess the ridge and soft tissue, noting any tenderness, masses, or displacement of the bone. Assess for patency by placing a finger on the side of the nose and occluding one naris at a time while asking the adolescent to breathe in and out with the mouth closed. Repeat this procedure on the other side. Normal nasal breathing should be quiet and easy.

Inspect the inside of the nose using a nasal speculum with good light. Tilt the child's head back slightly, then gently insert the first quarter of the speculum into the vestibule of each naris, inspecting the mucosa for color, discharge, masses, and lesions. Also inspect the turbinates for color and swelling; you will only be able to observe the inferior and middle turbinates. Inspect the nasal septum for alignment, perforation, and bleeding. The nasal mucosa should be moist and dark pink in color. The mucosa in the nose is a darker pink than the mucosa in the mouth. Increased redness may be associated with an upper respiratory infection.

The turbinates should be the same color as the surrounding tissue and firm in consistency. If turbinates are pale with a grayish color and a boggy, swollen appearance, they are usually associated with chronic rhinitis and/or allergies. You may observe polyps, which are elongated masses projecting into the nasal cavity. The nasal septum should be midline and straight without signs of perforation, bleeding, or lesions. Adolescents who frequently use cocaine intranasally may present with septal perforations that occur due to vasoconstriction, which leads to a decreased supply of nutrients to the underlying cartilage. These perforations may also occur due to the chemical irritants that damage the nasal mucosa (Romo, Yalamanchili, Presti, & Pearson, 2010).

The procedure for testing the sense of smell is described in Chapter 13 on the central nervous system.

Palpation of the Sinuses

Infants
Sinuses are not assessed in the infant because the sinuses of the skull are not pneumatized at this age.

School-Age Children
Sinusitis can cause various symptoms for children of different ages. Sinusitis in the young child generally presents the same as a cold, including runny nose and low-grade fever. If it persists for greater than 10–14 days, it could indicate sinusitis or another infection such as otitis media or a lower respiratory tract infection such as pneumonia. An important point is that many parents associate a headache that is a symptom of a cold with a sinus infection, but the sinuses in the forehead or the frontal sinuses are not fully pneumatized until early adolescence. Sinusitis in the school-age child usually presents the same as an upper respiratory infection, or the common cold, with the same symptoms of fever, cough, and greenish-yellow nasal discharge. However, the symptoms persist for approximately 10–14 days, which signals the presence of a sinus infection, particularly in the older child or adolescent.

Palpation of the sinuses in the school-age child and the adolescent is similar to the assessment in the adult. Start by inspecting the frontal and maxillary sinus areas for dark shadows or circles under the eyes, which could indicate fluid in the sinuses. When palpating the frontal sinuses, use your thumbs and press up under the cheekbones or maxillary sinuses on each side of the face. Next, using your thumbs, palpate the frontal sinuses below the eyebrows. When palpating, apply firm pressure. Signs of sinusitis or infection will be associated with tenderness or pain on palpation.

Adolescents

In an adolescent, sinusitis presents the same as in the adult, with facial pain, low-grade fever, dental pain, pain behind the eyes, nasal congestion, and daytime cough, all of which persist for greater than 10–14 days.

Remember, when assessing the sinuses, sinusitis in older children frequently involves the maxillary and ethmoid sinuses, which are present at birth but are not functional until 6 months of age. The frontal sinus does not become clinically significant until adolescence when it becomes pneumatized. In children 5 years of age and older, you may elicit tenderness on gentle percussion or palpation over the maxillary or frontal sinuses or between the eyes over the ethmoid sinuses. Although the ethmoid sinuses are difficult to palpate due to their location, they are most commonly affected.

Transillumination is generally unrewarding in evaluating sinusitis in children. It may be performed in the adolescent as it is done in the adult. The AAP recommends that the diagnosis of sinusitis in children be based on clinical symptoms. A runny nose, postnasal drip, and a cough that worsens at night and lasts for approximately 10–14 days suggest the diagnosis of sinusitis. The AAP notes that a shorter duration of symptoms might still indicate a sinus infection if the symptoms are severe, including 3–4 days of fever (greater than 102°F) and a child who appears ill.

Examination of the Mouth and Throat

Inspection

Inspection of the mouth and throat varies according to the child's age.

Infants

Inspection of the lips and exterior mouth may be done with minimal intrusion and basic inspection. Infants and young children will find assessment of the mouth and oral cavity including the posterior pharynx to be uncomfortable, so it is always helpful to save this part of the exam until the end. (Through experience, I have found that after examining the ears if the child is crying is a good time to assess the mouth and posterior pharynx. You can quickly shine the otoscope's light into the oral cavity and use a tongue depressor to displace the tongue to inspect the buccal mucosa, gingivae, dentition, and tonsils.)

For inspection of the mouth, wear gloves to protect both the child and yourself; remember to use a powder-free glove. For children of all ages, start by inspecting the lips for color, dryness, cracking, lesions, and fissures. Common lesions include cheilosis, which is cracking at the corners of the mouth often caused by a yeast infection. Other lesions to note are herpetic lesions, which present as vesicles, and impetigo, which presents as crusting lesions. The area where the lips meet the facial tissue is called the vermillion border. While inspecting the lips, note the philtrum, which is the median groove above the upper lip and below the nose. In children with fetal alcohol syndrome, the philtrum is longer and flat without the median groove.

The mouth is the first part of the digestive system. In newborns, use the light from the otoscope and a tongue depressor. The buccal mucosa and gingivae should be moist and pink. A normal finding in an infant is the sucking tubercle, a small pad in the middle of the upper lip caused from friction of breast- or bottle-feeding. In some infants, you may note small, hard, white lesions or pearly papules on the gum line that are often mistaken for teeth. They are retention cysts, or Epstein pearls, and disappear in 1 to 2 months. Tonsils are not visible in infants, gradually enlarging during childhood. In infants, there may appear to be increased drooling, particularly at 3 months of age when salivation increases. Because there is an inappropriate swallowing reflex and the infant has not yet learned to swallow the saliva, there is constant drooling. In addition, the infant does not have bottom teeth, which help to keep saliva in the mouth. Insert your finger into the mouth to elicit the suck reflex, which persists up to 12 months of age.

While inspecting the tongue, which is pink and moist, note that it is composed of numerous projections, called papillae, which assist in working food around in the mouth. While looking farther back on the tongue, you will note larger projections, which are the taste buds. Observe movement of the tongue. It should be freely moveable and move in all directions without quivering or trembling. A large tongue, or macroglossia, may be a sign of hypothyroidism. Down syndrome is also associated with a large tongue, although there is question whether it is because the oral cavity is small in these children or whether hypotonia also contributes to a large flaccid tongue. In the infant, tonsils may be difficult to visualize.

School-Age Children and Adolescents

For school-age children, ask them to touch the roof of the their mouth with their tongue. Note the ventral surface, which should be smooth and glossy with veins easily visible. While inspecting under the tongue, note the frenulum. In some children, the frenulum, which is a small mucous

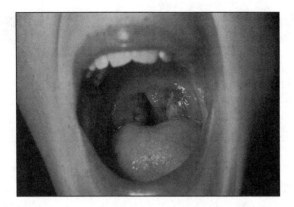

Figure 8-16 Tonsilitis (See Color Plate)

membrane that extends from the floor of the mouth to the underside of the tongue, may extend almost to the tip of the tongue. It may also be short, limiting the child's ability to stick out the tongue, although there is no evidence in the literature that partial ankyloglossia (tongue tie) causes speech defects, difficulty breast-feeding, or dental problems. The tip of the tongue normally grows until 4 years of age, and ankyloglossia gradually improves. Also while inspecting the tongue, you may observe a whitish coating. To determine if this is due to milk, use a tongue depressor to gently remove it. If it cannot be easily scraped away, the infant has oral candidiasis, or thrush.

In an ill child, check the tongue for a "strawberry tongue," which is associated with scarlet fever. This condition presents with a red tongue with prominent papillae, a beefy, red uvula, and palatal petechiae. Another lesion on the buccal mucosa is Koplik spots, which are an early sign of measles. They are small white spots that resemble a grain of sand; in the center of each is a bluish white speck. They occur before the skin eruptions of measles and therefore are considered a pathognomonic sign of the disease. If you see a blue or green tongue, always ask what color candy the child was eating.

On further assessment of the mouth, inspect the posterior pharynx, noting the size, position, symmetry, and appearance of the tonsils. Tonsils, which are masses of lymphoid tissue, are the largest between 8 and 16 years of age, and then gradually shrink. They are graded on a scale from 1+ to 4+. See **Figure 8-17**.

The tonsils are not encapsulated; therefore, squamous epithelium overlying them invaginates deep into their structure forming crypts. See **Figure**

TABLE 8-1
1+ is visible 2+ is halfway between the tonsillar pillars and the uvula 3+ is touching the uvula 4+ is touching each other (kissing tonsils)

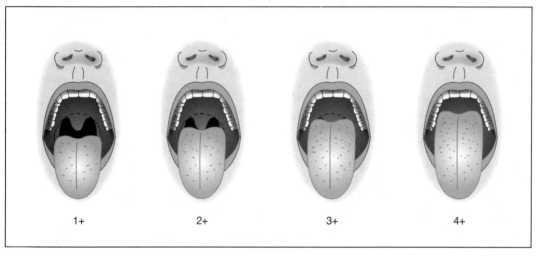

Figure 8-17   Tonsils Graded 0–4+

Source: Adapted from Mallampati SR, et al. *Can Anaesth Soc J.* 1985;32:429–434; and Samsoon GLT, Young JRB. *Anesthesiology.* 1987;42:487–490.

8-18. These openings trap bacteria and particulate matter or food, which *does not indicate disease.* Common infections of the tonsils include streptococcal pharyngitis, which typically presents with white exudates on the tonsils, a beefy, red uvula, and palatal petechiae. Peritonsillar abscess presents with asymmetric enlargement of the tonsils and with lateral displacement of the uvula to the noninfected side. See **Figure 8-20.**

Another infection of the posterior pharynx is epiglottitis, which is infrequently observed today due to immunization against *Haemophilus influenzae* type B. It can be seen at the base of the posterior tongue and pharynx. The epiglottis should be pink and moist without redness or edema. When evaluating for this disorder, examination of the throat is contraindicated because of potential laryngeal obstruction when opening the mouth.

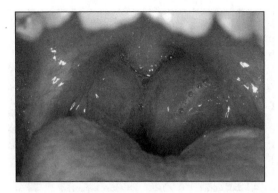

Figure 8-18   Kissing Tonsils (See Color Plate)

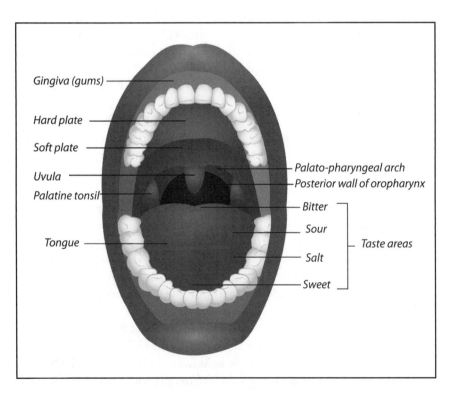

Figure 8-19   Tonsils, Uvula Tongue

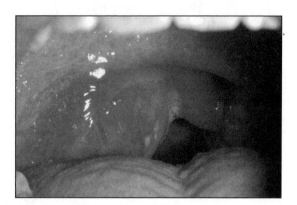

Figure 8-20 Peritonsillar Abscess

Further examination of the pharynx is assessment of exudates, which can be seen as white patches associated with both viral and bacterial infections. You may note yellow-green drainage high up in the posterior pharynx, which is sinus drainage, also called catarrh. In conjunction with sinus drainage and allergic rhinitis, you may note cobblestoning, which is a sign of follicular hypertrophy of mucosal lymphoid tissue secondary to chronic nasal infection.

In assessment of the uvula, note whether there is a bifid uvula (split or cleft uvula), which is a normal variation. See **Figure 8-21**. It results from failure of complete fusion of the medial nasal and maxillary processes. In some parts of Africa, such as Ethiopia, it is tradition to remove the uvula to allegedly prevent throat infections.

If the child is cooperative, have the child say "ahh" when examining the back of the throat. This is an important maneuver because on phonation the soft palate and the uvula rise symmetrically, allowing you to observe whether the uvula is midline and to better visualize the tonsils and posterior pharynx. In a child who resists this part of the exam, singing or playing singing games is always a good way to gain the child's cooperation. If the child says "ahh," you may not need to elicit the gag reflex, as you can assess movement of the palate that would be observed by using the tongue blade. If you need to use the tongue blade, ask the child to open his or her mouth and at the same time shine the light from the otoscope at the back of the throat. Touch the posterior third of the tongue with the tongue blade to elicit the gag reflex. Be gentle and quick, as most children dislike this part of the exam and may attempt to pull your hand away. Always explain what

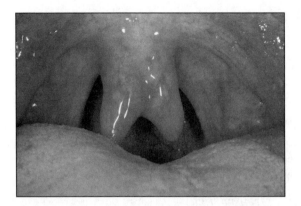

Figure 8-21   Bifid (Cleft or Split) Uvula at the Back of the Mouth

you are going to do before you do it. Be honest and let the child know if something is going to hurt or feel weird or uncomfortable.

Dentition
The teeth are in sockets called alveoli in the gum margins of the mandible and maxilla. Primary dentition consists of the deciduous teeth, also called baby teeth or milk teeth. These first teeth generally appear at around 6 months of age, and the lower central incisors are the first to erupt. Additional teeth erupt in pairs at 1- to 2-month intervals. By 24 months of age, a child will have all 20 deciduous teeth. Between the ages of 6 and 12 years, the permanent teeth develop roots and emerge. At the same time, the deciduous teeth are reabsorbed, which causes them to loosen and fall out. Generally, by the end of adolescence, all the permanent teeth have erupted, except the third molars, also called the wisdom teeth, which emerge generally between 17 and 25 years of age. Teeth are classified according to their shape and function as incisors, canines, premolars, and molars. The chisel-shaped incisors are adapted for cutting. The eyeteeth, or fanglike canines, are used for tearing and piercing. The premolars and molars have broad crowns with rounded tips and are best suited for grinding or crushing.

Palpation
For all age groups, palpation of the mouth is performed if there are lesions on the lips or oral cavity that require further assessment. Always use a glove when examining this area.

Common Abnormalities of the Ear, Nose, and Throat

Common abnormalities of the ear, nose, and throat will be discussed separately according to age group.

The Ear

Infants and Toddlers

OTITIS MEDIA is the most common infection in children 6 months to 2 years of age. It presents with fever, pain in the affected ear, and, on exam, a red tympanic membrane.

OTITIS MEDIA WITH EFFUSION presents with decreased mobility and a dark gray drum or amber-colored drum without a light reflex. If this is an acute process, the tympanic membrane may be red in color with decreased mobility.

PERFORATION OF THE EAR DRUM generally appears as an oval or round hole in the ear drum. It can be caused by middle ear infections if the pressure behind the drum causes the eardrum to rupture. Traumatic tympanic membrane perforations are also common, such as from sticking objects in the ear (e.g., bobby pin, pencil). Many times, visualization of the drum is difficult due to drainage in the ear canal.

School-Age Children

OTITIS MEDIA is the same as in the younger child. Otitis media with effusion occurs less frequently because the eustachian tube is better able to drain; therefore, there is less fluid buildup behind the tympanic membrane.

OTITIS EXTERNA is commonly known as "swimmer's ear" or inflammation of the ear canal. It presents as pain when tugging on the pinna and is associated with serous drainage from the external ear canal. It generally presents in children older than 5 years of age, often in conjunction with water-related sports.

CERUMEN IMPACTION occurs when earwax blocks the ear canal, occluding visualization of the tympanic membrane. This impaction can be corrected with irrigation of the ear canal.

FURUNCLE/ABSCESS is a reddened, infected hair follicle in the ear. It generally occurs on the tragus, or the dorsal end of the ear canal. It is tender and painful.

The Nose and Sinuses

Infants and Toddlers

FOREIGN BODIES in both the ear and nose are most frequently found in children ages 1–4 years. Symptoms range from obstruction to purulent nasal secretions. Commonly, there will be purulent secretions and possibly an odor from only one naris where a foreign object has occluded the passageway.

COMMON COLD is an acute, self-limited respiratory illness caused by a virus. Preschool-age children are more likely to develop cold symptoms as a result of frequent direct exposure from large aerosol droplets. Symptoms may include fever, rhinorrhea, anterior cervical adenopathy, and cough.

School-Age Children/Adolescents

EPISTAXIS is the result of repetitive habitual nose picking, which results in the formation of friable granulation tissue that bleeds easily, especially when traumatized.

ALLERGIC RHINITIS, as with other antigen–antibody reactions, involves antigen-specific IgE. It presents with vasodilatation and edema, which produce increased rhinorrhea and sneezing. *Allergic salute* is a specific gesture frequently performed by children with allergies, particularly allergic rhinitis. With their fingers pointed upward and the palm facing outward, children rub the back of the hand upward along the front of the nostrils, thus wiping away the rhinorrhea that continuously flows from the nose. As a result, a horizontal crease develops near the lower end of the nose, referred to as a transversal nasal crease.

SINUSITIS is infection of the lining of sinuses. It presents with a daytime cough, low-grade fever, increased congestion, dental pain, facial pain, tenderness on palpation/percussion of frontal and/or maxillary sinuses for greater than 10–14 days. Occasionally, there may also be pain behind the eyes.

NASAL ABNORMALITIES, either anatomic or vasculature, are often secondary to drug abuse, such as cocaine inhalation, or topical nasal drugs, such as phenylephrine hydrochloride. They may also be due to nasal trauma.

The Throat

Infants and Toddlers

CANDIDA ALBICANS, or thrush, is most frequently found during the first 2 months of life. It appears as whitish plaques on the buccal mucosa, the tongue, and the oral pharynx.

GINGIVOSTOMATITIS is very common in infants and young children between 1 and 3 years of age. It presents as painful erosions, ulcers, and blisters, affecting the lips, buccal mucosa, tongue, and posterior pharynx. It often presents as small pustules with an erythematous base. It is viral in etiology.

BOTTLE MOUTH is dental decay secondary to prolonged exposure of the teeth to milk or juice. See **Figure 8-22**. It generally occurs between the ages of 18 months and 3 years. Tooth decay results from the erosion of enamel due to the acid buildup in dental plaque.

School-Age Children

BRUXISM is grinding of the teeth, primarily at night. It often occurs in children between the ages of 6 and 12 years. It occurs as the permanent dentition erupts and can result in moderate wear of the primary canines and molars leading to temporomandibular joint (TMJ) pain.

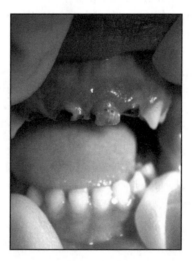

Figure 8-22   Bottle Mouth

GROUP A BETA-HEMOLYTIC STREPTOCOCCI (GABHS) PHARYNGITIS presents with the triad of associated symptoms: headache, vomiting, and abdominal pain. Onset of symptoms is precipitous versus gradual, as it is in viral pharyngitis. Sandpaper rash may also be associated with GABHS infection. There is a characteristic mouth odor associated with streptococcal infections.

VIRAL PHARYNGITIS presents with cough, low-grade fever, conjunctivitis, nasal congestion, and sore throat. Symptoms of viral pharyngitis generally progress gradually.

MUMPS is a viral illness with characteristic swelling of the parotid salivary glands that are located in front of the ears. It presents with fever, headache, and body ache. The characteristic swelling appears 1–2 days later. It is rare today due to the immunizations for mumps, measles, and rubella. It is spread by direct contact and airborne droplets.

COXSACKIE VIRAL INFECTION refers to type A viruses that cause herpangina (painful blisters in the mouth, throat, hands, and feet). It is also referred to as *hand, foot, and mouth disease* and usually occurs in young children to adolescents. It presents with fever and vesicular or ulcerated lesions on the soft palate, palms of the hands, and soles of the feet. It can also present with a generalized body rash, although the distinguishing features are the lesions on palms, soles, and soft palate.

Adolescents

MONONUCLEOSIS is a viral illness caused by the Epstein-Barr virus. It presents with fever, pharyngitis, nontender posterior cervical lymphadenopathy, involvement of other lymph node groups, fatigue, malaise, possible enlargement of the liver, and usual enlargement of the spleen (Fox, 2002).

VIRAL PHARYNGITIS presents the same in adolescents as in younger children.

GROUP A BETA-HEMOLYTIC STREPTOCOCCI (GABHS) PHARYNGITIS in adolescents generally presents with a sore throat of varying degrees. It also presents with enlarged, tender anterior cervical lymphadenopathy, a low-grade fever, headache, and malaise. When looking into the posterior pharynx, you will observe a red throat with petechiae and whitish exudate.

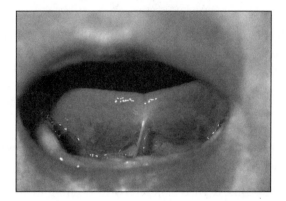

Figure 8-23 Tongue-Tied—Ankyloglossia

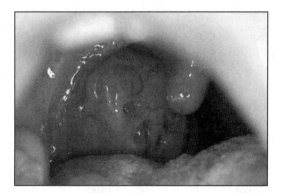

Figure 8-24 Enlarged Tonsil

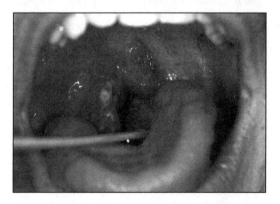

Figure 8-25 Tonsil Exudate (See Color Plate)

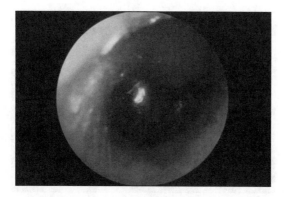

Figure 8-26   Acute Otitis Media (See Color Plate)

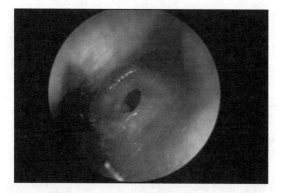

Figure 8-27   Perforation of Tympanic Membrane (See Color Plate)

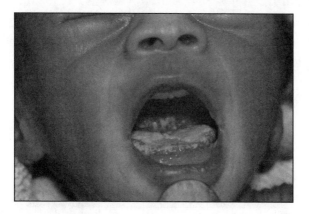

Figure 8-28   Thrush—Candidiasis

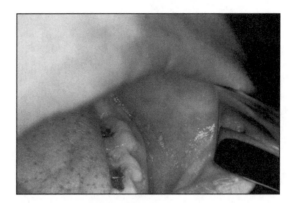

Figure 8-29 Measles, Koplik Spots

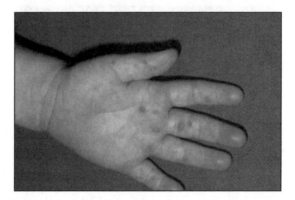

Figure 8-30 Coxsackie Virus Infection Image B

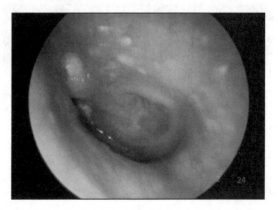

Figure 8-31 Congenital Cholesteatoma (See Color Plate)

Red Flags

Findings to worry about when examining the ears include the following:

- *MASTOIDITIS*, an inflammation or infection of the mastoid bone that is usually a complication of otitis media. The mastoid consists of air cells that drain the middle ear, and there is the possibility of abscess formation and extension into the surrounding structures in the brain. This condition is rare today because of frequent treatment of otitis media.

- *PERFORATION OF THE TYMPANIC MEMBRANE* and drainage into the external ear canal. In the classic scenario, the child complains of ear pain the previous evening. The next morning, the child denies ear pain, although there is serosanguinous discharge on the pillow case. Drainage in the ear canal usually signals perforation of the tympanic membrane: The pressure behind the drum builds and is released through a rupture of the drum, with subsequent fluid draining into the ear canal. When this rupture occurs, the middle ear is unprotected and is vulnerable to infection, requiring urgent treatment.

- *CHOLESTEATOMA*, a benign tumor of squamous epithelium that can grow and alter normal structure and function of surrounding soft tissue and bone in the ear. It requires immediate referral.

- *DELAYED SPEECH*. If a child is 18 months or 2 years and has no expressive language, referral is necessary. If a child has attained appropriate developmental milestone for speech acquisition and is gradually losing the ability to speak, immediate referral to neurology is necessary.

A finding of concern when examining the mouth is peritonsillar abscess, which is the most common deep neck infection in children and adolescents, although it occurs more frequently in adolescents (Wald, 2010). It presents with a severe sore throat that is usually unilateral, "hot potato" or muffled voice, and pooling or drooling of saliva.

Write-Up of the Ears, Nose, and Throat

EXAMPLE FOR INFANTS:

> ➤ *EARS*: Evenly aligned and symmetric in shape, external canal pink without lesions, tympanic membrane gray in color with diffuse light reflex.

> *NOSE/SINUSES*: Nares patent bilaterally.
> *THROAT*: Lips moist without fissures or cracking, oral mucosa pink and moist, tongue pink and moist without coating, posterior pharynx without erythema or exudates, tonsils not visualized, positive gag reflex, uvula rises midline.

EXAMPLE FOR SCHOOL-AGE CHILDREN AND ADOLESCENTS:
> *EARS*: Evenly aligned and symmetric in shape; external canal pink with small amount of cerumen, without lesions or discharge; tympanic membrane gray, translucent, and mobile with light reflex; bony landmarks present.
> *NOSE/SINUSES*: Nares patent bilaterally, turbinates pink and moist, septum midline. Sinuses without tenderness on palpation.
> *THROAT*: Lips moist without fissures or cracking, oral mucosa pink and moist without lesions, dentitions in good repair without gross malocclusion, tonsils 2+ without erythema and without exudates, positive gag reflex, uvula rises midline.

Case Study: Adolescent Boy Presenting with Ear, Nose, and Throat Symptoms

William is a 15-year-old male who presents to your office with a history of sore throat, headache, and low-grade fever of 38.1°C (100.7°F) for the past 4 days. He reports feeling tired, with malaise and loss of appetite. He has missed the past 3 days of school. He reports to you that he has taken ibuprofen with some relief of his headache.

His past medical history is noncontributory. He has no known allergies and takes no medications. On examination:

- *Skin*: Clear without rash
- *Neck*: Bilateral anterior cervical lymphadenopathy
- *Throat*: Posterior pharynx injected and tonsillar exudate
- *Lungs*: Clear to auscultation
- *Abdomen*: Hepatosplenomegaly

Questions

1. Which laboratory tests would be most helpful in determining this patient's diagnosis?
2. What conditions are considered in the differential diagnosis for exudative pharyngitis?
3. What are presenting signs and symptoms of GABHS pharyngitis?

Answers

1. A rapid strep test is used to determine whether a child with a sore throat has a group A streptococci infection. If the test is negative, a throat culture should be performed to confirm the result.

    The heterophile antibodies test, also called the monospot (agglutination slide), is used to diagnose infectious mononucleosis. Note, these antibodies may not be detectable until *7–14 days* of the illness. In addition, a complete blood count (CBC) with greater than 10% atypical lymphocytes and greater than 50% lymphocytosis supports the diagnosis of mononucleosis in conjunction with a positive monospot.

2. Disorders characterized by exudative pharyngitis include adenovirus, GABHS, and infectious mononucleosis. In some cases, pharyngeal gonorrhea should be considered based on the patient's sexual history.

3. Presenting signs and symptoms of GABHS include erythema of the posterior pharynx, exudative tonsillitis, palatal petechiae, tender and enlarged anterior cervical nodes, dysphagia, headache, abdominal pain, vomiting and fever, and a skin-colored sandpaper-type rash. Early treatment of GABHS prevents complications from rheumatic fever and poststreptococcal glomerulonephritis, as well as suppurative retropharyngeal abscess and cervical adenitis.

References

Ball, J., Bindler, R., & Cowen, K. (2010). *Child health nursing.* Upper Saddler River, NJ: Pearson.

Burns, C., Dunn, A., Brady, M., Starr, N., & Blosser, C. (2000). *Pediatric primary care: A handbook for nurse practitioners* (3rd ed.). St. Louis, MO: Saunders.

eMedicine. (n.d.). Preauricular cysts, pits, and fissures. Retrieved July 5, 2010, from *WebMD* Web site: http://emedicine.medscape.com/article/845288-overview

Fox, J. A. (2002). *Primary health care of infants, children and adolescents.* Boston: Mosby.

Ipp, M. (n.d.). *Preauricular skin tags.* Retrieved July 5, 2010, from *Primary Care Pediatrics* Web site: www.utoronto.ca/kids/eartag.htm

Jarvis, C. (2004). *Physical examination and health assessment* (5th ed.). St. Louis, MO: Elsevier.

Marieb, E. (2000). *Human anatomy and physiology* (3rd ed.). Redwood City, CA: Benjamin/Cummings Publishing Company.

Roizen, N. (2010). Clinical features and diagnosis of down syndrome. Retrieved from http://www.uptodate.com

Romo, T., Yalamanchili, H., Presti, P., & Pearson, J. M. (2010). Septal deviation: Surgical aspects. Retrieved July 5, 2010, from *WebMD* Web site: http://emedicine.medscape.com/article/878817-overview

Sanford, B., Weber, P. (2010). Evaluation of hearing impairment in children. Retrieved from http://www.uptodate.com

Vaile, L., Williamson, T., Waddell, A., & Taylor, G. (2006). Interventions for ear discharge associated with grommets (ventilation tubes). *Cochrane Database of Systematic Reviews, 19*(2):CD001933.

Wald, E. (2010). Peritonsillar cellulitis and abscess. Retrieved from http://www.uptodate.com

Resources

Bickley, L. (2003). *Bates' guide to physical examination and history taking* (8th ed.). New York: Lippincott Williams & Wilkins.

Estes, M. (1998). *Health assessment and physical examination*. Albany, NY: Delmar Publishers.

Hansen, M. (1998). *Pathophysiology: Foundations of disease and clinical intervention*. Philadelphia: Saunders.

Potts, N., & Mandleco, B. (2007). *Pediatraic nursing* (2nd ed.). Victoria, Australia: Thomson, Delmar Learning.

Tortora, G. J., Grabvowski, S. R. (2003). *Principles of anatomy and physiology* (10th ed.). New York: Wiley.

Examination of the Lungs and Thorax

Anatomy and Physiology

The respiratory system consists of the nasal cavity, pharynx, larynx, trachea, bronchi, and lungs. It is further divided into the upper respiratory tract, which includes the nasal cavity and pharynx, and the lower respiratory tract, which includes the larynx, trachea, bronchi, and lungs. This chapter will deal with only those components located in the thorax.

The thorax is cone shaped and narrower at the top, or apex. It is made up of the sternum and 12 pairs of ribs anteriorly, and the spinal column and 12 thoracic vertebrae posteriorly. The bottom, or floor, of the thorax is defined by the diaphragm, which separates the thoracic cavity from the abdomen. The first seven ribs are attached directly to the sternum via the costal cartilages and are called the vertebrosternal ribs. Ribs 8, 9, and 10 are attached to the costal cartilage just above them, and ribs 11 and 12 are free (or floating) and do not articulate at their anterior ends. All of the ribs articulate posteriorly to the vertebral column. The point at which the ribs attach to the sternum is called the costochondral junction, which is an area composed of cartilage. The area between each rib is called the intercostal space.

Within the thorax is the sternum, also called the breastbone. Landmarks on this bone are helpful in identifying specific structures in the thorax. The sternum is divided into three sections—the manubrium, or the upper bone of the sternum, which articulates with the clavicles, and the first pair of ribs. At the top of the manubrium is the suprasternal notch, which is a U-shaped depression. Inferior to the suprasternal notch is the body of the manubrium, and at the bottom is the angle of Louis. The identification of landmarks such as the angle of Louis is helpful when starting to count the ribs in the process of localizing specific respiratory findings.

Another identifying landmark that corresponds with the angle of Louis is the bifurcation of the trachea into the right and left main bronchi. This landmark lies above the fourth vertebrae on the spinal column and is in line with the upper border of the atrium of the heart. This portion of the manubrium also articulates with the body of the sternum and is continuous with the second set of ribs. At the base of the sternum is the xiphoid process, which is cartilaginous and does not articulate with the ribs. The xiphoid process is identified during cardiopulmonary resuscitation (CPR) so that hand compressions do not occur over this area, thus avoiding direct trauma

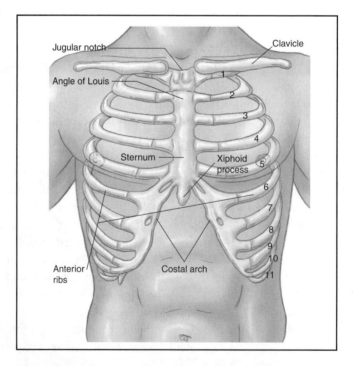

Figure 9-1(a) Rib Cage—Anterior View

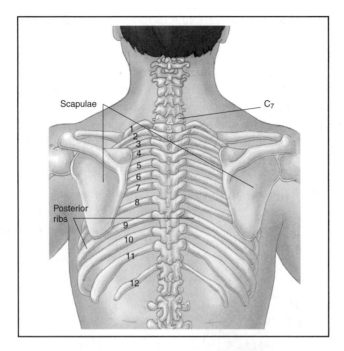

Figure 9-1(b)   Rib Cage—Posterior View

such as fracture or cartilage injury. At the base of the ribs are the right and left costal margins that meet at the xiphoid process, approximately in a 90-degree angle.

The lungs are the body's major organs of respiration, and their main function is to deliver oxygen to the lungs, remove carbon dioxide, and maintain homeostasis through acid–base balance.

Development of the Lungs

At 4 weeks of gestation, the lung is a groove on the ventral wall of the gut. It gradually evolves and matures from a simple sac to an involuted structure of tubules. The distal portion of this structure divides into two lung buds, which grow into the epithelial lining of the bronchi and lungs. As the lung buds develop, they branch repeatedly and develop into the bronchial tubes. After month 6 of gestation, the terminal portion of the bronchial tubes develops into the alveoli. Surfactant production begins at 28 weeks of gestation and the lungs are among the last of the fetal organ systems to mature.

The lungs are located on each side of the chest within the rib cage and are separated by the heart and the mediastinum. They are cone-shaped organs, with the apex of each lung extending into the lowest part of the neck and just above the level of the first rib. The base of the lungs extends down to the diaphragm, which separates the chest from the abdominal cavity. The lungs are further divided into upper and lower lobes. The right lung is broader than the left because of the position of the heart; it is shorter than the left lung because of the upward displacement of the diaphragm by the liver. The right lung is composed of three lobes—the upper, middle, and lower lobes. The left lung has two lobes and is narrower than the right lung because of the positioning of the heart. The lobes in both lungs are further divided by grooves, or fissures, that run obliquely. They are important in identifying the location of bronchopulmonary findings.

Each lung is encased in the pleural membrane, or serous sac, which protects the lung. The parietal pleura, or superficial layer, lines the thoracic wall and the superior surface of the diaphragm. The visceral pleura lines

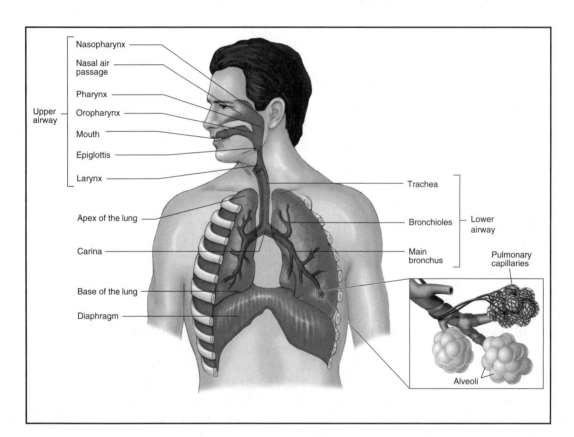

Figure 9-2 System of Air-Conducting Passages

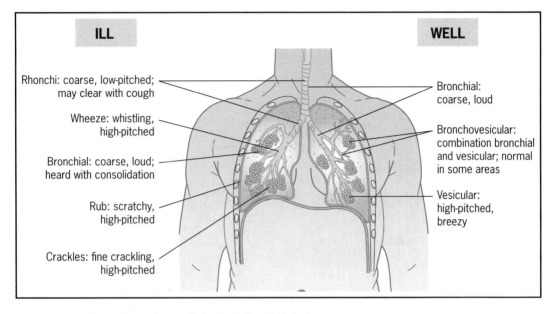

ILL

Rhonchi: coarse, low-pitched; may clear with cough

Wheeze: whistling, high-pitched

Bronchial: coarse, loud; heard with consolidation

Rub: scratchy, high-pitched

Crackles: fine crackling, high-pitched

WELL

Bronchial: coarse, loud

Bronchovesicular: combination bronchial and vesicular; normal in some areas

Vesicular: high-pitched, breezy

Figure 9-3   Schema of Breath Sounds in the Well and Ill Patient

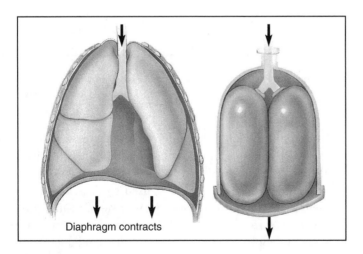

Diaphragm contracts

Figure 9-4(a)   Lungs and Oxygen Cycle With in Alveoli

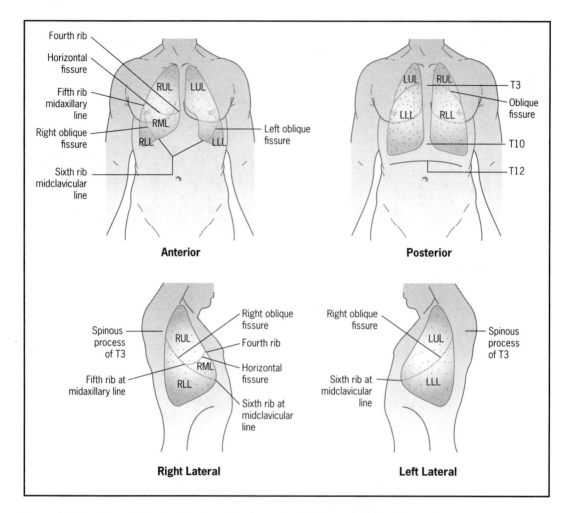

Figure 9-4(b) Thoracic Landmarks—Anterior, Posterior Right Lateral and Left Lateral

the external surface of the lungs themselves. Between these two layers is the pleural cavity, which contains a lubricating fluid that lines the pleural cavity and allows the lungs to glide easily over the thorax wall during respiration. Inflammation of the pleural membrane caused by decreased pleural fluid causes the pleural surfaces to become dry and rough, resulting in friction and stabbing pain. *Pleurisy*, which is inflammation of the pleural membrane, is frequently seen in adolescents and presents with stabbing chest pain and shortness of breath. When there is excess fluid accumulation in the pleural space, pleural effusion results. All of these conditions ultimately result in decreased lung expansion and difficulty breathing.

Tracheobronchial Tree: Respiratory Differences Between Children and Adults

One of the major anatomic differences between the child and the adult in the upper tracheobronchial tree is the tongue. The child's tongue is larger in relation to the amount of space in the oropharynx. Due to this anatomic difference, there is more likelihood of airway occlusion in a child. The size of the tongue in relation to the size of the oropharynx in a child is thought to be one explanation for why children are obligate nose breathers.

The child's trachea is much more pliable and smaller in diameter and has immature tracheal rings. The adult's trachea is approximately 10–11 cm in length. It begins at the level of the cricoid cartilage and bifurcates just below the sternal angle into the right and left main bronchi. Posteriorly, tracheal bifurcation is at the level of T4 and T5. The right main bronchus is shorter, wider, and more vertical than the left. In children, the trachea is shorter and narrower. Of note, the infant's airway is approximately 4 mm in diameter, approximately the width of a drinking straw; the adult's trachea, in comparison, is 20 mm in diameter. Due to the infant's narrow airway, there is greater airway resistance, which causes a greater effort to move oxygen into the lungs. See **Figure 9-5**. This difference comes into play when a child develops a respiratory tract infection that leads to edema and swelling of the main stem bronchi of the trachea. The inflammation from the respiratory infection further narrows the lumen of the trachea, which results in increased airway resistance (Ball, 2010).

The adult's larynx is positioned at the level of the fourth or fifth cervical vertebra, whereas the child's larynx is at the level of the first or second cervical vertebra. This difference is important because if the pediatric larynx were lower, children would aspirate into the trachea during swallowing. The higher larynx is more anterior, and, therefore, aspiration is less likely. The main stem bronchi in young children have less of an angle than in adults. As a result, aspiration can occur in either the left or right main stem bronchi. As children grow, an increase in chest diameter causes the angle of the left bronchus to increase, which decreases the chance of aspiration as well. Remember, the trachea lies anterior to the esophagus and splits into the right and left main stem bronchi. Note, in infants the chest muscles are immature and the ribs are cartilaginous, making the chest wall more flexible. As a result, retractions are more easily observed in the child, particularly in the substernal and subcostal areas. When a child is in severe respiratory distress, accessory muscles such as the trapezius and sternocleidomastoid are used, and retractions are observed in the supraclavicular and suprasternal areas. **Figure 9-8** showcases retraction sites.

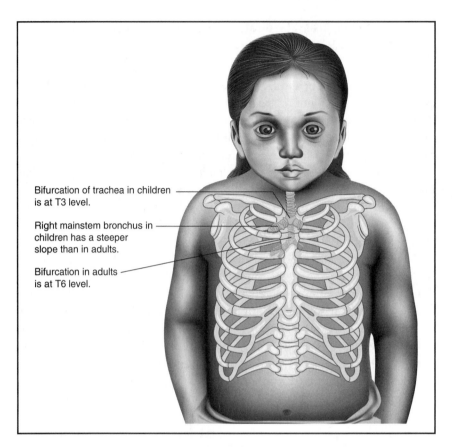

Bifurcation of trachea in children is at T3 level.

Right mainstem bronchus in children has a steeper slope than in adults.

Bifurcation in adults is at T6 level.

Figure 9-5   Diameter of an Child's Airway

The main stem bronchi are the major air passages from the trachea to the lungs and are similar to the trachea in tissue composition, which means they can easily become edematous due to bacterial or viral infection. The bronchi and bronchioles in the newborn are lined with smooth muscle, thus preventing the newborn from trapping airborne particles such as viruses or bacteria. By 5 months of age, the infant has more matured muscular development that protects him or her from ingestion of harmful organisms through the effect of bronchospasm and/or muscle contractions and cough.

Another important consideration is that oxygen consumption is higher in children than in adults due to their increased metabolic rate. When a child has a fever and is in respiratory distress, muscle glycogen reserves ultimately lead to more rapid muscle fatigue due to the child's extra effort and use of accessory muscles in breathing (Froh, 2006).

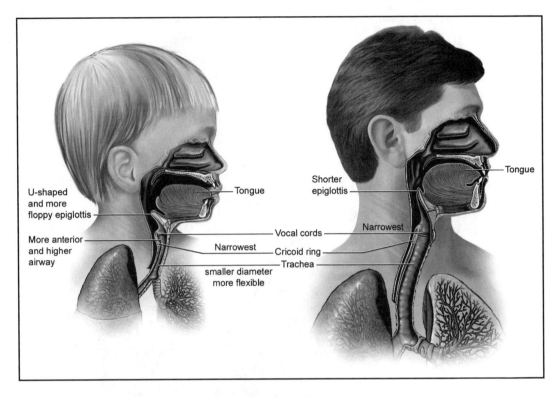

Figure 9-6 Comparison of Airway Structures

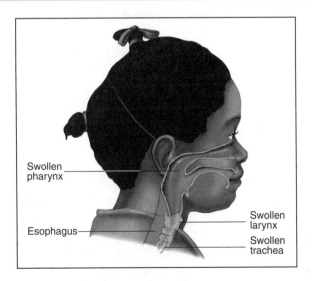

Figure 9-7 Airway Changes with Croup

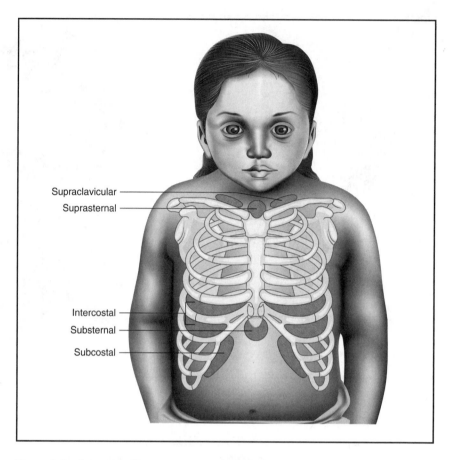

Figure 9-8   Retraction Sites

In the lower respiratory tree, there are also differences between the child and the adult. In the newborn, the lung tissue contains approximately 25 million alveoli, which are not fully developed until 8 years of age when the size and complexity of these air sacs increase. By adulthood, the alveoli increase to 300 million, which provides a large surface area for adequate gas exchange. During the toddler period, the intercostal muscles are immature and the child uses the diaphragm to breathe. By 6 years of age, the intercostal muscles have matured, allowing the child to more effectively use the intercostal muscles for breathing. Remember, newborns are obligate nose breathers and use the diaphragm to breathe because the intercostal muscles are too immature. In addition, the coordination of mouth breathing is controlled by neurologic pathways that do not mature adequately until approximately 2–3 months of age.

The diaphragm is the most important muscle of inspiration and forms the inferior border between the thorax and the abdominal cavity. It is innervated by the phrenic nerve. It is dome shaped in inspiration, but when it contracts on expiration, it flattens, increasing the volume of the thoracic cavity. This muscle is so important because during inspiration and expiration it causes pressure changes in the abdominal cavity, thus facilitating the return of venous blood to the heart. Note, by contracting (pushing down upon) the diaphragm, the pressure in the abdominal cavity is increased, which puts pressure on the pelvic organs, helping to evacuate urine and feces. This is referred to as a Valsalva maneuver.

Physiology of Respiration

The primary function of the respiratory system is the gas exchange of oxygen and carbon dioxide, which occurs in the alveoli, the smallest functional units of the respiratory system. Around the circumference of the alveolar ducts are numerous alveoli and alveolar sacs. There are two types of alveolar cells. Type I alveolar cells are squamous cells that form a lining of the alveolar wall; they are the main sites of gas exchange. Type II alveolar cells are epithelial cells that secrete alveolar fluid, which keeps the surface between the cells and the air moist. This alveolar fluid is surfactant, lowering the surface tension of the alveolar fluids and thus preventing the alveoli from collapsing. The actual exchange of oxygen and carbon dioxide occurs between the air spaces in the lungs and across the alveolar and capillary walls that form the respiratory membrane.

In newborns, particularly premature babies, there is not enough surfactant produced to keep the alveoli inflated. (Pulmonary surfactant is not produced until the last 2 months of fetal development.) When the amount of surfactant is inadequate, the surface tension forces collapse of the alveoli, requiring the alveoli to be reinflated during each inspiration. This process requires a tremendous amount of energy and subsequently leads to infant respiratory distress syndrome (IRDS). IRDS is treated with positive-pressure respirators that force air into the alveoli, thereby keeping them open between breaths.

The actual process of breathing is mediated by the respiratory center in the brainstem at the pons and medulla, and the stimulus to breathe is based on an increase of carbon dioxide in the blood called *hypercapnia*. In simple terms, air moves into the lungs (inspiration) when the air pressure inside the lungs is less than the air pressure in the atmosphere. Air moves out of the lungs (expiration) when the pressure inside the lungs is greater than the pressure in the atmosphere. During inspiration, when the diaphragm and external intercostal muscles contract, negative pressure is created in the thoracic cavity, forcing air into the lungs. (Pressure inside the alveoli must become lower than the atmospheric pressure.) During this process, the diaphragm lowers and the ribs elevate, thereby increasing the intrapulmonary volume and negative pressure.

During expiration, there is also a change in pressure gradient, although it is just the opposite of inspiration. The pressure in the lungs is greater than the pressure in the atmosphere, and expiration is a passive process that results from elastic recoil of the chest wall and lungs. As the diaphragm relaxes, its dome moves superiorly, and as the external intercostals relax, the ribs are depressed. These movements decrease the intrapulmonary volume, which in turn increases alveolar pressure. Air then moves out of the alveoli where the pressure is high into an area of lower pressure in the atmosphere.

Assessment Considerations: Subjective Information

The following sections present considerations for the assessment of the lungs and thorax.

Infants

- Was the infant born prematurely or with low birth weight? Ask the mother if there was ventilation assistance. If so, ask for how long, and whether the baby had respiratory distress syndrome or bronchopulmonary dysplasia. Premature and low birth weight infants are more prone to respiratory conditions. The most significant pathogen during this age is respiratory syncytial virus (RSV).
- Does the infant have a history of apnea episodes? Has an apnea monitor been used? Has the child experienced an apparent life-threatening event (ALTE)? Is there history of SIDS in a sibling?
- Does the infant have a history of feeding difficulty, such as tiring quickly, periods of cyanosis, diaphoresis during feeds, or inappropriate weight gain? These questions are associated with the possibility of cardiac abnormalities.
- Does the infant have a history of bronchiolitis or reactive airway disease?
- Does the infant have a history of frequent upper respiratory infections? Upper respiratory infections are more common during this period due to lack of acquired immunity to common pathogens, and also because of increased exposure frequency.

Toddlers and School-Age Children

- Has the child experienced sudden onset of coughing without cold symptoms? This condition may be associated with aspiration of a foreign object.
- Does the child have a history of nasal flaring or intercostal retractions associated with lower respiratory infections?
- Does the child have a history of frequent episodes of pneumonia?
- Has the child had croup (laryngotracheobronchitis)?
- Has the child been diagnosed with asthma, or does the child have a history of wheezing or tachypnea? Does the child have a history of allergies to pollens, dust, or other airborne irritants? Allergies to foods and/or drugs? Has allergy and pulmonary function testing been performed? If the child is younger than 2 years of age, ask what foods have been introduced and whether the child was breast- or bottle-fed.
- Has tuberculin testing been done? Do any close contacts or household members have tuberculosis, or are they currently being treated for tuberculosis? Are members of the household recent immigrants to this country? Has the family or a family member been living in a shelter or group home? Have any of the household members recently been in prison or any type of institutional setting?
- Does the child have a persistent cough (lasting more than 2 weeks), and is there sputum production?
- Does the child have a history of night sweats or recent weight loss?
- Does the child have a history of pain in the chest?
- Has the child received a flu shot this year or in the past?
- Is the parent concerned about chest wall abnormalities such as pectus excavatum (funnel chest) or pectus carinatum (pigeon breast)?

Adolescents

- In a preadolescent or adolescent male, is there concern of breast enlargement (gynecomastia)? It can be bilateral or unilateral and is generally hormonally related.
- Does the adolescent have a history of exercise-induced asthma? This condition often persists and leads to the question of whether medications are being properly used.
- Does the adolescent have a history of tobacco or cannabis use with resultant cough or dyspnea? There is also concern of exposure to

pulmonary irritants and carcinogens that may predispose to *chronic obstructive pulmonary disease* or cancer.

- Is there a complaint of episodic chest pain without radiation? If so, think of costochondritis, which is an inflammation of the cartilage that connects a rib to the sternum. It causes sharp pain in the costosternal joint.
- Does the adolescent have a history of chest trauma? The risk for chest trauma is highest among adolescents due to motor vehicle accidents and/or sports injuries.

Family History

During the subjective assessment, also consider the child's family history, including such considerations as the following:

- Is there a family history of tuberculosis, emphysema, allergies, asthma or atopic dermatitis, or chronic obstructive pulmonary disease?
- Does anyone in the household smoke?
- Is there a family history of cystic fibrosis?

Review of Systems

Review of systems with relevance to the respiratory system includes the following:

- *NOSE*: Consider the child's history of environmental allergies, discharge (serous or purulent), epistaxis, breathing difficulty, sinus pain, and mouth breathing.
- *EARS*: Consider the child's history of frequent otitis media secondary to upper respiratory infections.
- *THROAT*: Consider the child's history of frequent sore throats and viral illnesses associated with the posterior pharynx.
- *LUNGS*: Consider the frequency of upper respiratory infections; the history of asthma, cough, pneumonia, and croup; and presence of nasal flaring and retractions.
- *CARDIOVASCULAR*: Consider the child's history of shortness of breath and his or her endurance level during vigorous physical exercise. Assess for dyspnea and for cyanosis associated with crying, feeding, or exertion.

Assessment Considerations: Objective Information

Inspection

Inspection of the lungs varies by age group, as described in the following sections.

Infants

When inspecting the chest of the newborn, visual inspection is best performed by observing the pattern of breathing and counting the respiration, noting that newborns are abdominal breathers. If the child is quiet and sleeping on the parent's lap or resting in an alert quiet state, "seize the opportunity" to observe the child's breathing. The normal respiratory rate of the newborn is 30–60 breaths per minute. Periodic breaths with pauses less than 10 seconds are considered within normal. Pauses longer than 20 seconds are abnormal and should be monitored.

By unwrapping the infant or removing the clothes, you will initiate crying and disrupt a previously quiet state. You may need to give the child a pacifier or speak softly and in a soothing manner to quiet him or her again. Music from a wind-up toy is often helpful in quieting and distracting the child. Once the child has returned to a quiet state, inspect the appearance of the thorax. In infants, the thorax is rounded with the anteroposterior diameter equal to the transverse diameter.

The infant's chest circumference is 30–36 cm and is 2 cm smaller than the head circumference until 2 years of age (Estes, 2006; Jarvis, 2008). The chest wall in the infant is thin with little musculature, and the rib cage is cartilaginous, soft, and pliant. The xiphoid process may be seen protruding anteriorly at the apex of the costal angle. In the newborn, the breasts are often enlarged and engorged. There may be secretion of a white liquid called "witch's milk," which is physiologic galactorrhea and is due to the maternal hormone, estrogen. This secretion may last a week or two and resolves spontaneously.

A distance between the nipples of greater than 25% of the chest circumference (i.e., widespread nipples) may be associated with congenital disorders such as Turner syndrome. Also, supernumerary nipples are a common congenital malformation. They present as small and poorly formed in addition to the two nipples normally present on the chest. They generally follow the milk line curving from the axilla, through the nipples, and then vertical toward the midline just below the umbilicus.

Toddlers and School-Age Children

Inspection of this age group can be done from a distance without intruding into the child's space. If the child is sitting with a hospital gown on, *seize the opportunity* and observe from the posterior, noting the respiratory rate and the shape of the thorax. From the anterior angle, you can observe if the child is in respiratory distress by evidence of supraclavicular or suprasternal retractions, or nasal flaring. Also note skin color, including cyanosis or mottling, or increased or decreased color to the skin. Note if the child is perspiring or evidences a cough, assessing the sound, type of cough, and location of the cough.

For anterior inspection, you will have to open the hospital gown in the front to further inspect the chest for *pectus excavatum* (funnel chest), which may present with a marked depression in the lower portion of the sternum and marked midsubsternal retractions with normal respirations. Also observe for *pectus carinatum*, also called pigeon breast, in which the sternum is displaced anteriorly, increasing the anteroposterior diameter. Grooves in the chest wall accentuate this deformity.

To identify and describe specific areas within the chest during physical examination, draw imaginary lines on the anterior and posterior chest. **Figure 9-9** shows the topographic landmarks of the thorax.

Thoracic cage landmarks are described as follows:

1. The midsternal line is drawn vertically down to the midline of the sternum.
2. The midclavicular lines are drawn through the middle points of the clavicles and parallel to the midsternal line.
3. The anterior axillary lines are vertical lines drawn along the anterior axillary folds parallel to the midsternal line.
4. The midaxillary lines are drawn from each vertex of the axillae parallel to the midsternal line.
5. The posterior axillary lines are parallel to the midsternal line and extend vertically along the posterior axillary folds.

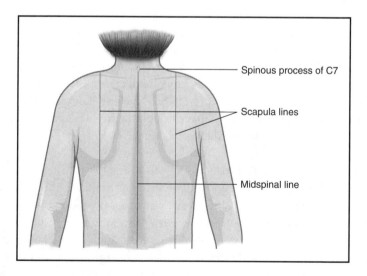

Spinous process of C7

Scapula lines

Midspinal line

Figure 9-9   Topographic Landmarks of the Thorax

6. The midspinal line is a vertical line that passes through the posterior spinous processes of the vertebrae.
7. The scapular lines are parallel to the midspinal line and pass through the inferior angles of the scapulae.

These topographic landmarks of both the anterior and posterior thorax apply to the child, the adolescent, and the adult. They are useful when palpating for tenderness, masses, or other abnormalities, as well as for identifying the location of adventitious breath sounds heard during auscultation. See Figure 9-9.

Adolescents

Inspection of the thorax in the adolescent is the same as in the adult. Start by inspecting the chest for respiratory movement, size, shape, and deformity. Note nipple placement in the male, and assess for gynecomastia. Note that the shape and configuration of the chest wall will be dependent upon the age of the adolescent and the stage of pubertal development. Younger adolescents in the early stages of puberty will have less definition and muscular development of the thorax. For the more physically mature adolescent, note that the thorax should be symmetric in an elliptical shape with downward-sloping ribs. The anteroposterior diameter should be less than the transverse diameter, and the ratio of anteroposterior to transverse diameter is from 1:2 to 5:7 (Jarvis, 2008, p. 449). On the posterior thorax, inspect the spinous processes, as they should appear in a straight line, and the scapula should be symmetrically placed.

Palpation

When palpating the thorax, it is important to identify key landmarks. The following landmarks, starting at the neck, are used to describe findings:

1. *SUPRASTERNAL NOTCH*: Starting at the most proximal point, which is at the base of the neck, use the pad of your index finger and feel in the midsternal line above the manubrium. This depression is the suprasternal notch.
2. *CLAVICLES*: Also referred to as the collarbone, they are slender, doubly curved long bones that can be palpated horizontally across the superior thorax. They attach to the manubrium.
3. *ANGLE OF LOUIS*: It is also called the manubriosternal junction or sternal angle. With your finger pads, feel for the suprasternal notch and move your finger pads down the sternum until they reach a horizontal ridge (the junction of the manubrium and the body of the sternum). This is the angle of Louis. The second rib articulates with this landmark and acts as a reference point for counting the ribs and intercostal

s p a c e s .
(Remember, the first rib is difficult to palpate.)

4. *COSTAL ANGLE*: This is the angle formed by the costal margins at the sternum. It is generally less than 90 degrees, with the ribs inserted at a 45-degree angle. Place your right finger pads on the bottom of the child's anterior left rib cage, which is the 10th rib; then place your left finger pads on the bottom of the right rib cage (10th rib), and move both hands horizontally toward the sternum until they meet at the midsternal line. This is the costal angle.

5. *VERTEBRA PROMINENS*: This spinous process of C7 and T1 can be seen when the child's head is bent forward. Ask the child to flex his or her neck forward, and palpate the posterior spinous processes. You may palpate two processes: The superior one is C7, and the inferior one is T1.

6. *NIPPLES*: They are located lateral to the proximal end of the sternum, just superior to the xyphoid process.

Infants

When palpating the chest of an infant, be gentle, and be sure to warm your hands before placing them on the child's chest..Use your fingers pads to gently palpate the entire chest wall, both anterior and posterior, being aware of any areas of tenderness and noting skin temperature and moisture. Also palpate for any superficial lumps or masses, or for skin lesions noted on inspection.

Palpating the infant's chest can further be performed by assessing for tactile fremitus. Vocal fremitus can be heard when you listen to the chest and lungs. When the child cries, vibrations can be felt on the chest and are termed tactile fremitus. Cries or speech sounds are conducted from the larynx through the tracheobronchial tree to the lung parenchyma and the chest wall. By placing your hands on the chest and feeling for vibrations, you can assess information regarding the density of the underlying lung tissue. Consolidation, increased fluid, or a mass that increases the density of the lung and makes it more solid will increase the transmission of vibrations and will therefore increase tactile fremitus.

When palpating the chest of an infant, simply place your hands on the infant's chest when he or she is crying. There will be increased vibrations felt with tactile fremitus if there is any kind of consolidation such as fluid or a mass. Remember, the infant's chest is hyperresonant throughout; therefore, it is often difficult to assess for abnormalities. Another technique used to assess for tactile fremitus is to place your hands (with particular emphasis on your finger pads) over each side of the infant's chest.

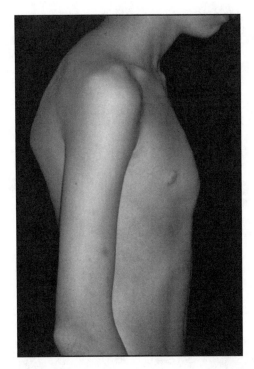

Figure 9-10(a)   Pectus Carinatum (Pigeon Chest)

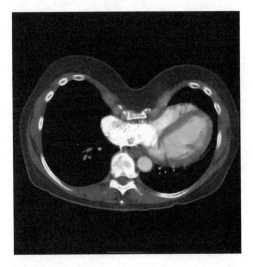

Figure 9-10(b)   Pectus Excavatum (Funnel Chest)

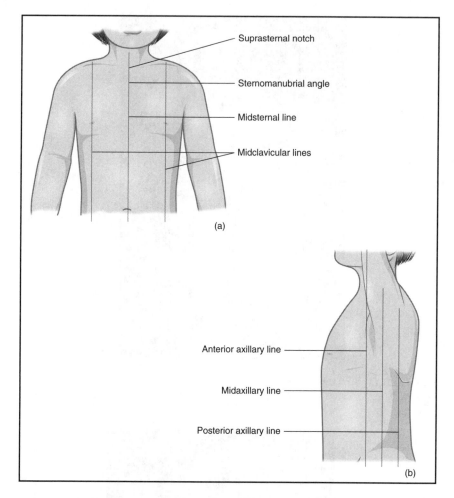

Figure 9-11 Thoracic Cage Landmarks

During crying or other noises, you can feel for symmetry in the transmitted vibrations.

Toddlers and School-Age Children

Palpation in the toddler is similar to that of infant. In the school-age child who can sit on the table, you can assess for tactile fremitus by placing your hands on the child's back starting at the second intercostal space, at the level of the bifurcation of the bronchi. If the child is cooperative, you can ask him or her to say "ninety-nine" or "blue moon," which generates strong vibrations, or simply ask the child questions so that he or she is speaking to you. During palpation, increased vibrations will be elicited if there is a marked density in the lungs and if there is a sufficiently large consolidation of lung tissue. In children with small areas of early pneumonia, increased vibrations will not be felt. When assessing for tactile fremitus, you may note that vibrations feel stronger on the right side than on the left. This is because the right side is closer to the bronchial bifurcation. Also, vibrations are generally more prominent between the scapulae and around the sternum where the major bronchi are closest to the chest wall. Fremitus decreases as you move downward on the chest because more and more tissue impedes sound transmission.

Remember that conditions that increase the density of lung tissue make a better conducting medium for sound vibrations and consequently increase tactile fremitus.

Adolescents

Palpation of the adolescent's thorax is the same as that in the adult. Start with the adolescent in an upright position. To perform posterior palpation, place your finger pads on the apex of the right or left lung, approximately at the level of T1. Using light palpation, initially assess the skin of the throax, then move your finger pads down to the first thoracic vertebra and palpate by proceeding down over each vertebra, assessing for tenderness, bulges, depressions, or masses. Repeat this procedure from top to bottom of the posterior chest, palpating between the intercostal spaces on both the right and left side, assessing for tenderness, masses, or lumps.

Thoracic expansion assesses the extent of chest wall expansion and is determined by standing behind the child and placing both your thumbs at the level of the 10th spinal vertebra. With your palms lightly on the posterolateral thorax, ask the child to take a deep breath, and observe the movement of your thumbs, noting the distance they separate. Your thumbs should separate an equal distance from the spinal column on each side. The normal distance for the thumbs to separate during thoracic expansion is 3–5 cm (Estes, 2006, p. 388). Lack of expansion or decreased expansion occurs with pneumothorax, pneumonia, atelectasis, and pleural effusion.

To assess for *tactile fremitus*, ask the adolescent to sit in an upright position and stand behind him or her. Three different aspects of the hand can be used to assess tactile fremitus—the palmar bases of the fingers, the ulnar aspect of the hand, or the ulnar aspect of the closed fist. Start by placing the ulnar aspect of both hands or palmar bases on the adolescent's posterior chest just above the scapulae, and position your hands on each side of the spinal column. Instruct the child to say "ninety-nine" or "one, two, three." You are feeling for any vibration on the ulnar aspect of your hand as the patient speaks. Compare vibrations on both sides of the posterior chest.

Move your hands down 2 to 3 inches and repeat the process until you are at the base of the lungs.

During this procedure, you should feel a buzzing or vibration on the ulnar aspect of your hand or the palmar surface. The vibrations will be more pronounced near the major bronchi and the trachea and will be less palpable in the periphery of the lungs. If there is a consolidation due to pneumonia or atelectasis, you will feel increased tactile fremitus because a compressed lung or consolidation will conduct sound better than air. If there is decreased tactile fremitus, think of more porous lung tissue associated with emphysema, asthma, or pneumothorax. In an obese child, you will note decreased tactile fremitus because the sound waves are dampened as they pass through adipose tissue, creating a greater distance.

Percussion

Infants
Percussion is generally not performed in the infant. Hyperresonance is heard throughout the infant's chest, making it difficult to detect abnormalities through percussion.

Toddlers and School-Age Children
If the child is cooperative, percussion is performed while the child is sitting on the parent's lap or on the table. The technique of percussion is to tap on a surface to determine the underlying structure. The sound produced from tapping on a child's chest wall is dependent upon the air–tissue ratio. Percussion over a solid organ, such as the liver, produces a dull, low-amplitude sound without resonance. Percussion over an area containing air within the tissue, such as the lung, produces a resonant, higher-amplitude sound. Percussion over a hollow, air-containing structure, such as the upper part of the stomach, produces a tympanic, high-pitched hollow sound. Percussion over a solid mass, such as the scapula, produces a flat sound. In a child with pneumonia, when the lungs are filled with fluid and are, therefore, denser, resonance is replaced by dullness. Hyperresonance is a sound heard by percussing over hyperinflated lungs, such as in emphysema in the adult or possibly asthma in the child.

To perform percussion on the school-age child, the child needs to be sitting straight up on the examining table. You cannot percuss adequately through clothing, so the child should be in a hospital gown that opens in the back. If the child is fearful or evidencing concern, demonstrate what you will be doing. Show the child how to percuss by using the table or even percussing on the child's leg. Tell the child it does not hurt and makes a funny sound like a drum. In examining the child, use the middle finger

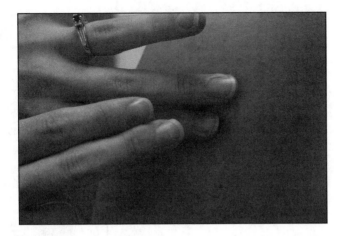

Figure 9-12   Technique of Percussion

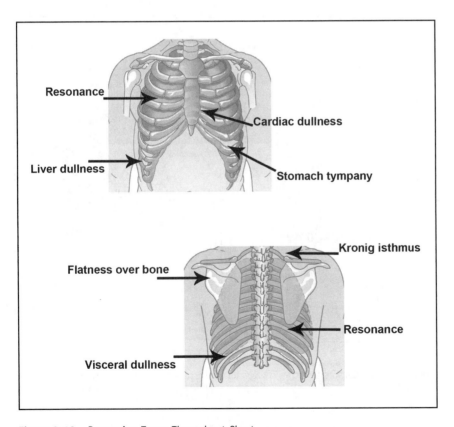

Figure 9-13   Percussion Tones Throughout Chest

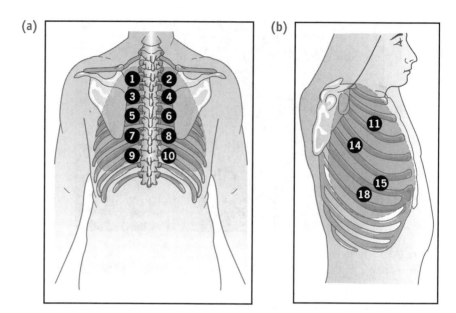

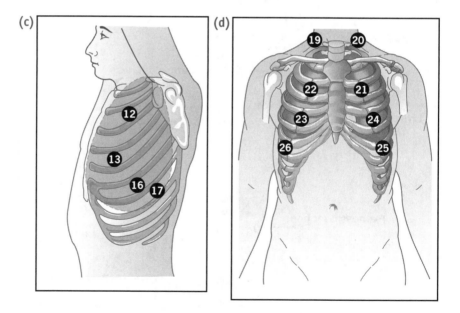

Figure 9-14 Suggested Sequence for Systematic Percussion and Auscultation of the Thorax

of your left hand and place it firmly against the child's chest wall parallel to the ribs in an interspace, with palm and other fingers held off of the chest. The tip of the right middle finger strikes a quick sharp blow with the terminal phalanx of the left finger on the chest wall. Note that to perform percussion correctly, the motion of the striking finger should come from the wrist and not from the elbow. When percussing, start with the posterior chest at the level of the apices, and move your hands symmetrically down along each side, alternating between the left and right sides, and percussing in the interspaces and making a side-to-side comparison over the lung region. The sounds produced during percussion are resonant—low-pitched, clear, hollow sounds. If necessary, percussion can be performed on the anterior upper chest wall.

Adolescents

Percussion in the adolescent follows the same pattern as that of the adult. Start with the adolescent in an upright position leaning slightly forward and with the arms folded across the chest. Percuss the apex of either the left or right lung located along the top of the shoulder. Two to three percussion strikes should be adequate. Repeat this process on the other side, noting the sound produced from each percussion strike. If the sound is not resonant, then pathology should be suspected. Move down the posterior chest approximately 5 cm or every other intercostal space and percuss in each area. Be sure to percuss in the intercostal space, not on the rib, as that will produce a flat sound.

Remember, normal lung tissue produces a resonant sound, although in a thin adolescent hyperresonance may be normal. Continue to percuss down the entire back, alternating side to side, in the same position on the contralateral side to the base of the lungs. Percussion of the anterior chest is performed in the same manner. If assessing an adolescent female, percuss the upper chest, then percuss over the lateral sides of the anterior chest.

Auscultations

The following table presents normal respiratory rates by age (Ball, Bindler, & Cowen, 2010):

Age	Breaths/min
Newborn	30–60
1 year	20–40
3 years	20–30
10 years	16–22
17 years	12–20

Characteristics of Normal Breath Sounds

As air moves through the tracheobronchial tree, different breath sounds are generated. These sounds are characterized by their pitch, intensity, and quality, and by the relative duration of inspiration and expiration. Normal breath sounds are classified as vesicular, bronchovesicular, and bronchial.

An important note is that in infants and toddlers, all sounds may sound like bronchovesicular and you may not hear much differentiation. In the school-age child and adolescent, differentiation of characteristic breath sounds is more clearly audible.

- *BRONCHIAL BREATH SOUNDS* are the loudest and highest in pitch and sound like air rushing through a tube or blowing through the trees. Expiratory sounds last longer than inspiratory sounds.
- *BRONCHOVESICULAR SOUNDS* are easily heard, but not quite as loud or harsh as bronchial sounds, and inspiratory and expiratory sounds are approximately equal in length.
- *VESICULAR BREATH SOUNDS* are the softest and lowest-pitched sounds. They are heard through inspiration and continue without pause through expiration.

When auscultating for breath sounds it is always helpful before placing the stethoscope on the chest to ask child to cover his or her mouth and "give a big cough" in order to clear any mucus from their bronchial tree. Also ask him or her to breathe with their mouth open and in slow deep breaths. Breathing through their mouth versus their nose decreases the potential of confusing upper airway noise that may be confused with adventitious sounds. If the child has an upper respiratory infection, nasal congestion, or allergies, sounds through the nose may be coarse, increased, and harsh sounding.

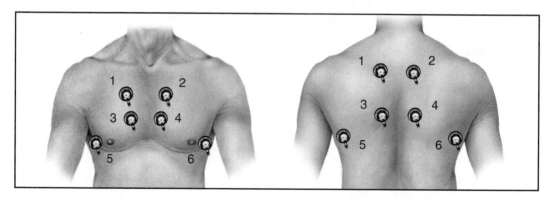

Figure 9-15 Breath Sounds

Characteristics of Adventitious Breath Sounds

In children it may be more difficult to distinguish normal from adventitious breath sounds such as *crackles*, *wheezes*, and *rhonchi.*, and '*stridor*' These abnormal breath sounds are the same as those heard in the adult patient.

- *CRACKLES* or *RALES* are short, discontinuous nonmusical sounds heard mostly during inspiration. They indicate the opening of a collapsed airway and collapsed alveoli. They are caused by the passage of air through the small airways in the lungs that have become sticky and adherent due to the presence of fluid and/or mucus, as in cystic fibrosis, lower respiratory tract infections, congestive heart failure, or pneumonia. They are often described as sounding like the noise made by rubbing hair next to the ear or the noise made when Velcro is opened.
- *WHEEZES* are continuous, musical, high-pitched sounds heard primarily during both inspiration and expiration. They are produced as the result of narrowing of the bronchi. The narrowing of the lumen of the bronchi may be due to bronchospasm associated with asthma, or inflammation and increased secretions associated with lower respiratory tract infections such as bronchiolitis or bronchitis. Localized or unilateral wheezes may be audible with ingestion of a foreign body that is lodged in a specific area of the bronchial tree. A tumor compressing a part of the bronchial tree can also create a consistent wheeze at the site of the compression.
- *RHONCHI* are lower-pitched sonorous sounds. They are caused by air passing through an airway obstructed with thick secretions and mucus plugging. An important point in differentiating rales from rhonchi and wheezes is that after coughing and clearing secretions from the bronchial tree, rhonchi and wheezes may have resolved, but rales will not clear after coughing. Rales are associated with a consolidation such as in pneumonia.
- *STRIDOR* is a high-pitched inspiratory sound associated with ingestion of a foreign object, or heard with croup (laryngotracheobronchitis). It generally can be heard without the stethoscope.

In conjunction with adventitious sounds are coughs, which are a common symptom of a respiratory problem. Coughs are reflexive responses to an irritant in the tracheobronchial tree. They are described based on the following characteristics: moisture, frequency, regularity, and quality.

- *MOIST COUGHS* are associated with infections and are usually accompanied by sputum production. In children, a productive cough can easily be heard, although actual production of the mucus rarely occurs. As children cough and the mucus reaches the back of the throat, it is automatically swallowed. Infants and toddlers with moist, productive coughs will cough, bringing the mucus to the back of their throat and initiating their gag reflex. This in turn ultimately causes vomiting. In young children with lower respiratory tract infections, vomiting may be the only way they can effectively clear their tracheobronchial tree. Parents are often disturbed by the vomiting and call for medical assistance. On questioning, it is evident that the vomiting is not due to a gastrointestinal problem, but rather is due to an overabundance of loose secretions in the tracheobronchial tree.

- *FREQUENCY* of the cough may increase in the presence of allergens. Children with environmental allergens may have an increased cough while outside or in the presence of the irritant. Children with asthma will have increased coughing while in the presence of specific triggers such as cigarette smoke or animal dander.
- *REGULARITY* of a cough may be associated with pertussis, which is evident in the paroxysmal nature of the cough.
- *QUALITY* of a cough is heard in a child with croup, which produces a dry, squeaky, seal-like or barking cough.

Infants

When auscultating the infant's lungs, an important note is to "seize the opportunity" to examine the lungs and heart when the child is sleeping or comfortably resting on the parent's shoulder. Start by gently placing a warmed stethoscope on the child's back without causing too much disturbance. The child is generally quiet and comfortable while being held by a

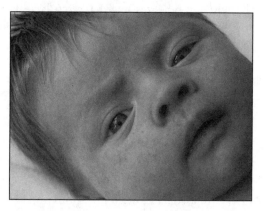

Figure 9-16(a)   Nasal Flaring

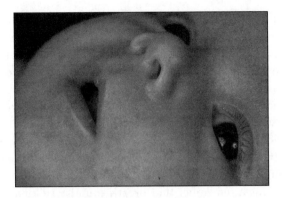

Figure 9-16(b)   Normal Nostrils

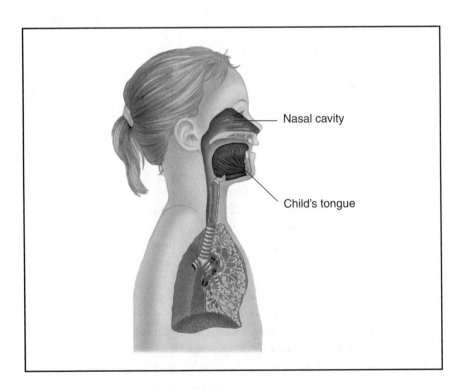

Figure 9-17   The Nasal Cavity in a Child

parent. It is always helpful if you can auscultate lung sounds when the child is not crying in order to maximize auscultation in the localization of findings. In this position, auscultate the posterior chest and then gently come around to the anterior chest as well. If the child is crying, the deep inspirations between cries will actually provide you with enhanced breath sounds.

While listening to the anterior chest, *seize the opportunity* to also auscultate heart sounds. (Heart sounds are addressed in Chapter 10.) It is particularly difficult to listen to the heart when a child is crying. It is hard enough to differentiate respiratory sounds from cardiac sounds in a baby, but this becomes even more difficult when the child is crying. While listening to the lungs, remember that breath sounds are louder and harsher than in the adult because the chest wall is thinner with less adipose tissue and muscle, and you are closer to the origin of the sounds. As mentioned earlier, breathing in newborns is usually intermittent with slow and shallow breaths, then rapid and deep breaths. When auscultating the infant's chest, you will hear primarily bronchovesicular breath sounds throughout due to the thin chest walls and underdeveloped musculature.

When auscultating the infant's thorax, start with the posterior chest and hold the diaphragm of the stethoscope firmly on the child's chest wall. Remember, the stethoscope generally has two heads, the bell and the diaphragm. The bell is used to detect low-pitched sounds, and the diaphragm is better at detecting higher-pitched sounds. When using the diaphragm, it is firmly applied to the skin, whereas the bell is loosely applied to the skin. If it is pressed too tightly, the skin will act as a diaphragm, and the lower-pitched sounds will be filtered out. Try to listen to one full respiration (one inhalation and one exhalation) in each location. Side-to-side comparison is most important. In infants, it is easy to confuse background noise with lungs sounds, such as heart sounds, bowel sounds, and, more importantly, upper airway sounds that come from the nasopharynx. These sounds are typically coarser, harsher, and louder. In the infant, it is not unusual to hear fine crackles and transient hoarseness. After auscultating the posterior chest, come around to the anterior chest and follow the same pattern; start at the apex of the lungs and auscultate going down from side to side. Also, it is important to listen at the axillary chest wall.

Remember, in the infant the small chest cavity allows sound waves to travel more quickly, making the location and differentiation of adventitious lung sounds more difficult to hear. Using a stethoscope with a pediatric diaphragm will help in decreasing ambient noise. It takes practice in listening to lung sounds in children to differentiate what you hear.

Toddlers and School-Age Children

When examining toddlers and/or school-age children, remember to approach them cautiously and *do not* immediately place your stethoscope on their chest. This will only frighten the child and lead to crying and an uncooperative patient. If the child is sitting on the parent's lap, pull up a stool so you are eye level. Let the child play with your stethoscope by placing it on his or her chest. You may even have to place it on the parent's arm or chest and slowly move it toward the child. Another technique is to encourage the child to place the stethoscope on his or her chest while you place your hand over the child's. Slowly move it from side to side with the child moving the diaphragm along with you. This technique generally works and provides you with a quiet, cooperative patient and the opportunity to listen to breath sounds, both inspiratory and expiratory, that are clear of crying or other extraneous noise.

If you are examining young school-age children, you may find it helpful to ask if they want to listen to their lungs first. If they say yes, gently place the earpieces of the stethoscope in their ears and place the stethoscope on their chest so they can hear their lung sounds. Some children will then place the stethoscope on your chest as well, imitating the role of the provider. School-age children and adolescents will often require more explanation as to why the assessment is necessary. In preadolescents and adolescent females, the concern of modesty becomes an issue. Always respect the needs of the child whose body is changing during preadolescence and adolescence, and be sensitive in moving and/or removing clothing. If possible, keep the child covered, while gently placing the stethoscope under the child's clothing to listen. An important point is to not listen over clothing. Doing so only increases friction and ambient noise, making it more difficult to discern adventitious from normal breath sounds.

Adolescents

Auscultation of the adolescent's lungs follows the same pattern as that of the adult. Start by having adolescents sit upright, then ask them to cover their mouth and cough to clear any mucus from the bronchial tree before you begin. Ask adolescents to bend their head forward slightly and cross or fold their arms in front of themselves in order to enlarge the lung area that is auscultated. Start by placing the diaphragm over the apex of the lungs on either the right or left side of the posterior chest. The apex is located along the top of the shoulder. Then, using the diaphragm, alternate from side to side, from top to bottom of the posterior chest. Be sure to listen for one complete respiratory cycle (one inhalation and one exhalation). Continue to move the stethoscope down approximately 5 cm or every other intercostal space, comparing contralateral sides until the entire posterior lung has been assessed. Remember to ask the adolescent to breathe in and out through the mouth, thus decreasing air turbulence that can interfere with interpretation of breath sounds (Estes, 2006, p. 389).

Auscultation of the anterior chest follows the same pattern. If you are assessing an adolescent female with large breasts, listen to the upper chest area, then auscultate along the lateral sides of the anterior chest.

Common Respiratory Disorders in Children

Infants

BRONCHIOLITIS is a lower respiratory tract infection that presents in children younger than 2 years of age. It is characterized by wheezing and airway obstruction. It is caused by a viral infection resulting in inflammation of the

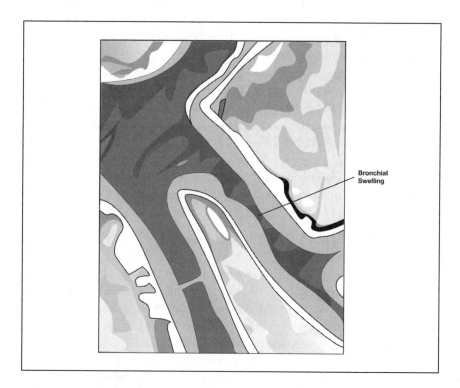

Bronchial Swelling

Figure 9-18 Swelling of the Bronchiole Walls

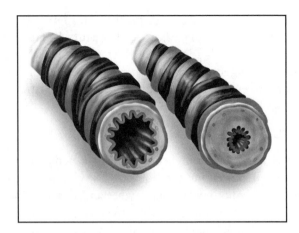

Figure 9-19   Lungs and Inflamed and Normal Bronchial Tubes

small airways/bronchioles (Piedra, 2010). The most common pathogen is RSV. It typically is seen in late fall and winter and is the most common cause of lower respiratory tract infections in children.

SIDS (SUDDEN INFANT DEATH SYNDROME) is the leading cause of mortality for children between 1 month and 1 year of age in the United States. It is defined as the sudden death of an infant younger than 1 year of age, which remains unexplained after a thorough case investigation, including performance of a complete autopsy, examination of the death scene, and review of the clinical history (CDC, 1996).

ALTE (APPARENT LIFE-THREATENING EVENT) is an acute, unexpected change in an infant's breathing behavior that was frightening to the infant's caretaker and that included some combination of the following features: (1) apnea, usually involving no respiratory effort (central) or sometimes involving effort with difficulty (obstructive); (2) color change that is usually cyanotic or pallid; (3) marked decrease in muscle tone resulting in limpness; and (4) choking or gagging.

BRONCHOPULMONARY DYSPLASIA presents in premature births requiring positive-pressure ventilation for respiratory failure. Clinical manifestations include persistent signs of increased respiratory effort, including tachypnea, nasal flaring, grunting, retractions, and irritability. There may also be pulmonary edema, wheezing and crackles, bronchospasms, and mucus plugging (Ball et al., 2010).

RESPIRATORY DISTRESS SYNDROME presents in premature infants generally less than 36 weeks of gestation. It occurs because the infant's underdeveloped lungs lack adequate surfactant to keep the alveoli open. With inadequate oxygen, premature infants develop dyspnea, hypoxia, and cyanosis that require oxygen administration and often mechanical ventilation.

School-Age Children and Adolescents

ASTHMA is the most common chronic illness in pediatric patients. It is defined as a chronic, inflammatory lung disease characterized by chronic inflammation, with symptoms of cough, wheezing, dyspnea and chest tightness, bronchoconstriction, and bronchial hyperresponsiveness to a variety of stimuli such as animal dander, cigarette smoke, or pungent fumes.

CROUP, also called laryngotracheobronchitis, is a viral respiratory illness characterized by inspiratory stridor, cough, and hoarseness. These symptoms result from inflammation in the larynx and subglottic airway. A barking cough is the hallmark of croup among infants and young children. Hoarseness presents more commonly in adolescents. Croup is usually a mild and self-limited illness (Woods, 2009).

BRONCHITIS (lower respiratory tract infection) is inflammation of the trachea and bronchi. The presenting symptom is a dry, hacking cough with increased severity at night (Ball et al., 2010).

UPPER RESPIRATORY INFECTION, one of the most common viral illnesses of early childhood, presents with nasal congestion, rhinorrhea, poor appetite, irritability, decreased activity level, fever, and congested cough.

PNEUMONIA can result from either a bacterial or viral infection associated with an acute inflammation of the pulmonary parenchyma and consolidation of the alveoli. In infancy and early childhood, pneumonia is usually caused by viruses, such as RSV, influenza, and adenovirus. In children older than 5 years, bacteria are more commonly the cause, such as *Streptococcus pneumoniae* and *Mycoplasma pneumoniae*. Regardless of the etiology, symptoms include fever (lower with viral pneumonia), crackles, wheezes, cough, dyspnea, and tachypnea.

FOREIGN BODY ASPIRATION is the inhalation of a solid, liquid, or object into the respiratory tract. It occurs most commonly while a toddler is crawling and putting small objects in their mouth Although most prevalent during toddlerhood, it can occur at any age in childhood.

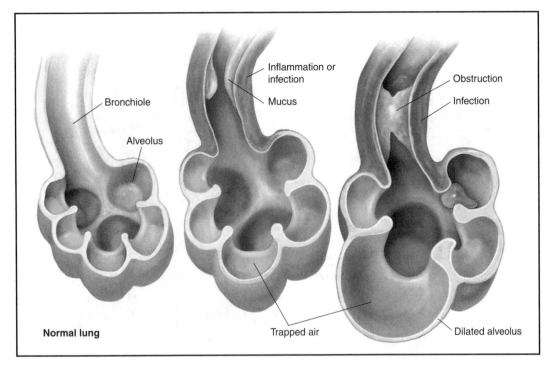

Figure 9-20   What Can Cause an Asthmatic Episode?

The following respiratory signs warrant prompt action if noted in a child. Aggressive intervention should be instituted as quickly as possible to prevent the child from going into cardiopulmonary arrest (Krost, Mistovich, & Limmer, 2006).

- Respiratory rate greater than 60 breaths/min
- Significant hemorrhage
- Respiratory distress or failure
- Significant trauma
- Nasal flaring
- Alterations in mentation
- Uncorrected noisy respiration
- Seizures

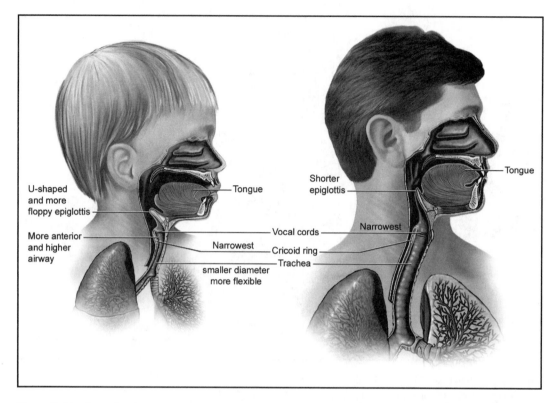

Figure 9-21 Croup Syndrome

- Cyanosis
- Fever or history of fever with a global rash
- Mottling
- Heart rate greater than 180 beats/min
- Pallor
- Heart rate less than 60 beats/min

Other red flags to be aware of are *epiglottitis,* which is a medical emergency. It is inflammation and swelling of the supraglottic structures and may progress to complete airway obstruction. It is less frequently seen today due to *Haemophilus* influenzae b vaccine. Another medical condition requiring immediate referral is the school-age child or adolescent who presents with an *asthma exacerbation* without response to his or her bronchodilator or steroids and with O_2 saturation levels below 90%.

Write-Up of the Chest Exam

EXAMPLE FOR INFANTS/TODDLERS: Chest is symmetric and expansion equal with respiration, no retractions, AP diameter approximate to transverse diameter. Chest is normal to palpation, without lumps, masses, or tenderness. Equal fremitus with crying, bronchovesicular breath sounds heard bilaterally, no adventitious breath sounds auscultated.

EXAMPLE FOR SCHOOL-AGE CHILDREN AND ADOLESCENTS: AP diameter < lateral with 1:2 ratio. Muscle and respiratory effort symmetric without use of accessory muscles, trachea midline, tactile fremitus symmetric, lungs resonant to percussion bilaterally, lungs clear throughout without adventitious sounds.

Case Study: Adolescent Girl Presenting with Respiratory Symptoms

Rebecca is a 16-year-old who presents with a 1-week history of recurrent wheezing, dry cough, shortness of breath, and tightness in her chest. Her past medical history indicates that she has a 3-year history of asthma that is exacerbated by upper respiratory infections. She tells you that she has been using her beta-2 agonists (albuterol HFA) more than the recommended three times per day and is not getting relief. She also admits that she frequently wakes during the night with asthma symptoms.

On examination, HEENT is normal. Her lung exam reveals diffuse expiratory wheezes, hyperresonance on percussion, and a prolonged expiratory phase. Her O_2 saturation was 90 on room air.

Questions
1. Based on her history, how would you characterize her asthma?
2. What would you initially do for this patient?
3. What is your plan of care for this patient?

Answers
1. Rebecca's asthma would be classified as moderate persistent based on the criteria established by the National Asthma Education and Prevention Program.
2. The treatment plan for Rebecca would include one of two long-term controller regimens for patients with moderate persistent asthma: either medium-dose inhaled glucocorticoids alone, or the combination of low-dose inhaled glucocorticoids and a long-acting beta agonist.

3. The educational plan for Rebecca should provide a personalized "asthma action plan," which describes how and when her medications should be used, as well as how to recognize an exacerbation and make appropriate adjustments in her medications (Peters, McCallister, & Pascual, 2008).

References

Ball, J., Bindler, R., & Cowen, K. (2010). *Child health nursing*. Upper Saddle River, NJ: Pearson.

Centers for Disease Control and Prevention. (1996). Sudden infant death syndrome—United States, 1983–1994. *Morbidity and Mortality Weekly Report, 45*(40), 859–863.

Estes, M. (1998). *Health assessment and physical examination*. Albany, NY: Delmar Publishers.

Froh, (2006). Alterations in pulmonary function in children. In K.I McCance & S.E. Huether (Eds.) Pathophysiology: The biologic basis for disease in adults and children (5th ed.). (1249–1278) St. Louis, MO: Elsevier/Mosby. From Ball, J., Bindler, R., Cowen, K. (2010). *Child health nursing*, (2nd ed.). Pearson.

Jarvis, C. (2004). *Physical examination and health assessment* (5th ed.). St. Louis, MO: Elsevier.

Krost, W. S., Mistovich, J. J., & Limmer, D. (2006). Retrieved July 10, 2010, from *EMSresponder.com* Web site: http://www.emsresponder.com/publication/bio.jsp?id=200&pubId=1

Peters, S., McCallister, J., & Pascual, R. (2008). Treatment of moderate persistent asthma in adolescents and adults. Retrieved July 7, 2010, from *Uptodate.com* Web site: http://www.uptodate.com/patients/content/topic.do?topicKey=~L6u86w4DzvF48

Piedra, P. A., Stark, A. R. (2010). Broncholitis in infants and children: Clinical features and diagnosis. *UpToDate*.

Woods, C. R. (2009). Patient Information: Croup in infants and children. *UpToDate*.

Resources

Bickley, L. (2003). *Bates' guide to physical examination and history taking* (8th ed.). New York: Lippincott Williams & Wilkins.

Hansen, M. (1998). *Pathophysiology: Foundations of disease and clinical intervention*. Philadelphia: Saunders.

Marieb, E. (2000). *Human anatomy and physiology* (3rd ed.). Redwood City, CA: Benjamin/Cummings Publishing Company.

Potts, N., & Mandleco, B. (2007). *Pediatraic nursing* (2nd ed.). Victoria, Australia: Thomson, Delmar Learning.

Tortora, G. J., & Grabvowski, S. R. (2003). *Principles of anatomy and physiology* (10th ed.). New York: Wiley.

Cardiovascular Examination

Anatomy and Physiology

The heart is located in the thoracic cavity between the lungs and above the diaphragm in the mediastinum. The uppermost portion of the heart, or the base, includes the left and right atria, the aorta, pulmonary arteries, and the superior and inferior venae cavae. These structures are situated behind the upper portion of the sternum. The lower portion, or apex, of the heart extends into the left thoracic cavity. The apex contacts the chest wall between the fifth and sixth ribs, and it is here that you can palpate the point of maximal impulse (PMI).

The heart wall has several layers. The pericardium is the tough fibrous double-walled sac that surrounds and protects the heart. It is composed of serous and fibrous layers, the outermost layer being the fibrous layer that is connected to the diaphragm and sternum by ligaments and tendons. During strenuous activity, the fibrous layer limits the stretching of the myocardial muscle. The serous layer is made up of two layers, the parietal layer and the visceral layer. Between these two layers is a small space called the pericardial cavity, which contains pericardial fluid that ensures smooth, friction-free movement of the heart muscle. If inflammation occurs in the pericardium secondary to bacterial pneumonia, pericarditis develops. This condition hinders production of serous fluid and in turn roughens the serous membrane, creating a rustling sound (pericardial friction rub). Pericarditis causes pain and shortness of breath, as these two layers stick together and impede contractility of the heart.

The other layer of the heart is the myocardium, which is the main muscular wall of the heart. It contracts and does the pumping. The endocardium is the thin layer of endothelium that lines the heart chambers and covers the connective tissue of the valves. This endocardium is continuous with the endothelial linings of the blood vessels leaving and entering the heart.

Chambers of the Heart

The heart is divided into two circuits—the right side, or the pulmonary circuit, and the left side, or the systemic circuit. The heart has four chambers—two superior atria and two inferior ventricles. The internal partition that divides the heart from the base to the apex is the interventricular septum. The atria receive blood returning to the heart through three veins: the superior vena cava, which returns blood from areas superior to the diaphragm; the inferior vena cava, which returns blood from areas below the diaphragm; and the coronary sinus, which collects blood draining from the myocardium itself. In addition, pulmonary veins enter the left atrium and transport blood from the lungs back to the heart.

The ventricles compose the larger portion of the heart. The right ventricle forms most of the heart's anterior surface, while the left ventricle dominates its inferior surface. The ventricles, due to their large muscular walls, are the pumping mechanism of the heart. When the right ventricle contracts, blood is pumped into the pulmonary vessels where it is directed to the lungs and gas exchange takes place. The left ventricle pumps blood into the aorta, which is the largest artery, and acts as a means to route systematic circulation throughout the body.

Within the four chambers are four valves. The first two, the atrioventricular (AV) valves, separate the atria and the ventricles and prevent backflow into the atria during contraction of the ventricles. The right AV valve, the tricuspid, has three flexible flaps of endocardium. The left AV valve, is called the bicuspid valve and also the mitral valve because of its resemblance to a bishop's hat. Chordae tendineae are tiny white collagen cords that are attached to the flaps of the valves, anchoring them to the ventricular wall. During circulation, when the heart is at rest (diastole), the AV valves are relaxed. Blood flows into the atria and then easily flows into the descending ventricle, also referred to as the filling phase. When the ventricle contracts, called the pumping phase (systole), the pressure inside increases, forcing blood up against the flap edges and closing them. The chordae tendineae come into play and act as anchors keeping the valve flaps in their closed position. If the chordae tendinae are malformed or damaged they will not close properly allowing blood to leak backward leading to valvular regurgitation.

The other two valves in the heart are the aortic and pulmonary semilunar valves. They function differently than the AV valves. During contraction, the semilunar valves—the pulmonic valve in the right side of the heart and the aortic valve in the left side of the heart—are forced open and their flaps (or cusps) are flattened against the arterial walls as the intraventricular pressure exceeds the pressure in the aorta and pulmonary vessels. Blood is then ejected or forced out of the heart, while back-flowing blood fills the valve cusps and closes the valves.

An important consideration is that occasionally valves are termed "leaky," or "impaired." This implies that an incompetent valve forces the heart to pump and repump the same blood as the valve does not properly close; subsequently there is blood backflow. For example, in untreated streptococcal pharyngitis, a common disorder in pediatrics, bacteria develop on the valve flaps, hampering them from closing properly and thereby causing the heart to contract more forcibly and ultimately leading to a weakened heart muscle.

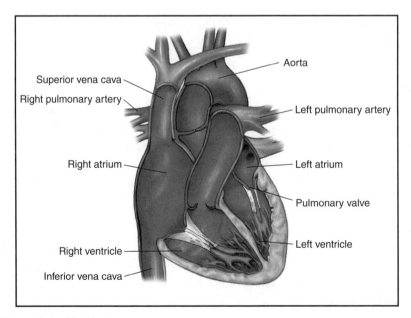

Figure 10-1   The Heart

Remember that there are no valves between the vena cava and the right atrium and between the pulmonary veins and the left atrium. Although not commonly seen in children, high blood pressure in the left side of the heart results in symptoms of pulmonary congestion such as congestive heart failure, and subsequent high blood pressure in the right side of the heart is evidenced by distention of the neck veins.

Circulation of Blood

Blood flows from an area of higher pressure to one of lower pressure, as follows (Jarvis, 2008, p. 485):

- Blood flows from the liver to the right atrium through the inferior vena cava.
- The superior vena cava drains venous blood from the head and upper extremities.
- From the right atrium, venous blood travels through the tricuspid valve to the right ventricle.
- From the right ventricle, venous blood flows through the pulmonic valve to the pulmonary artery. The pulmonary artery delivers unoxygenated blood to the lungs
- Lungs oxygenate the blood. Pulmonary veins return fresh blood to the left atrium.
- From the left atrium, arterial blood travels through the mitral valve to the left ventricle where it is ejected through the aortic valve into the aorta.
- The aorta delivers oxygenated blood to the body.

Heart Sounds

The rhythmic movement of blood through the heart constitutes the cardiac cycle. It has two distinct phases: diastole, when the ventricles relax and fill with blood, and systole, when blood is pumped from the ventricles and fills the pulmonary and systemic arteries. Two distinguishable sounds are heard in conjunction with closure of the heart valves. They are described as *lub-dub*. The first heart sound that occurs is the closure of the AV valves, which signifies the onset of systole, when ventricular pressure is higher than atrial pressure. This sound, termed S_1, is louder, longer, and more resonant than the second heart sound (S_2). The closure of the AV valves prevents any regurgitation of blood into the atria during contraction. The mitral component of this first heart sound slightly precedes the tricuspid valves as they close.

The second heart sound you hear is closure of the semilunar valves. After blood is ejected from the ventricles, pressure falls. When this pressure falls

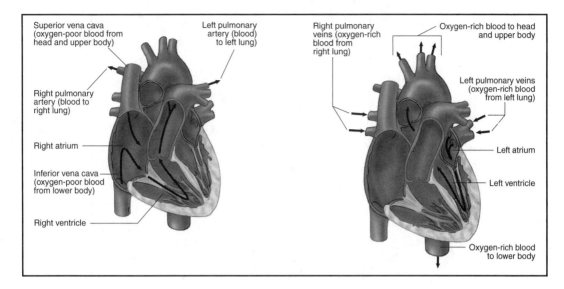

Figure 10-2 Heart–Blood Flow

below that in the aorta, some blood flows backward toward the ventricle, causing the aortic valve to close. As these valves close, you hear a short, sharp sound, S_2, that is softer and less resonant than S_1. The sound signals the beginning of ventricular diastole, or the end of systole. *When listening to the heart, S_1 is loudest at the apex, and S_2 is loudest at the base.*

Development of the Heart

By 22 days of gestation, the endothelial tubes that form the heart have fused to form a single chamber, or heart tube. Shortly afterward, the earliest heart chambers are evident, and gradually during the next 3 weeks, structural changes occur that convert the heart into a four-chamber pumping organ. By month 2 of gestation, few changes occur other than growth until birth.

During gestation, blood flows from the placenta to the fetus through the umbilical vein. Blood enters the right atrium of the heart through the ductus venosus, which is the fetal vascular channel between the umbilical vein and the inferior vena cava. The foramen ovale, which connects the two atria, allows blood to flow from the right to the left atrium and into the left ventricle, thus bypassing the pulmonary circuit and the nonfunctional fetal lungs. The ductus arteriosus is the fetal vascular channel between the pulmonary artery and the descending aorta, another fetal circulatory bypass

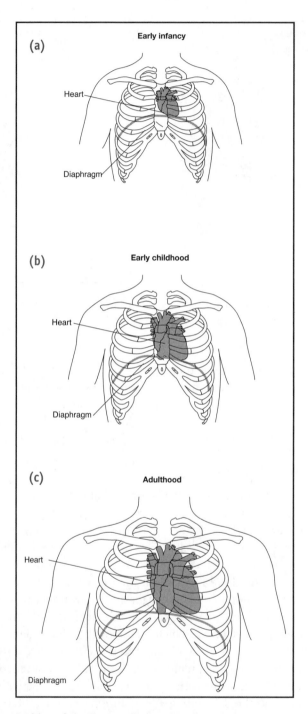

Figure 10-3 Position of the Heart at Various Ages

that closes shortly after birth. Blood eventually returns to the placenta by way of the umbilical arteries.

During fetal circulation, blood with the highest oxygen content is circulated to the heart and the brain. Because systemic vascular resistance is low, blood flows easily to the extremities. At birth, when the umbilical cord is cut, the lungs inflate and the newborn quickly adapts to receiving oxygen from the lungs. (More detail on the transition from fetal to pulmonary circulation is provided in Chapter 4.)

Cardiovascular Differences in the Child

A number of cardiovascular changes occur in the child. Due to fetal circulation, the infant's heart is proportionately larger in relation to body size than an adult's. Because of high pulmonary resistance during fetal life, the right ventricle is larger than the left at birth. Once the transition to extrauterine life is complete, the pulmonary resistance drops, and within two months, the right ventricle reduces in size.

The higher systemic vascular pressure forces the left ventricle to quickly develop. The decrease in pulmonary vascular resistance at birth leads to thinning of the small pulmonary arteriole lining and, subsequently, increases in the diameter of these blood vessels. The pulmonary environment matures and develops in response to lung growth. With these changes, adult levels of pulmonary resistance are achieved by 2 months of age. In the infant, the muscle fibers of the heart are less developed and organized, and the heart is more sensitive to volume pressure overload, all of which lead to limited functional capacity, placing young babies at risk for developing heart failure. As the child grows, the heart muscle fibers develop, and by 9 years of age, the weight of the heart has increased by six times (Connor, 2006). By the time the child has reached puberty, the systolic blood pressure has risen to adult levels.

As the infant transitions from fetal to extrauterine life, the metabolic rate and oxygen requirements double. With this change, a higher heart rate is required to maintain an adequate cardiac output. For cardiac output to meet the necessary oxygen requirements, stroke volume is determined by the amount of blood yielded by the ventricles per contraction. Determinants of stroke volume are based on three factors: preload, afterload, and contractility. For more on this subject, refer to a text on cardiac physiology.

Performing a cardiac assessment on a child with a potential cardiac condition involves the assessment of many body systems and their interrelationships. **Table 10-1** provides guidelines to use in the assessment of children with potential cardiac problems.

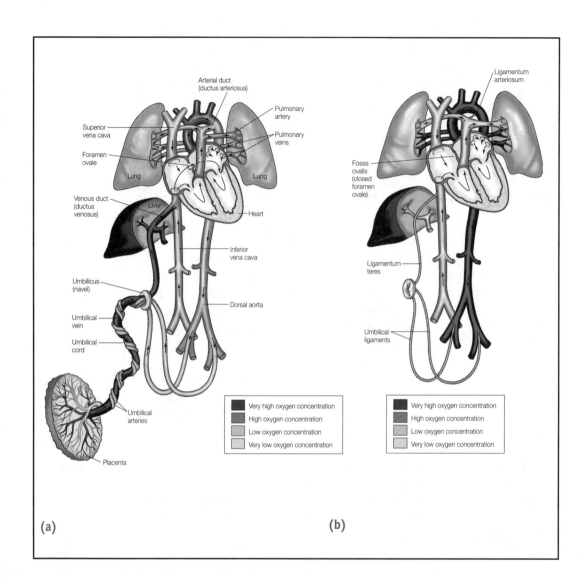

Figure 10-4 (a) Fetal Circulation Before Birth, (b) Fetal Circulation After Birth

TABLE 10–1 GUIDELINES FOR ASSESSMENT OF THE CHILD WITH A CARDIAC CONDITION

Characteristics to focus on include the following:

Respirations: Inspect the rate, depth, and respiratory effort. Note whether there are signs of increased respiratory effort, tachypnea, dyspnea, retractions, nasal flaring, and expiratory grunting. Auscultate breath sounds listening for adventitious sounds such as wheezes and or crackles. Note whether a cough is present.

Pulse Characteristics: Assess the pulse rate, rhythm, and quality. Compare pulse sites for strength and rate (apical to brachial or radial). Compare strength of pulse between the upper and lower extremities (brachial to femoral).

Blood Pressure: Compare the blood pressure to expected value for age, sex, and height percentile.

Color: Observe for overall color, noting pallor, cyanosis or dusky color. Compare the color in peripheral and central locations such nail beds to mucous membranes of the eyes and or mouth. Note whether the color improves or worsens with crying. Assess pulse oximetry.

Chest: Inspect the anterior and posterior chest for any skeletal abnormalities. Palpate the chest wall and over the heart for pulsations, heaves or vibrations. Using topographical landmarks, locate the joint of maximum intensity (PMI).

Heart Auscultation: Auscultate the heart fgor the heart sounds noting quality, loud versus weak, and distinct versus muffled.

Listen for extra heart sounds such as third or fourth heart sounds, murmurs. If a murmur is heard describe it by intensity, location, radiation, timing, and quality. Auscultate the heart with the child in both a sitting and reclining positions to detect differences in heart sounds.

Fluid Status: Observe for signs of periorbital, facial, or peripheral edema.

Observe for abdominal distention. Palpate the liver to detect hepatomegaly. Observe for signs of dehydration and acute illnesses. Assess for capillary refill.

Activity and Behavior: Determine if exercise intolerance is present or if the child tires with feeding. Observe for the presence of diaphoresis. Identify changes in activity level. Observe for abrupt behavior changes, restlessness, irritability, and lowered level of consciousness.

General: Assess pattern of growth.

Source: Adapted from Bickely, Lynn S., Bates' Guide to Physical Examination and History Taking, Lippincott Williams & Wilkins, 1999.

Assessment Considerations: Subjective Information

The following sections present considerations for the assessment of the heart and peripheral vascular system.

Infants

- Did the mother have any problems during pregnancy, including exposure to rubella, drug use, unexplained fevers, or use of any medications other than those prescribed?
- Does the child tire easily during feeding?
- Are there respiratory changes during feeding such as more rapid breaths, diaphoresis, or color change?
- Is there cyanosis in association with eating or crying?
- Is the child growing normally based on the growth chart?

Toddlers, School-Age Children, and Adolescents

- Does the child tire easily during play or have difficulty keeping up with other children?
- Does the child have to take extended rest periods or naps during the day?
- Does the child complain of leg pains during play or exercise?
- Does the child have unexplained joint pain or unexplained fevers?
- Does the child have frequent headaches or nosebleeds?
- Does the child have frequent respiratory infections? If so, how many per year, and how are they treated? Have any been streptococcal infections?

Family History

- Do any siblings have a history of congenital heart disease?
- Is there a family history of chromosomal abnormalities such as Down syndrome?

Review of Systems

Review of systems with relevance to the cardiac system includes the following:

- Start with consideration of height and weight and evidence of appropriate continued growth and development.
- Consider the *integument*, with questions regarding the overall color of the skin, assessing for pallor, dusky color, or cyanosis. Question extremities and nails for capillary refill, clubbing, color, and temperature. Also consider signs of peripheral or periorbital edema.
- Consider unusual facial characteristics such as microcephaly, cleft lip or plate, malformed ears, and wide-spaced eyes all of which may be

associated with chromosomal abnormalities or particular syndromes. Also consider polydactyly.

- Consider the *respiratory system*, regarding history of wheezing, nasal flaring, retractions, tachynea and prominent neck veins. Consider a history of a persistent cough.

Assessment Considerations: Objective Information

The cardiac examination is similar for all children in regard to the physical assessment techniques of inspection, palpation, and auscultation. What is different is your approach to the child, which is based on the child's age and development. As such, the following discussion is formatted differently than the objective assessment portions of previous chapters. Rather than listing a particular assessment method followed by a description of each age group, the age groups are discussed first, noting special considerations for each group. The assessment methods are then discussed without distinction between pediatric age groups. Finally, symptoms you may encounter during the assessment are discussed.

'Seizing the opportunity' when the child is quiet, comfortable, and cooperative will allow you to perform a comprehensive cardiac exam. In primary care, those children found to have complex cardiovascular disorders are referred to a pediatric cardiologist.

Infants and Toddlers

One of the first considerations when performing a cardiac assessment on an infant is to ensure that the room is quiet. The infant may lie quietly on the examination table or rest comfortably on the parent's shoulder. If the child is covered, keep the blanket on to avoid discomfort and maintain a sense of warmth and comfort, particularly in relation to physiologic changes associated with chilling. Observe the baby's color, respiratory effort, and general affect while the child is quiet. Being sensitive to the developmental stage of the child will allow you to perform a more comprehensive exam and in turn make the exam easier and less frightening for the child, and less disruptive for the parent as well.

If you are assessing a toddler, *seize the opportunity* while the child is sitting on the parent's lap or resting over the parent's shoulder to listen to heart sounds. Perform the assessment wherever the child is most comfortable. Allow the child to handle your stethoscope while you are getting the history and talking to the parent. Have a toy for distraction while you are listening, but do not use a musical toy, as it will interfere with your ability to concentrate on heart sounds. Using finger puppets keeps a child's attention while you focus on the exam.

School-Age Children

When assessing a school-age child, explain what you are going to do before you start the examination. Ask if the child has any questions and answer them honestly, but directly, without going into too much detail. Talk to the child about subjects he or she may be studying in school such as science, or sports, or whatever interests the child. Also ask the child about any symptoms he or she may be experiencing and the possible events surrounding them. For children who appear frightened or apprehensive, be reassuring and ask if they want to listen to their heart before you start. Place the earpieces gently in their ears and direct them where to place the diaphragm of the stethoscope. Explain that they will hear a *lub-dub* sound, but keep your descriptions simple. Giving a child a sense of control and some understanding of what to expect goes a long way in setting the tone for a successful visit.

Adolescents

When obtaining a history from an adolescent, direct your questions to the patient, be professional, and demonstrate sincere interest in his or her concerns. Generally, it is helpful if the parent is in the room when you are obtaining the history, as the parent can add family details that may be relevant and that the adolescent is not aware of. Ask the parent if he or she would prefer to wait in the waiting room while you do the examination. Remember, adolescents are particularly conscious about their body, so sensitivity to privacy while they are changing and while doing the exam is important. Assure the adolescent that the questions you ask while the parent is out of the room are confidential and that you will not relate that information to the parent unless it is life threatening to the patient. Again, be reassuring and sensitive to the adolescent's concerns and questions.

Inspection

When performing a cardiovascular examination on a child, evaluation begins as you first see the child and assess the child's overall health, nutritional state, and ease of respirations. During inspection, observation of unusual facies, including wide-spaced eyes, malformed ears, microcephaly, cleft lip, or polydactyly, may be associated with chromosomal abnormalities or a specific syndrome. Many syndromes have cardiac abnormalities associated with them.

The skin is assessed for central cyanosis and mottling. A means of assessing cyanosis is to inspect the lips, tongue, and nail beds for a ruddy red color, as well as distinguishing a pale, blue tone to the skin. Peripheral cyanosis, also called acrocyanosis, is noted around the mouth and on the extremities such as the hands or feet, particularly if the child is cold. Clubbing, a long-standing sign of cyanosis, can be seen in older children with a history of cardiovascular and pulmonary disease.

Accurate measurement of height and weight is an important assessment tool in the evaluation of growth and development. Children with heart disease frequently evidence poor weight gain and linear growth, as well as demonstrate delay in achievement of developmental milestones.

For children with a known heart murmur or history of cardiac disease, a comprehensive cardiac exam is paramount. In children, there are basically two types of cardiovascular disease—congenital heart disease and acquired heart disease due to infection.

> Symptoms of congenital heart disease present with decompensating characteristics such as cyanosis, peripheral edema, and dyspnea that are easily recognized. It is the subtle early signs that you must be continuously watchful for, such as:
>
> - The infant who becomes tired while sucking and rests periodically
> - The infant who has tachycardia and tachypnea while eating
> - The child who tires frequently during play
> - The child who is reported to "turn blue" during crying episodes
> - The child who requires several sleep or rest periods during the day that are not normal for the age
> - The child who repeatedly becomes short of breath while running
> - The child who complains of leg pains while running
> - The child who is falling behind the normal growth curve

Blood pressure readings are an important measurement as part of a routine physical examination of children 2 years and older, but particularly for the child in whom there is a question of cardiac disease. Selection of the correct blood pressure cuff is important, as a cuff that is too narrow can falsely elevate the blood pressure and a wider cuff can lower the blood pressure by interfering with proper placement of the stethoscope diaphragm over the artery (**Figure 10-5**).

Palpation

When performing a cardiac exam, palpate the chest to assess for precordial activity and femoral pulses. Gently place the pads of your fingers over the precordial area and palpate for the PMI. In infants and toddlers, the PMI is usually palpated an interspace higher than in the adult (around the third

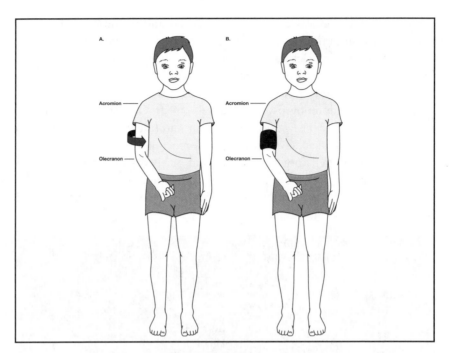

Figure 10-5 Determination of Proper Blood Pressure Cuff Size

or fourth interspace) because the heart lies more horizontally in the young child. Assess for thrills, a sensation caused by turbulence within the heart or great vessels representing blood rapidly flowing from high pressure to lower pressure. It can be related to the feel of a cat's purr. In assessing for thrills, using the palm of your hand allows you to better feel the rough vibrating quality. Moderate to severe pulmonic valve stenosis may cause a thrill at the upper left sternal border or may also result from aortic stenosis at the suprasternal notch. Increased precordial activity or thrills can also be palpated in children with increased right or left ventricular stroke volume. It can occur in infants with moderate or a large ventricular septal defect or significant patent ductus arteriosus (AAFP, 1999). Increased precordial activity may be due to anemia, hyperthyroidism, or anemia in an older child as well.

Next palpate both femoral pulses, comparing their strength and quality with those of the brachial pulses. You are assessing for coarctation of the aorta, which is a narrowing of the descending aorta or obstruction of the left subclavian artery. This defect is common, occurring in 5% of all children with congenital heart disease (Rome & Kretuzer, 2004). In assessing the femoral pulses, they are located in the midline just below the inguinal crease between the iliac crest and the symphysis pubis. In chubby babies, it can be difficult to detect the femoral pulses. Flex the child's thighs to the abdomen and then extend the legs, which will decrease the reflex flexion that occurs when you simply extend the legs. While palpating the femoral pulse, simultaneously palpate the right brachial pulse. The timing and intensity of the two pulses should be equal, and in conjunction with normal blood pressure in the right arm, coarctation of the aorta is unlikely.

Other pulses should be palpated as well in both the upper and lower extremities, noting character or strength. A thready pulse may indicate congestive heart failure or a narrowing such as aortic stenosis, where a bounding pulse may indicate patent ductus arteriosus. Evaluate the pulses for rate, regularity of rhythm, and strength, and compare bilaterally.

Pediatric heart rates are variable. Pulse points are no different in children than they are in adults, but there are some differences in the way these pulses are evaluated. The small anatomy of children, coupled with the lower palpable magnitude of pediatric cardiac output, makes palpation of pulses in certain anatomic regions impossible, or extremely difficult. In small children, it is recommended that peripheral pulses be obtained at the brachial artery (inside of the bicep) and central pulses be obtained at either the femoral or carotid arteries. If no pulses can be palpated, consider auscultating an apical pulse using a stethoscope. If a heartbeat can be heard, the child has a pulse; however, the presence of a pulse does not automatically indicate adequate perfusion. Capillary refill time is typically quite accurate in children and considered to be reliable in most cases. Healthy children do not have the vascular diseases of adults; therefore, their capillary blood flow is very responsive. Just as in the adult patient, environmental factors such as cold ambient temperatures can influence capillary refill times. Normal capillary refill time is less than 2–3 seconds.

Palpation of the liver and the spleen should be performed to assess for enlargement. A child with a liver palpated 1 cm below the costal margin raises a red flag for hepatomegaly, particularly in view of the child with suspected cardiac disease. In infants, the liver edges may be palpated below the costal margin, which is considered a normal finding.

Percussion

Percussion is generally not performed during examination of the heart.

Auscultation

Auscultation of the heart starts with assessment of the rate and rhythm and is followed by listening at the five noted areas for identification of heart

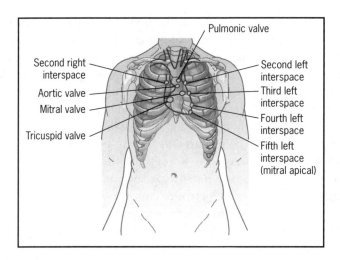

Figure 10-6   Areas for Auscultation of Heart

sounds and detection of murmurs. At each area, you should identify the first and second heart sounds (S_1 and S_2).

In assessing heart sounds, begin with the child in a sitting position and listen for S_1 at the lower left border of the sternum. As described earlier, S_1 is the result of closure of the mitral and tricuspid valves and is normally a single sound. S_2 is caused by closure of the aortic and pulmonic valves. The S_2 can have two components, or a split sound, heard during inspiration. The first component is closure of the aortic valve, and the second is closure of the pulmonic valve. Splitting of S_2 is referred to as physiologic splitting. This sound is more apparent during inspiration when the child takes a deep breath because as more blood returns to the right ventricle it causes the pulmonic valve to close a fraction of a second later than the aortic valve. To reassess physiologic splitting, auscultate over the pulmonic area while the child breathes normally and then also have the child take a deep breath. It is more easily auscultated after a deep breath. See **Figure 10-7**.

For a comprehensive cardiac examination, you should auscultate the child's heart in both a sitting and leaning forward and a reclining position. Different sounds can be heard with changes in position and depending on how close the heart is to the chest wall.

There are four heart sounds that represent specific events in the cardiac cycle. S_1 and S_2 represent normal heart sounds, and S_3 and S_4 represent abnormal heart sounds. Although not frequently heard in children, S_3 is

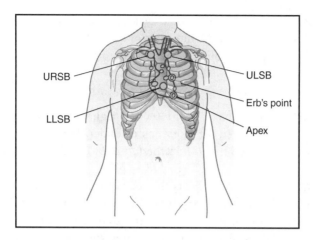

Figure 10-7 Traditional Auscultatory Areas for Clicks and Murmurs

associated with rapid ventricular filling. It is referred to as a "gallop" and is heard best at the apex with the bell of the stethoscope during early diastole. When combined with the normal S_1 and S_2, it sounds like the word "Kentucky." S_4 represents increased force of atrial contraction and ventricular distention and is always pathologic. The S_4 "gallop" sounds like the word "Tennessee" and is best heard in late diastole with the bell at the apex of the heart.

If you are having difficulty differentiating between S_1 and S_2, palpate the carotid pulse when auscultating the heart. The heart sound heard simultaneously with the carotid pulsation is S_1. By placing the diaphragm firmly against the chest wall during auscultation, you will hear the high-pitched sounds of S_1 and S_2, as well as murmurs of aortic and mitral regurgitation and pericardial friction rubs.

Auscultation of the entire precordium continues with auscultation at five distinct areas. Using a systematic approach with the child sitting upright, start at either the aortic area or the apex and carefully listen to heart sounds. After all areas have been examined, ask the child to lie in a supine position, and repeat the exam starting with the diaphragm of the stethoscope and then switching to the bell. Listening to all areas with both the diaphragm and the bell allows you to hear the variation in sound. If you are having difficulty isolating heart sounds from respiratory sounds, ask the child to hold his or her breath for several seconds so you can concentrate solely on S_1 and S_2. Closing your eyes while listening may help to eliminate distractions. Listen to several cardiac cycles at each position, describing the intensity of S_1 in all areas, the intensity of S_2 in all areas, the characterization of any extrasystolic sounds, and the characterization of any extradiastolic sounds.

The areas of assessment can be described as follows:

- *AORTIC AREA*, or base, is the second right intercostal space at the sternal border. Listen for S_2, which is louder than S_1 at this landmark and corresponds to the *dub* in the *lub-dub*. It indicates closure of the semilunar valves.
- *PULMONIC AREA*, or base, is the second left intercostal space at the sternal border. Listen for S_2, which is louder than S_1 at this landmark and corresponds to the *dub* in the *lub-dub*. It indicates closure of the semilunar valves. A normal physiologic splitting of S_2, if present, is heard best in this area.
- *ERB'S POINT* is the third left intercostal space at the sternal border. It is where both aortic and pulmonic sounds may be auscultated.
- *TRICUSPID AREA* is the fourth left intercostal space at the sternal border. Listen for S_1, which is louder than S_2 at this landmark. It indicates closure of the tricuspid valve and corresponds to the *dub* in the *lub-dub*.
- *MITRAL AREA*, or apex, is the fourth intercostal space at the midclavicular line; in school-age children and adolescents, it is the fifth intercostal space at the midclavicular line. This area is referred to as the apical area. Listen for S_1, which is louder than S_2 at this landmark. It indicates closure of the mitral valve and heralds the onset of systole.

When auscultating the heart, it is essential to follow a systematic procedure for listening to heart sounds. Start either at the apex and follow through to the base, or start at the base and end at the apex.

A child's heart rate decreases as the child becomes older. A child's need for more oxygen is accomplished by increasing the heart rate, referred to as sinus tachycardia. Stressors such as fever, exercise, and anxiety increase a child's metabolic rate and simultaneously create a need for more oxygen.

Assessing for Murmurs

A challenging aspect of the cardiac exam in children is assessing for murmurs. In an infant or young child, it is difficult to evaluate normal heart sounds at a rate of 70 to 120 beats/minute, as well as to distinguish an extra sound or differentiate background noise such as lung sounds or upper airway sounds. The majority of healthy children will at some point present with a functional or benign heart murmur, many times in conjunction with a febrile illness.

A functional murmur implies that there is no structural or functional heart disease. Children with innocent murmurs require no further intervention or specific follow-up, since these murmurs are sporadic and generally disappear with age. Activity restrictions are not necessary, and, most importantly, the child should be treated normally. As a provider, it is important to remember

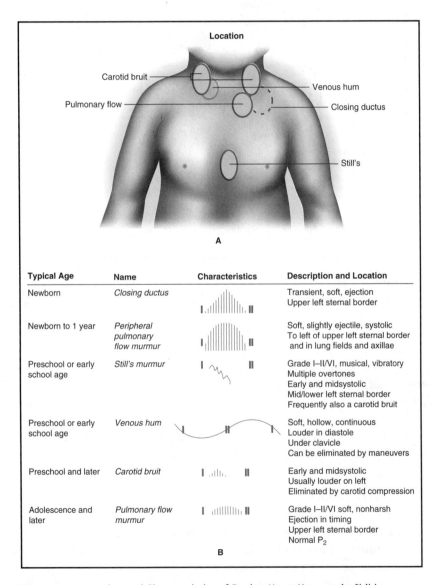

Figure 10-8 Location and Characteristics of Benign Heart Murmurs in Children

Source: This article was published in *Mosby's Guide to Physical Examination*, 6th edition, Seidel, Ball, Dains, and Benedict. Location and Characteristics of Benign Heart Murmurs in Children. Copyright Elsevier (2006).

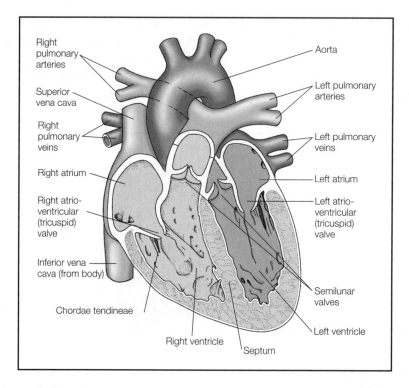

Figure 10-9 Heart

that the intensity of an innocent murmur will increase with fever, illness, or stress. Education of the family is crucial to dispel the notion that the child has heart disease. Children with serious heart disease or malformations will have signs and symptoms that were reviewed previously.

When listening to the heart, timing the murmurs to determine whether they are systolic or diastolic is critical. Questions to consider include the following:

- Does the systolic murmur begin with or after S_1? Does it end before, with, or after S_2? Does the murmur occupy the entire systolic period? These types of murmurs are referred to as holosystolic or pansystolic murmurs. They begin with S_1 and end after S_2. A systolic ejection murmur begins after S_1 and ends before S_2.

- When does the murmur occur? In early, mid, or late systole? Diastolic murmurs are heard after S_2 but before S_1; they always indicate cardiac pathology.
- Where is the murmur best heard? Is there radiation to the axilla, neck, or back?

When murmurs are heard, they are graded by intensity, from I to VI, according to the Levine scale:

- *GRADE I*: Low intensity that is difficult to hear in a quiet room
- *GRADE II*: Low intensity, but clearly audible
- *GRADE III*: Medium intensity and easy to hear, but without a palpable thrill
- *GRADE IV*: Medium intensity, with a palpable thrill
- *GRADE V*: Loud intensity and heard with the stethoscope barely on the chest, with a palpable thrill
- *GRADE VI*: Loudest intensity and audible without the stethoscope in direct contact with the chest, with a palpable thrill

After grading the murmur, the following characteristics are used to describe the murmur:

- *LOCATION*: Where is the murmur heard best and/or most loudly? Is the child sitting up or lying down? Are the characteristics altered when the child changes position?
- *RADIATION*: Is the sound transmitted to another part of the chest, including to the axilla or the back?
- *TIMING*: When is the murmur heard best, between S_1 and S_2, or between S_2 and S_1? Is it heard throughout the entire phase of S_1 and S_2 (holosystolic)?
- *QUALITY*: What does the murmur sound like? Words commonly used to describe murmurs include rumbling, blowing, machinery, harsh, scratchy, and musical.

Murmurs can be described as grade II/VI, grade IV/VI, or grade II–III/VI.

Table 10-3 outlines characteristics of benign heart murmurs, noting their location and key characteristics.

In toddlers and school-age children, the most common benign murmur is the *Still's murmur*. It is a low-pitched, grade II/VI early systolic ejection murmur. It is described as a classic vibratory or musical murmur. It is nonradiating, midsystolic, and is best heard at the left lower sternal border at the apex. It will increase in a supine position, with fever, and with anemia. It will decrease in a sitting or standing position and with a Valsalva maneuver.

Pulmonary flow murmur is a benign murmur heard in a wide range of children, from school-age children to adolescents. It is typically a low-intensity systolic ejection murmur and is heard best at the left upper sternal border (LUSB). It is increased with a fever or anemia. It will be decreased in a standing position with inspiration.

Physiologic peripheral pulmonic stenosis most often occurs in infants from birth to 6 months of age. It is a soft low-pitched systolic ejection murmur, blowing in quality. It is heard best at the left infraclavicular area, with radiation to the axillae and the back. It is increased in high-output states such as fever and/or anemia.

Assessing for Venous Hum

Many children with functional murmurs also have a venous hum, a finding common between the ages of 2 and 8 years. It is heard as a continuous low-pitched hum throughout the cardiac cycle, although it may be loudest during diastole and when the child stands. It is caused by the flow of venous blood from the head and neck into the thorax. The venous hum does not change with respirations, although the sound disappears when light pressure is applied over the jugular vein. Compressing the jugular vein or turning the head to the right will diminish the murmur. The venous hum will diminish completely when lying in a supine position. This is a common

---

TABLE 10-2   LOCATIONS OF PALPABLE PULSES

- Carotid pulse is located in the neck just medial to and below the angle of the jaw. Do not palpate both sides simultaneously.
- Brachial pulse is medial to the biceps tendon.
- Radial pulse is medial and on the ventral side of the wrist. Use gentle pressure.
- Femoral pulse is inferior to the inguinal ligament. If the child is obese, palpation of the femoral pulse is midway between anterior superior iliac spine and pubic tubercle. Press harder here than in most areas.
- Popliteal pulse is located in the popliteal fossae behind the knee. Press firmly.
- Dorsalis pedis pulse is on the medial side of the dorsum of the foot with the foot slightly dorsiflexed. Pulse may be difficult to palpate.
- Posterior tibial pulse is behind and slightly inferior to the medial malleolus of the ankle.

Source: Adapted from *Mosby's Guide to Physical Examination*, 6th edition, Seidel, Ball, Dains, and Benedict. Locations of Palpable Pulses, page 308. Copyright Elsevier (2006).

TABLE 10–3 CHARACTERISTICS OF HEART MURMURS

Timing and Duration:
- Early systolic begins with S_1, decrescendos, ends before S_2.
- Midsystolic begins after S_1 and ends before S_2.
- Late systolic begins mid to late systole, crescendos, ends at S_2. Often introduced by mid to late systolic clicks.
- Diastolic—Early diastolic begins with S_2
- Mid-diastolic begins at clear interval after S_2
- Late diastolic or (presystolic) begins immediately before S_1
- Holodiastolic begins with S_2, occupies all of diastole, land ends at S_1
- Continuous starts in systole, continues without interruption through S_2, into all or part of diastole; does not necessarily persist through out entire cardiac cycle
- Systolic murmurs are best described according to time of onset and termination;
- Diastolic murmurs are best classified according to time of onset only.

Pitch Intensity:
- Classification: high, medium, low depends on pressure and rate of blood flow
- Grade I is barely audible in quiet room
- Grade II is quiet but clearly audible
- Grade III is moderately loud
- Grade IV is loud, associated with a thrill
- Grade V is very loud, with a thrill and easily palpable
- Grade VI is very loud, audible with stethoscope not in contact with the chest, a thrill is palpable and visible

Pattern:
Crescendo with increasing intensity caused by increased blood velocity
Decrescendo with decreasing intensity caused by decreased blood velocity

Quality:
Harsh, raspy, machine-like, vibratory, musical blowing.
Quality depends o valve compromise, force of contractions, and blood volume

Location:
Anatomic landmarks (i.e., 2nd left intercostal space on sternal border)
The area of greatest intensity is usually the area to which valve sounds are normally transmitted

Radiation:
Identified by anatomic landmarks. (i.e., axilla)
The site farthest from location of greatest intensity at which the sound is still audible. The sound is usually transmitted in direction of blood flow.

Respiratory phase variations:
Intensity, quality and timing may vary. Venous blood return increases on inspiration and decreases on expiration.

Source: Adapted from *Mosby's Guide to Physical Examination*, 6th edition, Seidel, Ball, Dains, and Benedict. Locations of Palpable Pulses, page 308. Copyright Elsevier (2006).

finding and is not pathologic. Children with venous hums do not require referral to a cardiologist.

Assessing for Clicks

Ejection and nonejection clicks are viewed as extra heart sounds and are categorized as pulmonic or aortic. Overall ejection clicks are auscultated in early systole and sound like a split S_1. Pulmonic ejection clicks are high in frequency, vary with respirations, and disappear with inspiration. An aortic ejection click is constant in intensity and may be appreciated as a *snap* or a *click*. It is heard best at Erb's point. Nonejection clicks are heard best in midsystole, or halfway between S_1 and S_2. They are heard best at the apex and when the child is standing. They vary with respirations and are due to mitral valve prolapse (Burns, 2004, p. 777).

Common Cardiac Disorders in Children

The majority of cardiac disorders in children are congenital disorders such as congenital heart disease, ventricular septal defect, atrial septal defect, patent ductus arteriosus, transposition of the great vessels, tetralogy of Fallot, and coarctation of the aorta. The more common cardiac disorders seen in primary care are those that are acquired. These disorders can occur at any age, from infancy to adolescence.

HYPERTENSION in children is defined as systolic and/or diastolic pressure, based on repeated measurements (more than three occasions), above the 95th percentile for age, sex, and height. The incidence of hypertension in children has risen significantly over the past two decades. The increase is thought to be linked to increases in body weight, diets high in fat and cholesterol, and sedentary lifestyles. These factors not only raise the blood pressure to unhealthy levels, they increase a child's risk for developing type 2 diabetes mellitus. The updated classification of hypertension in children was published in August 2004 by the National Blood Pressure Education Program, Working Group on Children and Adolescents. See **Figures 10-14** and **10-15**.

KAWASAKI DISEASE is characterized by an acute generalized systemic microvasculitis with the potential for the formation of coronary artery aneurysms. The diagnostic criteria for Kawasaki disease is based on six findings: fever, bilateral conjunctival injection, polymorphous rash, red cracked lips, erythema of the palms and soles, and cervical lymphadenopathy. It is the most common cause of acquired heart disease in children in Japan and the United States (Burns, 2004).

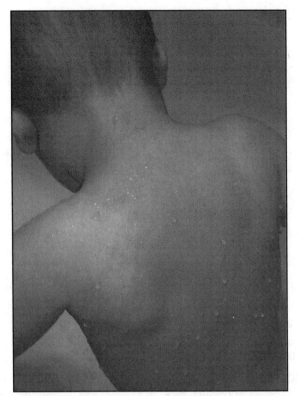

Figure 10-10 Infant with Kawasaki Disease with an Erythematous, Predominantly Truncal Rash (See Color Plate)

ACUTE RHEUMATIC FEVER is a systemic connective tissue disease. It results in inflammation of the heart, joints, and central nervous system. Diagnosis is based on minor and major manifestations of the Jones criteria for rheumatic fever. It classically occurs 10–20 days following an infection of streptococcal pharyngitis. It is the leading cause of acquired heart disease in children worldwide.

Major Manifestations
- Carditis
- Chorea
- Erythema marginatum
- Subcutaneous nodules

Minor Manifestations

- Arthralgia
- Fever
- Elevated acute-phase reactants
- Elevated erythrocyte sedimentation rate
- Elevated C-reactive protein
- Prolonged PR interval on ECG (Special Writing Group of the Committee on Rheumatic Fever, Endocarditis, and Kawasaki Disease of the Council on Cardiovascular Disease in the Young of the American Heart Association, 1992).

INFECTIVE ENDOCARDITIS is inflammation of the lining and valves of the heart. It is caused by bacterial, enterococcal, and/or fungal infections, and often occurs in children with preexisting heart defects. Diagnosis is made based on the Duke criteria and blood cultures. Acute manifestations include high fever, myalgias, night sweats, arthralgias, and increase in intensity of a preexisting murmur or new onset of a murmur. Treatment is based on high doses of antibiotics for 4–6 weeks.

MYOCARDITIS is inflammation of the muscular walls of the heart or the myocardium. It is the most common cause of heart failure in an otherwise healthy child. The most common causes in children are enterovirus (coxsackie group B) and adenovirus. The disease may go unrecognized in many children and resolve spontaneously, or it may lead to fulminant disease and

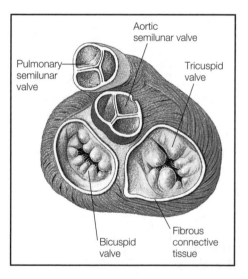

Figure 10-11 Rheumatic Fever

progress to chronic cardiomyopathy. Symptoms are secondary to reduced myocardial function, which leads to decreased muscle function and eventually enlargement of the heart with decreased contractility, leading to congestive heart failure (CHF).

DYSLIPIDEMIA refers to disorders of lipoprotein metabolism that result in high total cholesterol, high low-density lipoprotein cholesterol (LDL), low high-density lipoprotein cholesterol, (HDL) and high triglycerides. The process of atherosclerotic vascular changes is accelerated in children with risk factors such as obesity, hypertension, and diabetes mellitus, and with positive family history. The AAP (2008) recommends that a dyslipidemia risk assessment be performed beginning at 2 years of age if the child has designated risk factors as outlined by the AAP.

PERICARDITIS is inflammation of the pericardium, the sac that surrounds the heart. It presents as a sharp piercing pain over the center or left side of the chest that increases on inspiration. The most common etiology in children is viral, usually coxsackievirus or adenovirus. There is a film of serous fluid between the inner and outer layers of the pericardium. When the pericardium becomes inflamed, this fluid increases, compressing the heart and interfering with the heart's contractility. Presenting symptoms are low-grade fever, fatigue, and irregular heartbeat. A pericardial friction

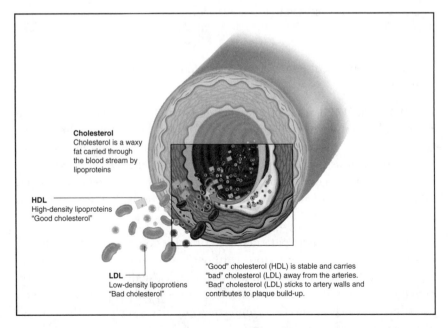

Cholesterol
Cholesterol is a waxy fat carried through the blood stream by lipoproteins

HDL
High-density lipoproteins "Good cholesterol"

LDL
Low-density lipoprotiens "Bad cholesterol"

"Good" cholesterol (HDL) is stable and carries "bad" cholesterol (LDL) away from the arteries. "Bad" cholesterol (LDL) sticks to artery walls and contributes to plaque build-up.

Figure 10-12   Lipid Formation

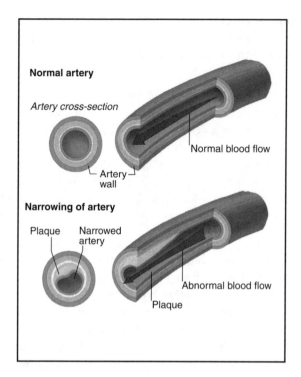

Figure 10-13 High Cholesterol—Vascular Changes

rub is heard on auscultation. It is most common in children younger than 2 years of age.

CARDIAC ARRHYTHMIAS, or heart conduction disturbances, result from abnormal impulse formation or conduction. In children without cardiac disease, sinus arrhythmia that increases with inspiration and decreases with expiration is benign and requires no treatment. Other arrythmias, such tachycardia, conduction disturbances, AV block, premature atrial contractions, and premature ventricular contractions, require referral to a pediatric cardiologist.

CHEST PAIN in pediatric patients is a common complaint, although it is generally not indicative of serious cardiovascular problems. The most frequent etiology of chest pain is musculoskeletal, usually related to athletic activity. The second most common cause of chest pain is pulmonary, such as asthma or pneumonia. Gastrointestinal problems such as reflux should also be considered in the differential diagnosis.

FIGURE 10-14 BLOOD PRESSURE LEVELS FOR BOYS BY AGE AND HEIGHT PERCENTILE

Age (Year)	BP Percentile	Systolic BP (mmHg) Percentile of Height							Diastolic BP (mmHg) Percentile of Height						
		5th	10th	25th	50th	75th	80th	95th	5th	10th	25th	50th	75th	80th	95th
1	50th	80	81	83	85	87	88	89	34	35	36	37	38	39	39
	90th	94	95	97	99	100	102	103	49	50	51	52	53	53	54
	95th	98	99	101	103	104	106	106	54	54	55	56	57	58	58
	99th	105	106	108	110	112	113	114	61	62	63	64	65	66	66
2	50th	84	85	87	88	90	92	92	39	40	41	42	43	44	44
	90th	97	99	100	102	104	105	106	54	55	56	57	58	58	59
	95th	101	102	104	106	108	109	110	59	59	60	61	62	63	63
	99th	109	110	111	113	115	117	117	66	67	68	69	70	71	71
3	50th	86	87	89	91	93	94	95	44	44	45	46	47	48	48
	90th	100	101	103	105	107	108	109	59	59	60	61	62	63	63
	95th	104	105	107	109	110	112	113	63	63	64	65	66	67	67
	99th	111	112	114	116	118	119	120	71	71	72	73	74	75	75
4	50th	88	89	91	93	95	96	97	47	48	49	50	51	51	52
	90th	102	103	105	107	109	110	111	62	63	64	65	66	66	67
	95th	106	107	109	111	112	114	115	66	67	68	69	70	71	71
	99th	113	114	116	116	120	121	122	74	75	76	77	78	78	79
5	50th	90	91	93	95	96	98	98	47	48	49	50	51	51	52
	90th	104	105	106	108	110	111	112	65	66	67	68	69	69	70
	95th	108	109	110	112	114	115	116	69	70	71	72	73	74	74
	99th	115	116	118	120	121	123	123	77	78	79	80	81	81	82
6	50th	91	92	94	96	98	99	100	53	53	54	55	56	57	57
	90th	105	106	108	110	111	113	113	68	68	69	70	71	72	72
	95th	109	110	112	114	115	117	117	72	72	73	74	75	76	76
	99th	116	117	119	121	123	124	125	80	80	81	82	83	84	84

(continues)

FIGURE 10-14 BLOOD PRESSURE LEVELS FOR BOYS BY AGE AND HEIGHT PERCENTILE

Age (Year)	BP Percentile	Systolic BP (mmHg) Percentile of Height							Diastolic BP (mmHg) Percentile of Height						
		5th	10th	25th	50th	75th	80th	95th	5th	10th	25th	50th	75th	80th	95th
7	50th	92	94	95	97	99	100	101	55	55	56	57	58	59	59
	90th	106	107	109	111	113	114	115	70	70	71	72	73	74	74
	95th	110	111	113	115	117	118	119	74	74	75	76	77	78	78
	99th	117	118	120	122	124	125	126	82	82	83	84	85	86	86
8	50th	94	95	97	99	100	102	102	56	57	58	59	60	60	61
	90th	107	109	110	112	114	115	116	71	72	72	73	74	75	76
	95th	111	112	114	116	118	119	120	75	76	77	78	79	79	80
	99th	119	120	122	123	125	127	127	83	84	85	86	87	87	88
9	50th	95	96	98	100	102	103	104	56	57	58	59	60	60	61
	90th	109	110	112	114	115	117	118	72	73	74	75	76	76	77
	95th	113	114	116	118	119	121	121	76	77	78	79	80	81	81
	99th	120	121	123	125	127	128	129	84	85	86	87	88	88	89
10	50th	97	98	100	102	103	105	106	58	59	60	61	61	62	63
	90th	111	112	114	115	117	119	119	73	73	74	75	76	77	78
	95th	115	116	117	119	121	122	123	77	78	79	80	81	81	82
	99th	122	123	125	127	128	130	130	85	86	86	88	88	89	90
11	50th	99	100	102	104	105	107	107	59	59	60	61	62	63	63
	90th	113	114	115	117	119	120	121	74	74	75	76	77	78	78
	95th	117	118	119	121	123	124	125	78	78	79	80	81	82	82
	99th	124	125	127	129	130	132	132	85	86	87	88	89	90	90
12	50th	101	102	104	106	108	109	110	59	60	61	62	63	63	64
	90th	115	116	118	120	121	123	123	74	75	75	76	77	78	79
	95th	119	120	122	123	125	127	127	78	79	80	81	82	82	83
	99th	126	127	129	131	133	134	135	86	87	88	89	90	90	91

FIGURE 10-14   BLOOD PRESSURE LEVELS FOR BOYS BY AGE AND HEIGHT PERCENTILE

Age (Year)	BP Percentile	Systolic BP (mmHg) Percentile of Height							Diastolic BP (mmHg) Percentile of Height						
		5th	10th	25th	50th	75th	80th	95th	5th	10th	25th	50th	75th	80th	95th
13	50th	104	105	106	108	110	111	112	60	60	61	62	63	64	64
	90th	117	118	120	122	124	125	126	75	75	76	77	78	79	79
	95th	121	122	124	126	128	129	130	79	79	80	81	82	83	83
	99th	128	130	131	133	135	136	137	87	87	88	89	90	91	91
14	50th	106	107	109	111	113	114	115	60	61	62	63	64	65	65
	90th	120	121	123	125	126	128	128	75	76	77	78	79	79	80
	95th	124	125	127	128	130	132	132	80	80	81	82	83	84	84
	99th	131	132	134	136	138	139	140	87	88	89	90	91	92	92
15	50th	109	110	112	113	115	117	117	61	62	63	64	65	66	66
	90th	122	124	125	127	129	130	131	76	77	78	79	80	80	81
	95th	126	127	129	131	133	134	135	81	81	82	83	84	85	85
	99th	134	135	136	138	140	142	142	88	89	90	91	92	93	93
16	50th	111	112	114	116	118	119	120	63	63	64	65	66	67	67
	90th	125	126	128	130	131	133	134	78	78	79	80	81	82	82
	95th	129	130	132	134	135	137	137	82	83	83	84	85	86	87
	99th	136	137	139	141	143	144	145	90	90	91	92	93	94	94
17	50th	114	115	116	118	120	121	122	65	66	66	67	68	69	70
	90th	127	128	130	132	134	135	136	80	80	81	82	83	84	84
	95th	131	132	134	136	138	139	140	84	85	86	87	88	88	89
	99th	139	140	141	143	145	146	147	92	93	93	94	95	96	97

BP, blood pressure

Source: www.nhlbi.nih.gov/guidelines/hypertension/children

FIGURE 10-15   BLOOD PRESSURE LEVELS FOR GIRLS BY AGE AND HEIGHT PERCENTILE

Age (Year)	BP Percentile	Systolic BP (mmHg) Percentile of Height							Diastolic BP (mmHg) Percentile of Height						
		5th	10th	25th	50th	75th	80th	95th	5th	10th	25th	50th	75th	80th	95th
1	50th	83	84	85	86	88	89	90	38	39	39	40	41	41	42
	90th	97	97	98	100	101	102	103	52	53	53	54	55	55	56
	95th	100	101	102	104	105	106	107	56	57	57	58	59	59	60
	99th	108	108	109	111	112	113	114	64	64	65	65	66	67	67
2	50th	85	85	87	88	89	91	91	43	44	44	45	46	46	47
	90th	98	99	100	101	103	104	105	57	58	58	59	60	61	61
	95th	102	103	104	105	107	108	109	61	62	62	63	64	65	65
	99th	109	110	111	112	114	115	116	69	69	70	70	71	72	72
3	50th	86	87	88	89	91	92	93	47	48	48	49	50	50	51
	90th	100	100	102	103	104	106	106	61	62	62	63	64	64	65
	95th	104	104	105	107	108	109	110	65	66	66	67	68	68	69
	99th	111	111	113	114	115	116	117	73	73	74	74	75	76	76
4	50th	88	88	90	91	92	94	94	50	50	51	52	52	53	54
	90th	101	102	103	104	106	107	108	64	64	65	66	67	67	68
	95th	105	106	107	108	110	111	112	68	68	69	70	71	71	72
	99th	112	113	114	115	117	118	119	76	76	76	77	78	79	79
5	50th	89	90	91	93	94	95	96	52	53	53	54	55	55	56
	90th	103	103	105	106	107	109	109	66	67	67	68	69	69	70
	95th	107	107	108	110	111	112	113	70	71	71	72	73	73	74
	99th	114	114	116	117	118	120	120	78	78	79	79	80	81	81
6	50th	91	92	93	94	96	97	98	54	54	55	56	56	57	58
	90th	104	105	106	108	109	110	111	68	68	69	70	70	71	72
	95th	108	109	110	111	113	114	115	72	72	73	74	74	75	76
	99th	115	116	117	119	120	121	122	80	80	80	81	82	83	83

FIGURE 10-15 BLOOD PRESSURE LEVELS FOR GIRLS BY AGE AND HEIGHT PERCENTILE

Age (Year)	BP Percentile	Systolic BP (mmHg) Percentile of Height							Diastolic BP (mmHg) Percentile of Height						
		5th	10th	25th	50th	75th	80th	95th	5th	10th	25th	50th	75th	80th	95th
7	50th	93	93	95	96	97	99	99	55	56	56	57	58	58	59
	90th	106	107	108	109	111	112	113	69	70	70	71	72	72	73
	95th	110	111	112	113	115	116	116	73	74	74	75	76	76	77
	99th	117	118	119	120	122	123	124	81	81	82	82	83	84	84
8	50th	95	95	96	98	99	100	101	57	57	57	58	59	60	60
	90th	108	109	110	111	113	114	114	71	71	71	72	73	74	74
	95th	112	112	114	115	116	118	118	75	75	75	76	77	78	78
	99th	119	120	121	122	123	125	125	82	82	83	83	84	85	86
9	50th	96	97	98	100	101	102	103	58	58	58	59	60	61	61
	90th	110	110	112	113	114	116	116	72	72	72	73	74	75	75
	95th	114	114	115	117	118	119	120	76	76	76	77	78	79	79
	99th	121	121	123	124	125	127	127	83	83	84	84	85	86	87
10	50th	98	99	100	102	103	104	105	59	59	59	60	61	62	62
	90th	112	112	114	115	116	118	118	73	73	73	74	75	76	76
	95th	116	116	117	19	120	121	122	77	77	77	78	79	80	80
	99th	123	123	125	126	127	129	129	84	84	85	86	86	87	88
11	50th	100	101	102	103	105	106	107	60	60	60	61	62	63	63
	90th	114	114	116	117	118	119	120	74	74	74	75	76	77	77
	95th	118	118	119	121	122	123	124	78	78	78	79	80	81	81
	99th	125	125	126	128	129	130	131	85	85	86	87	87	88	89
12	50th	102	103	104	105	107	108	109	61	61	61	62	63	64	64
	90th	116	116	117	119	120	121	122	75	75	75	76	77	78	78
	95th	119	120	121	123	124	125	126	79	79	70	80	81	82	82
	99th	127	127	128	130	131	132	133	86	86	87	88	88	89	90

(continues)

FIGURE 10-15 BLOOD PRESSURE LEVELS FOR GIRLS BY AGE AND HEIGHT PERCENTILE

Age (Year)	BP Percentile	Systolic BP (mmHg) Percentile of Height							Diastolic BP (mmHg) Percentile of Height						
		5th	10th	25th	50th	75th	80th	95th	5th	10th	25th	50th	75th	80th	95th
13	50th	104	105	106	107	109	110	110	62	62	62	63	64	65	65
	90th	117	118	119	121	122	123	124	76	76	76	77	78	79	79
	95th	121	122	123	124	126	127	128	80	80	80	81	82	83	83
	99th	128	129	130	132	133	134	135	87	87	88	89	89	90	91
14	50th	106	106	107	109	110	110	62	62	62	63	64	65	66	66
	90th	119	120	121	122	124	125	125	77	77	77	78	79	80	80
	95th	123	123	125	126	127	129	129	81	81	81	82	83	84	84
	99th	130	131	132	133	135	136	136	88	88	89	90	91	91	92
15	50th	107	108	109	110	111	113	113	64	64	64	65	66	67	67
	90th	120	121	122	123	125	126	127	78	78	78	79	80	81	81
	95th	124	125	126	127	129	130	131	82	82	82	83	84	85	85
	99th	131	132	133	134	136	137	138	89	89	90	91	91	92	93
16	50th	108	108	110	111	112	114	114	64	64	65	66	66	67	68
	90th	121	122	123	124	126	127	128	78	78	79	80	81	81	82
	95th	125	126	127	128	130	131	132	82	82	83	84	85	85	86
	99th	132	133	143	135	137	138	139	90	90	90	91	92	93	93
17	50th	108	109	110	111	113	114	115	64	65	65	66	67	67	68
	90th	122	122	123	125	26	127	128	78	79	79	80	81	81	82
	95th	125	126	127	129	130	131	132	82	83	83	84	85	85	86
	99th	133	133	134	136	137	138	139	90	90	91	91	92	93	93

BP, blood pressure

Source: www.nhlbi.nih.gov/guidelines/hypertension/children

When auscultating the heart, findings that need to be referred to a pediatric cardiologist include the following:

- Diastolic murmurs, nonfunctional murmurs (such as a pansystolic murmur), continuous murmurs that cannot be suppressed, and systolic clicks
- Extra heart sounds such as S_3 and S_4
- A murmur associated with a syndrome known to have a high incidence of congenital heart disease such as Down syndrome
- An infant with suspected symptoms of congestive heart failure, cyanosis, poor growth and development, and poor feeding
- In an older child, the complaint of dyspnea, chest pain with exertion, dizziness, shortness of breath, and abnormal vital signs

Write-Up of the Cardiovascular Exam

The write-up is the same for all age groups.

EXAMPLE OF A NORMAL CARDIAC EXAM: Inspection without pulsations, edema, cyanosis, or clubbing. Femoral pulses full and equal, apical impulse palpable at 4th intercostal space MCL, no thrills. S_1 and S_2 heard without splitting, no murmurs, S_1 heard best at mitral and tricuspid areas, S_2 heard best at pulmonic and aortic areas, NSR.

EXAMPLE OF AN ABNORMAL CARDIAC EXAM: Inspection without pulsations, edema, cyanosis, or clubbing. Femoral pulses full and equal, apical impulse palpable at 5th intercostal space MCL, no thrills. S_1 and S_2 heard without splitting, grade II/VI SEM (systolic ejection murmur) vibratory in quality, heard in LLSB without radiating. Heard both sitting up and in supine. S_1 heard best at mitral and tricuspid areas. S_2 heard best at pulmonic and aortic areas. NSR.

Case Study: Infant Presenting with Difficulty Feeding

A 3-month-old infant named Jason is brought to your office by his mother, who informs you that her son is having difficulty taking his bottle. She reports that when he feeds, he sucks for a short while and then becomes pale and diaphoretic. She has noticed this for the past 2 weeks. She denies that he has fever, nasal congestion, cough, vomiting, or diarrhea.

His perinatal history is unremarkable. His physical exams have been unremarkable except for a heart murmur that was noted at the 1-month well-child checkup.

On examination, Jason's weight is in the 5th percentile, and his length is in the 25th percentile. He is afebrile, his heart rate is 170 beats/min, and his respirations are shallow at 65 breaths/min without evidence of distress. His skin is pale and slightly diaphoretic. Further findings are as follows:

- *HEAD AND NECK*: Normal without venous distention.
- *ORAL PHARYNX*: Mucosa is pink and moist.
- *LUNGS*: Clear without adventitious sounds.
- *HEART*: The precordium is hyperdynamic, and a prominent systolic murmur is audible at the left lower sternal border.
- *ABDOMEN*: Liver edges are palpable 4 cm below the right costal margin in the right midclavicular line. The spleen is not palpable.
- *PULSES*: Normal pulses without edema.

Questions

1. What are the signs of congestive heart failure in children?
2. What are the primary symptoms associated with left-sided (left-to-right shunt) congestive heart failure?
3. What are some underlying disorders in children contributing to congestive heart failure?

Answers

1. Signs of congestive heart failure in an infant include tiring easily during feeding, weight loss or lack of normal weight gain, diaphoresis, irritability, and frequent infections. In older children, there may be signs of exercise intolerance, dyspnea, abdominal pain or distention associated with hepatomegaly, and peripheral edema. There may also be tachycardia, diminished pulses, hypotension, capillary refill time greater than 2 seconds, pallor, cool extremities, and oliguria.
2. Signs of left-sided congestive heart failure are predominantly respiratory symptoms. (Right-sided failure is associated with venous congestion and peripheral edema.)
3. Left-to-right shunts: Acyanotic congenital heart disease such as atrial septal defect, ventricular septal defect, patent ductus arteriosus. Right-to-left shunts: Cyanotic congenital heart disease such as transposition of the great arteries, tetralogy of Fallot, and tricuspid atresia.

References

AAFP. (1999). *Caring for infants with congenital heart disease and their families.* Jackson, MS: Saenz, R.B. , Beebe, D.K., Triplett, L.C.

American Academy of Pediatrics. (2008). Lipid screening and cardiovascular health in childhood. *Pediatrics, 122,* 198–208.

Burns, C., Dunn, A., Brady, M., Starr, N., & Blosser, C. (2004). *Pediatric primary care: A handbook for nurse practitioners* (3rd ed.). St. Louis, MO: Saunders.

Connor, S.M. (2006). Newborn infants for critical congenital heart disease. *Pediatrics, 118,* 1478–1485.

Jarvis, C. (2004). *Physical examination and health assessment* (5th ed.). St. Louis, MO: Elsevier.

Rome, J.J., Kreutzer, J. (2004). Pediatric interventional catheterization: Reasonable expectations and outcomes. *Pediatric Clinic North America, 51,* 1589–1610.

Special Writing Group of the Committee on Rheumatic Fever, Endocarditis, and Kawasaki Disease of the Council on Cardiovascular Disease in the Young of the American Heart Association. (1992). Guidelines for the diagnosis of rheumatic fever. *Journal of the American Medical Association, 268*(15), 2069–2073.

Resources

Ayoub, E. (2001). *Acute rheumatic fever.* In Allen H et al. *Moss and Adams' heart disease in infants, children and adolescents.* (6th ed.). Philadelphia: Lippincott, Williams & Wilkins.

Ball, J., Bindler, R., & Cowen, K. (2010). *Child health nursing.* Upper Saddle River, NJ: Pearson.

Bickley, L. (2003). *Bates' guide to physical examination and history taking* (8th ed.). New York: Lippincott Williams & Wilkins.

Estes, M. (1998). *Health assessment and physical examination.* Albany, NY: Delmar Publishers.

Hansen, M. (1998). *Pathophysiology: Foundations of disease and clinical intervention.* Philadelphia: Saunders.

Marieb, E. (1995). *Human anatomy and physiology* (3rd ed.). Redwood City, CA: Benjamin/Cummings Publishing Company.

Potts, N., & Mandleco, B. (2007). *Pediatraic nursing* (2nd ed.). Victoria, Australia: Thomson, Delmar Learning.

Tortora, G. J., & Grabvowski, S. R. (2003). *Principles of anatomy and physiology* (10th ed.). New York: Wiley.

Examination of the Abdomen

Anatomy and Physiology

The abdomen is the largest cavity in the body. It is located between the diaphragm at the top and the symphysis at the bottom. It contains several of the body's vital organs. The posterior wall of the abdomen includes the lumbar vertebrae, the sacrum, and the coccyx. The sides of the abdominal cavity are shaped by the iliac bones and the lateral portion of the ribs. These bony structures are held together by four pairs of flat muscles that are important in supporting and protecting the abdominal viscera. They play an important role in promoting movement flexion and lateral bending of the vertebral column. These muscles include the rectus abdominis, which is the medial superficial muscle pair; the external oblique, which is the largest and most superficial of the three lateral muscles; the transverse abdominis, which is the deepest, or innermost, muscle of the abdominal wall; and the internal oblique, which is composed of fibers that fan upward and forward and are at right angles to those fibers of the external oblique. The linea alba is a tendinous seam that extends from the sternum to the symphysis pubis and prevents the vertical muscles from bowstringing, or protruding anteriorly.

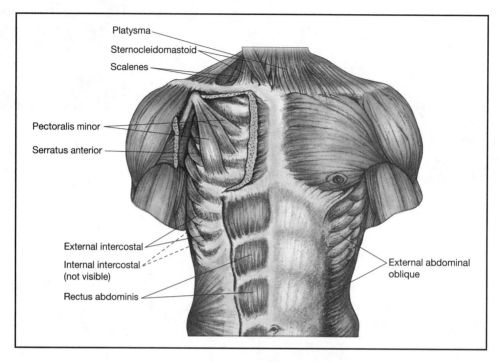

Platysma
Sternocleidomastoid
Scalenes
Pectoralis minor
Serratus anterior
External intercostal
Internal intercostal (not visible)
Rectus abdominis
External abdominal oblique

Figure 11-1 Abdomen

    Inside the abdominal cavity, the endothelial lining consists of the peritoneal serous membranes. The serous layer that lines the walls of the cavity is called the parietal peritoneum, and the lining that covers the organs is called the visceral peritoneum. The space between the two layers is called the peritoneal cavity. In the male, this cavity is completely closed, whereas in the female, openings exist for the fallopian tubes. The organs within the peritoneum are held in place by mesentery and consist of the spleen, gallbladder, stomach, liver, bile duct, small intestine, and large intestine. These organs are referred to as intraperitoneal organs. The organs behind the peritoneum are not held in place by mesenteric attachment and consist of the pancreas, kidneys, ureters, and bladder. They are referred to as the retroperitoneal organs.

Abdominal Vasculature

The largest artery in the body is the aorta, which extends from left of midline below the level of the diaphragm into the abdominal cavity. It is referred to as the descending aorta and becomes the abdominal aorta. At the fourth vertebra and approximately 2 cm below the umbilicus, the aorta bifurcates into the right and left common iliac arteries, which become the femoral arteries in the groin area. The abdominal aorta gives rise to arterial vasculature that supplies the abdominal wall and gastrointestinal (GI) organs with blood. You may palpate the aorta pulsations in the upper anterior abdominal wall, as well as the femoral arteries at a point halfway between the anterior superior iliac spine and the symphysis pubis.

In examination of the abdomen, anatomic mapping serves as a frame of reference during examination. The abdominal cavity is divided into quadrants based on imaginary vertical and horizontal lines that intersect and coincide with nine anatomic locations. It is important to be able to pinpoint the location of abdominal organs during palpation and percussion of the abdomen.

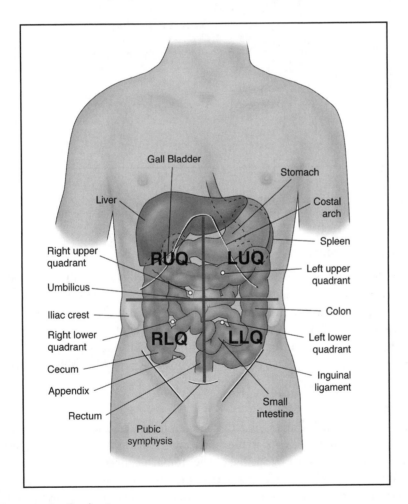

Figure 11-2   Quadrants

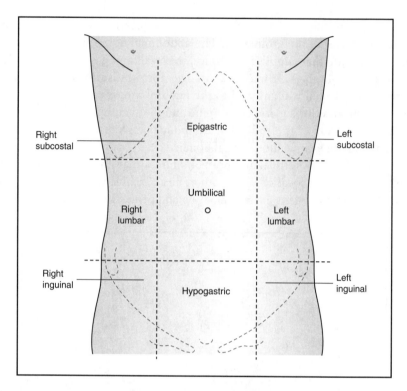

Figure 11-3

Abdominal Organs

The abdominal organs are reviewed next. Included are solid viscera and hollow viscera. The solid viscera are those organs that maintain a characteristic shape, such as the liver, pancreas, spleen, adrenal glands, kidneys, ovaries, and uterus. The hollow viscera that are not palpable include the stomach, gallbladder, small intestine, colon, and bladder. Typically, the colon and bladder are hollow organs, although they may be palpable if full with feces or urine.

Stomach

The stomach is a J-shaped, pouchlike organ located in the left upper quadrant of the abdomen inferior to the diaphragm. It lies to the right of the spleen and is partially covered by the liver. The stomach connects the esophagus to the duodenum, which is the first part of the small intestine. It functions as a reservoir for the complex process of digestion. The digestion of starch, which starts in the mouth, continues, and the digestion of proteins and triglycerides occurs. This semisolid bolus, or chyme, is converted to a liquid in which certain substances are absorbed. Digestive enzymes and hydrochloric acid are secreted by the stomach to aid in the digestive process. Chyme is released into the first part of the small intestine, the duodenum, for further digestion and absorption.

A detailed description of the pathophysiology of the GI system is beyond the scope of this text. Refer to a text on human anatomy and physiology for more information.

Small Intestine

The small intestine is where the major events of digestion and absorption occur. The small intestine is a tubular-shaped organ extending from the pyloric sphincter to the ileocecal valve at the opening of the large intestine. The small intestine is divided into three regions—the duodenum, the jejunum, and the ileum. The duodenum is the shortest region; it starts at the pyloric sphincter of the stomach and extends about 25 cm where it merges with the jejunum. The duodenum plays a major role in digestion as hormonal secretions are released, and both the common bile and main pancreatic ducts open into the duodenum. The jejunum is the second component and is about 1 m (3 ft) long; it is the longest part of the small intestine and extends to the ileum. It is composed of circular folds that enhance absorption by increasing the surface area and causing the chyme to spiral, rather than move in a straight line, as it passes through the small intestine. The last section is the ileum, which joins the large intestine at the ileocecal valve. This last section of the small intestine absorbs bile salts and vitamin B_{12}.

Large Intestine

The large intestine is the terminal portion of the GI tract and is divided into four regions—the ascending, transverse, descending, and sigmoid portions. It is a tubular-shaped organ extending from the ileocecal valve to the anus. It has a greater diameter than the small intestine and can vary in length, depending upon the size of the individual.

Hanging inferior to the ileocecal valve is the cecum, which is a blind pouch. Attached to the cecum is the appendix, a twisted, coiled tube approximately 8 cm in length. Also attached to the cecum is the ascending colon located in the right lower quadrant of the abdomen. The ascending colon ascends on the right side of the abdomen to the inferior surface of the liver and turns to the left to form the right colic flexure. The colon continues across the abdomen to the left side, where it is referred to as the transverse colon. It curves beneath the inferior portion of the spleen and is the left colonic, or splenic, flexure. From here, it passes inferiorly to the level of the iliac crest as the descending colon. The sigmoid colon begins near

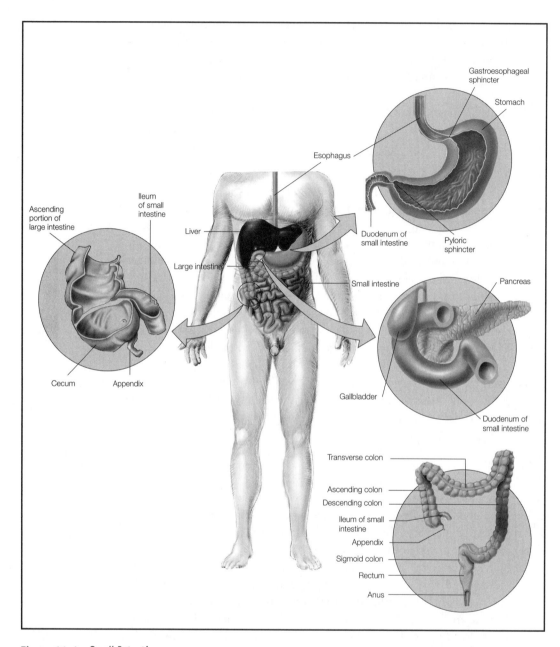

Figure 11-4 Small Intestine

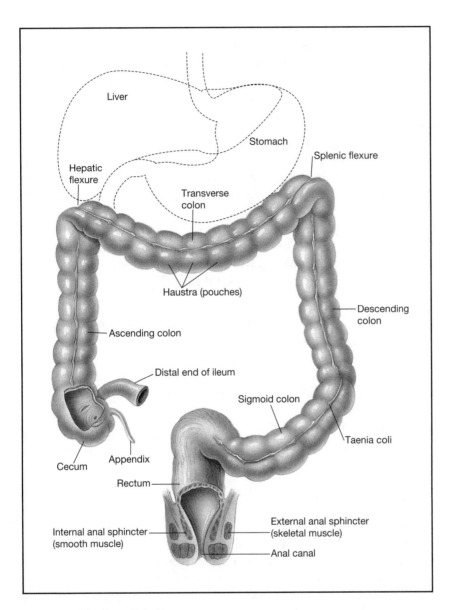

Liver

Stomach

Splenic flexure

Hepatic flexure

Transverse colon

Haustra (pouches)

Descending colon

Ascending colon

Distal end of ileum

Sigmoid colon

Taenia coli

Cecum

Appendix

Rectum

Internal anal sphincter (smooth muscle)

External anal sphincter (skeletal muscle)

Anal canal

Figure 11-5(a)   Large Intestine

the left iliac crest, projects medially to the midline, and terminates as the rectum. The rectum is the last 20 cm of the GI tract; it progresses to the anal canal, which is surrounded by internal and external sphincter muscles. The large intestine has limited digestive function; its primary function is water absorption.

Liver

The liver is the second largest solid organ in the body after the skin. It is located in the right upper quadrant inferior to the diaphragm and extends across the midline to the left upper quadrant. In the right upper quadrant, the superior aspect of the liver is at the fifth rib. The lower border generally does not extend more then 1 cm below the right costal margin. The liver is divided into two principal lobes, the large right lobe and smaller left lobe. The liver performs many functions, one of the main ones being secretion of bile, which is needed for absorption of dietary fats.

Other functions of the liver include (Marieb, 1995):

- Carbohydrate metabolism, which is important in maintaining a normal blood glucose level. When blood glucose is high, the liver converts glucose to glycogen and triglycerides for storage.
- Lipid metabolism
- Protein metabolism
- Detoxification and filtration of drugs such as alcohol or excretion of drugs such as penicillin
- Excretion of bilirubin
- Synthesis of bile salts
- Storage
- Phagocytosis
- Activation of vitamin D

Gallbladder

The gallbladder is a pear-shaped sac located in a depression of the posterior surface of the liver in the right upper quadrant of the abdomen. Its primary function is to store and concentrate bile produced by the liver. Bile consists mostly of water and bile acids, bile salts, cholesterol, and a phospholipid plus bile pigments. It is a yellow, brownish, or olive-green liquid. As the gallbladder contracts, the bile is released through the cystic duct into the common bile duct, which drains into the duodenum.

Pancreas

The pancreas is located posterior to the curvature of the stomach, where it lies in a transverse position along the posterior abdominal wall. It is both an exocrine gland and an endocrine gland. As an exocrine gland, it secretes

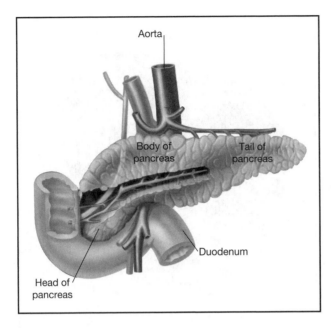

Figure 11-5(b) Pancreas

bicarbonate and pancreatic enzymes that aid in digestion and create the proper pH level for the action of digestive enzymes in the small intestine. It also functions as an endocrine gland that secretes the hormones insulin, glucagons, and gastrin.

Spleen

The spleen is the largest organ of lymphatic tissue in the body. It is located behind the fundus of the stomach, inferior to the diaphragm and superior to the left kidney and splenic flexure. It lies obliquely with its long axis behind and parallel to the 10th rib, lateral to the midaxillary line. It is generally not palpable, although if it becomes enlarged, it moves downward and toward the midline. The spleen is part of the reticuloendothelial system and functions in the body as a filter for old and destroyed red blood cells and platelets. It also serves as a reservoir by contributing needed red blood cells to the circulation during times of vasoconstriction, such as hemorrhage or exercise.

Vermiform Appendix

The appendix is a fingerlike appendage that extends off the lower cecum in the right lower quadrant. Due to obstruction of the lumen by a fecalith, foreign body, or digestive materials, the appendix becomes distended and is subject to infection, leading to ischemia and necrosis.

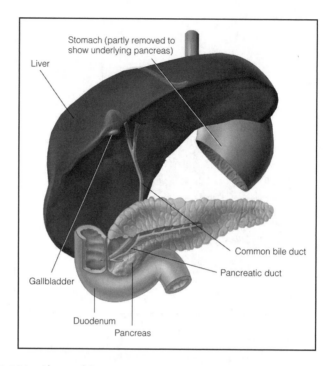

Figure 11-5(c) Liver and Pancreas

Kidneys, Ureters, and Bladder

The kidneys are bean-shaped organs that lie against the posterior abdominal wall where they are protected by the posterior ribs. The 12th rib forms an angle with the vertebral column, the costovertebral angle. The left kidney is slightly larger and lies at the level of the 11th and 12th rib. Because of the superior placement of the liver over the right kidney, it rests 1 to 2 cm lower than the left and at times may be palpable between the 12th and 13th rib. The kidneys' main function is to rid the body of waste products. The kidneys also maintain homeostasis through regulation of fluid and electrolyte balance, acid–base balance, and arterial blood pressure.

Anatomic Map

The anatomic location of the organs are described by quadrants based on a vertical and a horizontal line bisecting the umbilicus.

The right upper quadrant (RUQ) includes the:

- Liver
- Gallbladder
- Duodenum
- Head of the pancreas

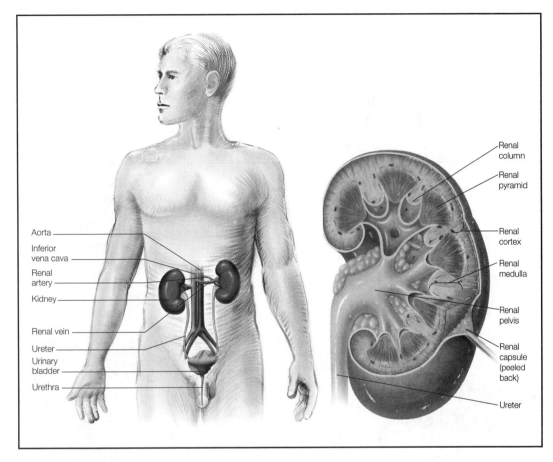

Figure 11-5(d)   Kidneys

- Right kidney and adrenal gland
- Hepatic flexure of the colon
- Ascending and transverse colon (in part)

The left upper quadrant (LUQ) includes the:

- Stomach
- Spleen
- Left lobe of the liver
- Body of the pancreas
- Left kidney and adrenal gland
- Splenic flexure of the colon
- Transverse and descending colon (in part)

The right lower quadrant (RLQ) includes the:

- Cecum
- Appendix
- Right ovary and tube
- Right ureter
- Right spermatic cord

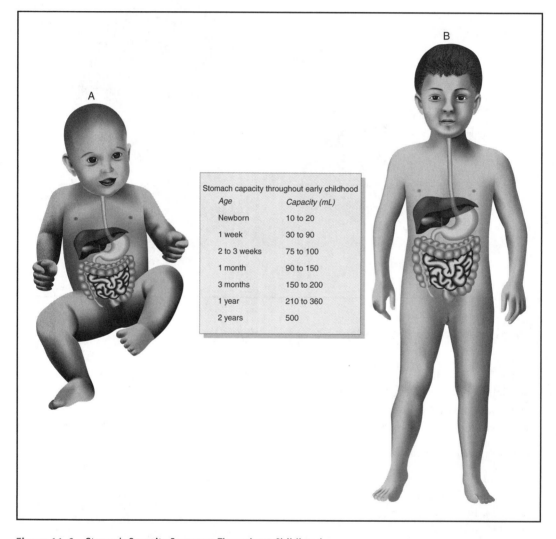

Stomach capacity throughout early childhood	
Age	*Capacity (mL)*
Newborn	10 to 20
1 week	30 to 90
2 to 3 weeks	75 to 100
1 month	90 to 150
3 months	150 to 200
1 year	210 to 360
2 years	500

Figure 11-6 Stomach Capacity Increases Throughout Childhood

Source: This article was published in *Mosby's Guide to Physical Examination*, 6th edition, Seidel, Ball, Dains, and Benedict. Stomach Capacity Increases Throughout Childhood, page 1128. Copyright Elsevier (2006).

The left lower quadrant (LLQ) includes the:

- Descending colon (in part)
- Sigmoid colon
- Left ovary and tube
- Left ureter
- Left spermatic cord

The midline area includes the:

- Aorta
- Uterus
- Bladder

Development of the Stomach

The stomach's main processes of absorption and excretion do not start to occur until after birth. In utero the GI system is immature, and the placenta provides nutrients and removes wastes from the fetus. In the neonate, the stomach is small and the process of peristalsis or intestinal mobility is greater than in the toddler. Because of the small capacity of the stomach, and the increased peristalsis, the infant requires small, frequent feedings and has frequent soft bowel movements. Because the infant's GI system is immature, the infant does not have adequate quantities of enzymes in the stomach; therefore, digestion primarily takes place in the duodenum. Because of the lack of intestinal enzymes, gas often builds up in the infant's stomach, and due to the relaxed cardiac sphincter, the infant may evidence reflux or regurgitate small amounts of feedings referred to as gastro esophageal reflux.

Enzymes necessary for digestion include amylase, which digests carbohydrates; lipase, which enhances fat absorption; and trypsin, which catabolizes protein into polypeptides and amino acids. All of these enzymes are not produced in sufficient quantity until 4–6 months of age, which explains why delaying the addition of solids until 4–6 months of life decreases the chances of GI problems in the infant.

In the newborn the liver is also immature which accounts for increased bilirubin levels. It takes two to three weeks of life for the liver to adequately conjugate bilirubin and excrete bile. This explains why bilirubin levels are monitored in the newborn period if there is any concern regarding jaundice. Due to the immaturity of the liver, the processes of gluconeogenesis which is the formation of glycogen from noncarbohydrates such as amino acids and glycerol portion of fats and deamination which is removal of amino radicals from an amino acid are not fully active until close to one year of age.

TABLE 11-1   LANDMARKS FOR ABDOMINAL EXAMINATION

Anatomic Correlates of the Four Quadrants of the Abdomen

Right Upper Quadrant (RUQ)	Left Upper Quadrant (LUQ)
Liver and gallbladder	Left lobe of liver
Pylorus	Spleen
Duodenum	Stomach
Head of pancreas	Body of pancreas
Right adrenal gland	Left adrenal gland
Portion of right kidney	Portion of left kidney
Hepatic flexure of colon	Splenic flexure of colon
Portions of ascending and transverse colon	Portions of transverse and descending colon

Right Lower Quadrant (RLQ)	Left Lower Quadrant (LLQ)
Lower pole of right kidney	Lower pole of left kidney
Cecum and appendix	Sigmoid colon
Portion of ascending colon	Portion of descending colon
Bladder (if distended)	Bladder (if distended)
Ovary and salpinx	Ovary and salpinx
Uterus (if enlarged)	Uterus (if enlarged)
Right spermatic cord	Left spermatic cord
Right ureter	Left ureter

Anatomic Correlates of the Nine Regions of the Abdomen

4 Right Hypochondriac	1 Epigastric	5 Left Hypochondriac
Right lobe of liver	Pyloric end of stomach	Stomach
Gallbladder	Duodenum	Spleen
Portion of duodenum	Pancreas	Tail of pancreas
Hepatic flexure of colon	Portion of liver	Splenic flexure of colon
Portion of right kidney		Upper pole of left kidney
Suprarenal gland		Suprarenal gland
6 Right Lumbar	**2 Umbilical**	**7 Left Lumbar**
Ascending colon	Omentum	Descending colon
Lower half of right kidney	Mesentery	Lower half of left kidney
Portion of duodenum and jejunum	Lower part of duodenum	Portions of jejunum and ileum
	Jejunum and ileum	
8 Right Inguinal	**3 Hypogastric (Pubic)**	**9 Left Inguinal**
Cecum	Ileum	Sigmoid colon
Appendix	Bladder	Left ureter
Lower end of ileum	Uterus (in pregnancy)	Left spermatic cord
Right ureter		Left ovary
Right spermatic cord		
Right ovary		

Source: This article was published in *Health & Physical Assessment*, 3rd edition, Barkauskas, Baumann, and Darling-Fisher. Landmarks for Abdominal Examination, page 526. Copyright Mosby (2002).

The processes necessary for digestion are complete by 2 years of age. At this time, the capacity of the stomach has increased sufficiently to accommodate a schedule of three meals per day.

In conjunction with development of the GI tract, structural anomalies associated with atresia (absence or closure of a normal body orifice) can occur during the first trimester, such as cleft lip and cleft palate. Both cleft lip with or without cleft palate is the fourth most common birth defect (Merritt, 2005). This disorder occurs during week 6 of gestation when there is failure of the maxillary and/or palatine processes to fuse. Union of the upper lip is normally complete by week 7, and fusion of the secondary palate occurs between weeks 5 and 12 of gestation. Both cleft lip and cleft palate may occur independently of each other. Cleft palate forms a continuous opening between the mouth and the nasal cavity, which may be unilateral or bilateral involving both the soft and hard palate. Cleft lip is readily apparent at birth and can include complete separation of the lip extending to the floor of the nose.

Assessment Considerations: Subjective Information

The following sections present considerations for the assessment of the stomach.

Infants and Toddlers

- Was the mother's pregnancy normal? Has the infant's growth been normal?
- Has the child had an imperforate anus or failure to pass meconium? Failure to pass meconium is associated with Hirschsprung disease, which is lack of parasympathetic innervation to part of the intestines resulting in inadequate motility and obstruction. Is there a history of difficulty feeding, cleft palate or lip, or prolonged jaundice?
- Is the infant breast- or bottle-feeding? If bottle-feeding, what formula is the child taking, and how does he or she tolerate it? If breast-feeding, are there any problems in digesting the milk?
- How often is the infant fed? Is the infant on a regular schedule or an on-demand feeding schedule?
- Does the child have a history of vomiting? If so, is it forceful or projectile? Does the child have a history of failure to gain weight? Are there concerns about reflux?
- Does the child have a history of colic, diarrhea, or weight loss?
- What table food has the parent introduced, and how does the child tolerate the food? Adding only one new food at a time to the child's diet helps in the identification of potential allergies.

- How does the parent describe the child's eating habits, including a 24-hour recall? What does the child eat for breakfast, lunch, and dinner, including snacks?
- Does the child drink milk, soda, juice, or water? If so, how much?
- Does the child eat nonfood articles such as dirt, paint, crayons, or paper? Pica is defined as the ingestion of nonfood products and is seen between the ages of 1 and 3 years. It is often associated with lead poisoning.
- Does the child have a history of constipation? How often does the child stool, and what is the character of the stool?
- Does the child take a bottle to bed at night?
- Does the child have a recent history of diarrhea? Has the child traveled out of the country? Has the child had any new exposures, such as to food or sick individuals?
- Has the child been on any medications, such as antibiotics? Is the child currently taking any new medication?

Toddlers and School-Age Children

- Does the child have a history of encopresis? When did it start, and was it in conjunction with toilet training?
- Does the child frequently complain of abdominal pain? Does it occur on the weekends or during vacation? Is it associated with certain foods? What time of day does it usually occur? Is there a pattern to it? Explore the possible stressors and response to stressors in the child's life. (Recurrent abdominal pain will be further addressed under Common Gastrointestinal Disorders.)
- Is the child overweight? If so, has this been a long-standing problem? Do other family members have obesity problems? How does the child deal with this weight issue?
- How does the parent describe the child's diet? What are the child's favorite foods? Does the child eat what is prepared for dinner?
- Does the child have a history of nausea, vomiting, and diarrhea? If so, explore the possibility of family members or close friends with similar symptoms.
- Has the child traveled outside of the country? Has the child had any new exposures? Is the child taking any new medications?

Adolescents

- What is the adolescent's dietary pattern? How many meals per day does the adolescent eat?
- Does the adolescent eat breakfast? Does the adolescent eat lunch at school? What does the adolescent eat for dinner?

- What does the adolescent eat for snacks?
- Does the adolescent exercise on a regular basis? What type of exercise?
- Is the adolescent happy with his or her weight? Does the adolescent want to gain or lose weight?
- Is sports participation dependent upon the adolescent's weight?
- Does the adolescent take medication to control his or her weight?
- Does the adolescent take dietary supplements such as vitamins, protein powders, or herbal remedies?
- Are the female patient's menstrual cycles regular?
- Does the adolescent have a history of an eating disorder? Ask the patient questions regarding anorexia nervosa and bulimia.
- Has the adolescent experienced a recent onset of vomiting, diarrhea, or associated symptoms? Is so, ask if family members or close friends have similar symptoms. Has the adolescent traveled outside of the country? Has the adolescent had any new exposures? Is the adolescent taking any new medications?

Family History

- Is there a family history of allergies to certain foods?
- Is there a history of gallbladder disease or ulcers?
- Do other family members have dietary issues such as food intolerance?
- Is there a family history of obesity?
- Is there a history of malabsorption syndrome, such as cystic fibrosis or celiac disease?
- Is there a history of inflammatory bowel disease such as ulcerative colitis or Crohn disease?
- Is there a history of colon cancer?

Review of Systems

Review of systems with relevance to the abdomen and the digestive process includes questions regarding dietary intake and the child's response to specific foods. Allergic reactions to foods can be evident through the integument in the form of a diaper rash, urticaria, hives, or even anaphylaxis. Also include questions regarding the pulmonary system and a history of wheezing and/or bronchial constriction secondary to ingestion of certain foods.

Assessment Considerations: Objective Information

When examining the abdomen, the order of assessment techniques is altered. Inspection is performed first, followed by auscultation, then percussion and palpation. Assessment of the abdomen is the only time that auscultation follows inspection. It is performed in this order to avoid disrupting the internal organs, particularly when listening for discrete bowel sounds.

Inspection

Infants

When inspecting the abdomen of the newborn, visual inspection is best performed by observing the infant in a supine position. The abdomen will be protuberant in an infant due to underdevelopment of the abdominal musculature. Intestinal peristalsis will be easily observable due to the thin musculature, as well as blood vessels in the abdominal wall.

An important consideration in inspection of the abdomen is the infant's *umbilical cord.* There are normally two umbilical arteries and one umbilical vein. The vein is located at the 12 o'clock position. Congenital anomalies are associated with a single umbilical artery. In the newborn, the umbilicus is surrounded by mucoid connective tissue called Wharton's jelly. This umbilical stump dries up and falls off within 2 weeks. The remainder is the cutaneous portion, which retracts to become flush with the abdominal wall. In newborns, an umbilical granuloma may be observed at the base of the navel. It is the development of pink granulation tissue that is formed during the healing process. Always inspect the umbilicus and the area surrounding it for signs of infections such as redness, swelling, or drainage. A common finding in infants is *umbilical hernia,* which is due to an umbilical ring that does not close properly. It can be up to 6 cm in diameter, but any hernia larger than 2.5 cm should be referred. An umbilical hernia will become more protuberant when the baby is crying, straining, or coughing, but can be evident when the baby is lying quietly. Most often, umbilical hernias resolve by 1 year of age without intervention.

On further inspection of the infant's abdomen, you may notice a midline ridge called *diastasis recti.* This is separation of the two rectus abdominis muscles that cause the ridge running midline. It is more apparent on contraction of the abdominal muscles. It is a benign condition and resolves spontaneously by early childhood.

Toddlers and School-Age Children

In the toddler and school-age child, inspection is much the same as it is in the adult. Assessment is done noting any skin changes, or scars, and inspecting for any pulsations. In the toddler, the abdomen may still be quite protuberant, which is evident in both a supine and standing position. A protuberant abdomen, or potbelly, remains apparent in the standing position until after 4 years of age because of lumbar lordosis. Respiratory movements may also be visible, as children are abdominal breathers until approximately 7 years of age.

Print heart sounds

Abdo – inspect
– Ausc
– Pay .

view the abdomen from a lat-
stooping down to gaze across
face characteristics, noting any
ndary to weight gain or preg-
or; they turn silvery over time.
ation of the umbilicus, which
decorative umbilical rings may
infection, erythema, drainage,
r of the abdomen, noting sym-
peristalsis that may be visible in
pulsation of the aorta beneath
the skin in the epigastric area. Also, in both the male and the female adolescent, observe the pattern of pubic hair growth. In adolescent males at
Tanner stage 5, pubic hair growth assumes a diamond shape extending up
the abdomen toward the umbilicus; in females at Tanner stage 5, pubic hair
growth assumes an inverted triangle shape.

The contour can be described as flat, rounded, or scaphoid. A flat contour is observed in athletic adolescents, whereas a rounded or convex
contour is noted in adolescents who have poor muscle tone, are overweight, and get inadequate exercise. A scaphoid or concave abdomen can
be seen in thin adolescents, particularly those with eating disorders.

Auscultation

Infants

In the infant, auscultation is performed in all four quadrants, listening
for bowel sounds. The diaphragm of the stethoscope should be warm or
room temperature to avoid disturbing the infant. By gently placing the
stethoscope on the infant's abdomen, musical tinkling bowel sounds can
be heard every 10 to 30 seconds. This procedure is quite easily performed
without causing disruption or crying by using a pacifier or bottle if necessary. Hyperactive bowel sounds are heard in children with gastroenteritis
and diarrhea, whereas decreased or absent bowel sounds are noted with
appendicitis or intestinal obstruction. The absence of bowel sounds is
determined after 5 minutes of continuous listening (Seidel, 2007). In children with aortic stenosis or stenosis of the iliac, femoral, or renal arteries,
an audible abdominal bruit can be heard.

Toddlers and School-Age Children

By the time toddlerhood has been reached, the child has been examined
numerous times, often involving immunizations or other intrusive and
uncomfortable procedures. To auscultate the abdomen, allow the child

to first examine and inspect your stethoscope before placing it on his or her skin. Warm the diaphragm with your hands before placing it on the abdomen. Once you have gained the child's trust, listen in all four quadrants for tinkling bowel sounds, noting their frequency and character. Occasionally, you will hear loud gurgles called borborygmi, or stomach growling. These sounds may be heard in conjunction with gastroenteritis, early intestinal obstruction, or hunger.

Adolescents

Auscultation of the adolescent's abdomen starts by placing a warmed stethoscope on the patient's abdomen and listening in all four quadrants. As with the toddler and school-age child, you are listening for tingling sounds, noting their frequency and character. Also listen for borborygmi as well as the total absence of bowel sounds. Remember, bowel sounds are produced from the movement of air and fluid passing through the small intestine. The frequency of bowel sounds is dependent upon the time since eating. Typically, bowel sounds are irregular and can occur anywhere from 5 to 30 times per minute (Jarvis, 2008, p. 570). You do not need to count them, but document whether you hear normal, hypoactive, or hyperactive vowel sounds. In the adolescent, listen for vascular sounds or bruits over the aorta, renal arteries, and femoral arteries. Usually no sounds are audible.

Palpation

Infants

In children, palpation of the abdomen is beneficial in assessment of the liver and spleen and also for detecting abdominal masses. When palpating an infant's abdomen, flex the knees with one hand while palpating with the other. This technique helps to relax the infant while examining the abdomen. Also, offering the infant a pacifier if necessary will help to relax him or her.

In a newborn, because the liver is large and fills the majority of the RUQ, the liver edges are easily palpated 1–2 cm below the costal margin. Start by gently palpating the liver in the RLQ at the right midclavicular line 3–4 cm below the costal margin, and gradually move your fingers upward toward the costal margin. During inspiration, wait to feel a narrow mass touch your fingers, and as you do, move your fingers up along the midclavicular line toward the costal margin until the sensation is felt a little stronger. In infants and toddlers, liver edges may still be palpated 1–2 cm below the costal margin. By starting low in the abdomen, you are less likely to miss an enlarged liver. Hepatomegaly in an infant may be due to congestive heart disease, liver disease, or a glycogen storage disease. Pyloric stenosis is often identified by the almond-shaped mass palpated in the RUQ. A helpful technique is to sit the infant in your lap and fold the child's upper body gently against your hand. At the same time, palpate the upper abdomen, which brings the pyloric mass into opposition with your hand.

Palpate across the abdomen, feeling for any masses. Along the LUQ, you may be able to palpate the spleen tip. It feels much narrower and sharper than the liver and feels like the edge of a tongue. As you palpate downward in the LLQ, you will be able to feel the descending colon, which feels similar to a sausage-like mass when filled with stool. Assessment of abdominal tenderness and determining whether a child has a hard or soft abdomen is difficult if the infant is crying. *Seize the opportunity* when the child pauses to take a deep breath, and palpate the abdomen. The abdominal muscles relax during inspiration, and the abdomen should therefore be soft on palpation. A rigid or tense abdomen that is resistant to pressure may indicate peritoneal irritation or may be associated with increased gastric distention. Abdominal tenderness in an infant may be difficult to assess, although evidence of facial grimacing, a higher pitch in crying, drawing the knees up toward the chest, or refusal to suck or take a pacifier may be helpful clues or indicators.

Toddlers and School-Age Children

Palpation of the toddler or the school-age child's abdomen is basically the same, following the established pattern of inspection, auscultation, palpation, and percussion. The difference comes in the approach to the child. Being calm, gentle, and reassuring is helpful in developing rapport with the child. Speaking softly, approaching the child with slow, gentle movements, and taking time to interact with the child through play or through conversation helps build trust and cooperation, thus enabling you to perform a comprehensive abdominal examination.

Palpating the abdomen of a toddler requires a little more expertise because by the time he or she reaches toddlerhood, the child often associates an office visit with immunizations and other intrusive procedures. Gaining the child's cooperation is paramount. Start by warming your hands, then gently place them on the RUQ or LUQ and gently palpate the entire abdominal surface including all four quadrants. It is helpful to develop a pattern of palpation, such as always starting on the RUQ or LUQ and working in a circular motion until all aspects of the abdomen have been examined.

Palpation of abdominal organs assesses for size, shape, location, and consistency. Begin with light systematic palpation of all four quadrants by placing the palmar surface of four fingers lightly on the abdomen. With one hand, depress the abdominal wall approximately 1 cm using a light and even pressing motion. Avoid sharp quick movements or jabs. Continue palpation of all four quadrants in a clockwise movement. Repeat the same systematic assessment for deep palpation by using a bimanual technique with one hand on top of the other. With deep palpation, depress the abdominal wall approximately 4–6 cm. Again extending your four fingers and using the palmar surface, press deeply and evenly into the abdominal wall, at the same time moving your fingers back and forth over the abdominal contents. If the child is obese or very tense, deep palpation with the fingers of one hand applying pressure on top of the fingers of the other hand may be an alternate method for palpation. Many providers routinely perform light palpation followed in the same pattern with deep palpation. During deep palpation, you may be able to feel the borders of the rectus abdominis muscles, the aorta, and portions of the colon.

It is helpful to form an image in your mind of the abdominal contents and visualize what is under each quadrant as you palpate, distinguishing what you are feeling and noting any abnormal enlargement, tenderness, or masses. In children, abdominal organs are relatively easy to palpate due to the thin abdominal wall with minimal adipose tissue and muscle. If you

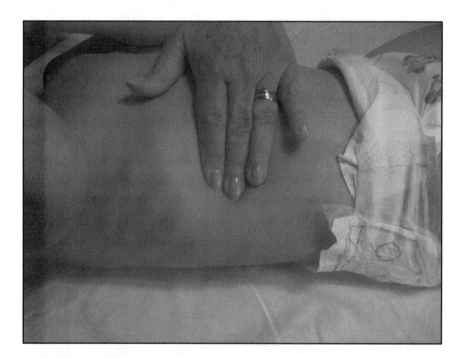

Figure 11-7 Light Palpation

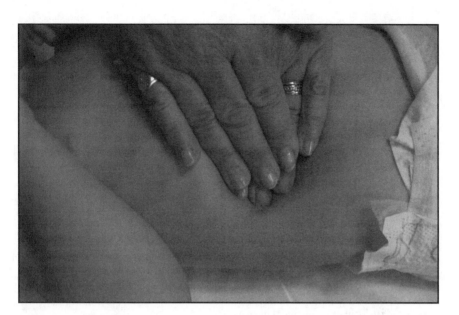

Figure 11-8 Deep Palpation

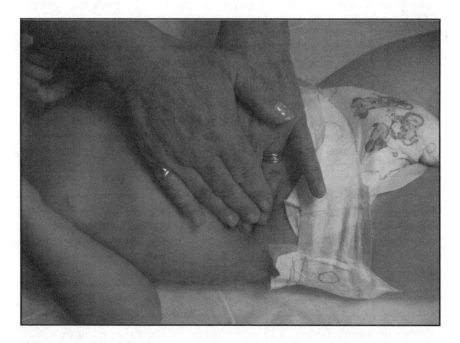

Figure 11-9 Deep Palpation

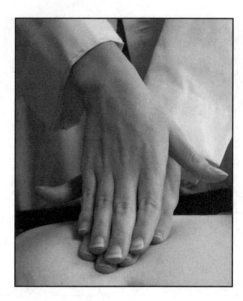

Figure 11-10 Palpation of the Abdomen

identify an enlarged organ or questionable mass, distinguish it by noting the following (Jarvis, 2008, p. 578):

- Location
- Size, shape, consistency (soft, firm, hard)
- Surface (smooth, modular)
- Mobility (including movement with respirations)
- Pulsibility
- Tenderness

If a toddler is frightened about lying on the exam table, *seize the opportunity* and have the child lie down on the parent's lap. Pull a stool up so you are eye level with the child, and gently place your warm hands on the child's abdomen. If putting on a hospital gown causes too much disruption, just moving up the shirt during the examination alleviates some of the child's discomfort and avoids crying. Having a conversation with the child will also help to distract him or her. While talking, you can accomplish a great deal, including palpating the liver and spleen as well as the rest of the abdomen. If the child is on the table and is particularly ticklish and/or frightened, place the child's hand underneath yours and place your fingers between the child's fingers. This way you can examine the abdomen with a somewhat relaxed and cooperative child; in a short time, you will be able to remove the child's hand and palpate the entire abdomen.

Ask a school-age child who is very tense to bend his or her knees by flexing at the hips. This position relieves the tension on the rectus abdominis muscles and allows you to palpate the abdomen more effectively. Continue by following the same pattern used for adults. Always start and palpate lightly across the abdomen. When assessing for the liver and spleen in a school-age child, the edges are normally not palpated below the costal margin. Occasionally, you may feel the liver edges, which are firm and solid and move easily when pushed upward during deep inspiration.

If a child complains of abdominal pain, it is important to ask the child to point to the area that hurts. When palpating, always leave the site of potential pathology for the end.

The presence of feces in the colon is a common finding in children, especially those with a history of constipation, and can be easily palpated as a soft, rounded, boggy mass in the ascending, descending, or sigmoid colon.

Palpating the Liver and Spleen

After palpating throughout the abdomen, next assess the liver and spleen. The technique is the same from toddlerhood through adolescence and is based on the technique used in the adult. Starting on the right side, place your left hand under the child's back and place your right hand on the RUQ with your fingers parallel to and just under the costal margin. If the child is cooperative, ask him or her to take a deep breath, and push deeply down and under the right costal margin. While the child is taking a deep breath, the diaphragm pushes down on the liver. See **Figure 11-11**. It is normal to feel the edges of the liver touch your fingertips during inhalation. The liver edges will feel firm and solid, without nodules or ridges. Usually, you will not be able to feel the liver edges.

Another method to assess the liver is the *hooking technique*. Standing lateral to the child's shoulders, hook your fingers over and under the costal margin. Ask the child to take a deep breath, and try to feel to the liver edges as it is pushed down by the diaphragm. See **Figure 11-12** and **Figure 11-13**. This technique is easy to perform on a thin child, as the costal margin is pronounced and easy to hook your fingers around.

Next, to assess for the spleen, remain standing on the right side, reach across the child's abdomen, and place your left hand under the child's back at the level of the 11th or 12th rib. With your right hand pointing toward the axilla, push your fingertips deeply down and under the left costal margin, asking the child to take a deep breath. In most cases, you will not feel the spleen. The spleen is not palpable unless there is a question of infection, such as mononucleosis, in which case both the liver and the spleen may be palpable. If the spleen is enlarged, it may become 2 to 3 times its normal size and may extend into the LLQ. An enlarged spleen is

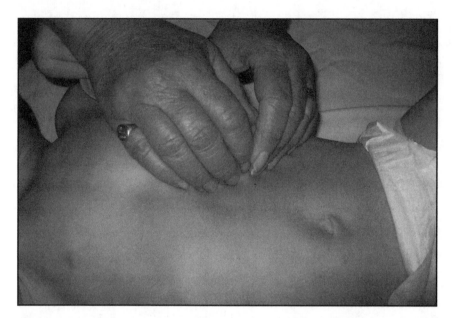

Figure 11-11 Hooking Technique

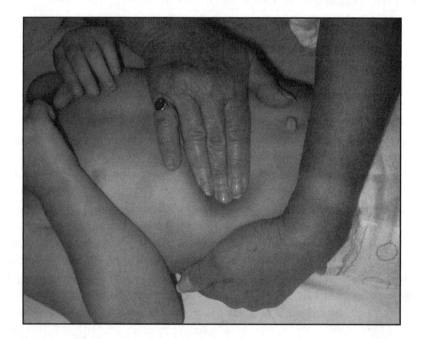

Figure 11-12 Palpation of Liver

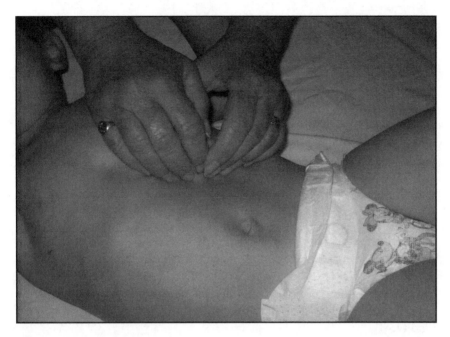

Figure 11-13 Hooking Technique

quite friable and can rupture with deep palpation. Assess the enlargement of the spleen based on centimeters below the costal margin.

During palpation, observe the child's behavior, noting any change in facial expression, rigidity, tensing, guarding, or wincing. These reactions are helpful in confirming areas of tenderness.

Palpating the Kidneys

Palpation of the kidneys in children is performed the same as in adults, with the child in supine position. For the *left kidney*, stand on the child's right side, reach across with your left hand as though you were going to palpate the spleen, and place your hand on the left flank. Place your right hand at the left costal margin, and ask the child to take a deep breath. At the same time, elevate the left flank with your left hand and palpate deeply with your right hand. You may feel the lower pole of the kidney with your fingertips as the child inhales. The left kidney is generally not palpable because of the retroperitoneal position.

To palpate the *right kidney*, stand at the child's right side, and place your left hand under the right flank and your right hand at the right costal margin. Perform the same maneuver as for the left kidney. Due to the position of the right kidney, the lower pole may be felt in a thin relaxed child.

Overall, kidneys are more easily palpable in young children due to less muscle tone and bulk and less adipose tissue. The kidney should feel firm, smooth, and without tenderness.

After palpating the kidneys, you can assess the costovertebral angle for tenderness. Start by asking the child to sit on the edge of the exam table. Place the palm of your hand over the right costovertebral angle over the area of the 12th rib, and strike that hand with the ulnar surface of the fist of your other hand. The same maneuver of indirect fist percussion is performed for the other kidney as well. Generally, the child will feel a thud but no pain. Pain is elicited when there is inflammation of the kidney such as with pyelonephritis.

Guarding

As you are palpating the abdomen, watch the child's face, noting any change in expression. Also watch for voluntary guarding. If the child has pointed out an area of the abdomen that hurts, tell the child you will not touch that area until last. Circulate the abdomen in a systematic manner as you palpate, observing for voluntary muscle guarding and/or involuntary rigidity.

 Voluntary guarding occurs when the child is ticklish, tense, afraid, or cold. As you touch the abdomen, the muscles constrict and will interfere with palpation. Involuntary rigidity presents as a board-like hardness of the muscles, which acts as a protective mechanism due to acute inflammation of the peritoneum.

Adolescents

Palpation of the abdomen in the adolescent is the same as in the school-age child, including light and deep palpation, palpation of the kidneys, assessment for costovertebral angle tenderness, and assessment of guarding.

Special Techniques Used for Assessment of the Abdomen

Rebound Tenderness Assessment

If you are concerned about tenderness or guarding during palpation, assess for rebound tenderness. Always save this for the end of the examination, as it may cause severe pain.

Iliopsoas Muscle Test and Obturator Test

In children and adolescents, appendicitis is the most common cause for emergency abdominal surgery (Kosloske, Love, Rohrer, Goldthorn, & Lacey, 2004). It is generally caused by an obstruction in the appendicle lumen caused by a fecalith. The most predictable signs of acute appendicitis

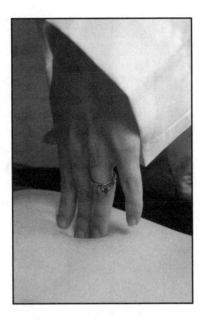

Figure 11-14   Eliciting Rebound Tenderness

Rebound tenderness is an abnormal finding associated with appendicitis or peritoneal inflammation. It is imperative to perform the test away from the site where pain is initially located. To perform this technique, hold one hand perpendicular to the abdomen, then push down slowly and deeply, lifting up quickly. If there is inflammation, the child will complain of sharp pain. With no pain on release of pressure, the response is normal or negative. The sharp pain is caused by the rebound effect of the organs or internal structures that are indented by this technique.

are pain in the RLQ, abdominal rigidity, and, most typically, migration of pain from the periumbilical region to the RLQ. In children, however, appendicitis can mimic many other intra-abdominal conditions, thereby making diagnosis difficult. The child may evidence difficulty climbing onto the examination table and may be reluctant to move around while lying down. Two tests performed in the assessment of possible appendicitis are the *iliopsoas muscle test* and the *obturator test*.

The *iliopsoas muscle test* is performed with the child in a supine position. Lift the child's right leg straight up, flexing it at the hip. As the child tries to hold the leg up, push down over the lower part of the right thigh. If the iliopsoas muscle is inflamed or is pushing on an inflamed appendix, pain is felt in the RLQ. If no pain is felt, the test is negative.

The *obturator test* is performed with the child in a supine position. Lift the child's right leg, flexing it at the hip and the knee to approximately a 90-degree angle. Holding the ankle, rotate the leg internally and externally. Pain in the RLQ indicates irritation of the obturator muscle and is a positive sign. Internal rotation of the right leg at the hip stretches the obturator muscle, which lies over the area of the appendix. If the child has an inflamed appendix, this movement will elicit pain.

Digital examination of the anterior rectal wall can also be performed in assessment of appendicitis and will elicit pain if there is inflammation. Digital examination may also elicit pain due to other pathologic conditions such as pelvic inflammatory disease and ovarian cyst, which can raise questions regarding the differential diagnosis.

Percussion

In both the young child and the adolescent, percussion is used to assess the size and density of the abdominal organs. Percussion sounds will vary depending upon the area being examined. Percussion over a solid organ, such as the liver, will produce a dull, low-amplitude sound, whereas percussion over the transverse colon, which is often air filled, will produce a tympanic sound.

The following is a review of percussion sounds:

- *DULLNESS* is a short, high-pitched note with little resonance. It is heard over solid organs.
- *RESONANCE* is a sustained note of moderate pitch. It is heard primarily over lung tissue.
- *TYMPANY* is a musical note of higher pitch than resonance. It is heard over air-filled viscera such as the transverse colon and the stomach.
- *HYPERRESONANCE* is a note that lies between tympany and resonance in pitch. It is heard best at the base of the lungs.

The following is a review of percussion technique:

1. Start by hyperextending the middle finger of one hand, and place the distal interphalangeal joint *firmly* against the child's abdomen.
2. With the end (not the pad) of the opposite middle finger, use a quick flick of the wrist to strike the first finger. See **Figure 11-15** for an example.
3. Categorize what you hear as normal, dull, or tympany.

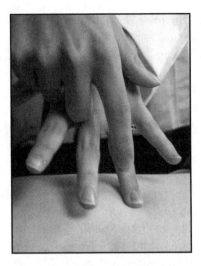

Figure 11-15 Percussion of the Abdomen

Infants
Percussion of the infant is rarely performed.

Toddlers and School-Age Children
Before you start percussion, explain what you are going to do and demonstrate to the child. You can show the child by placing your hand on the table and tapping. If the child is apprehensive, start percussion at a distal point, on an arm or leg, and gradually move more proximal until you reach the stomach. Make a game out of percussion by tapping on the child's abdomen and demonstrating the sound of a tom-tom. Once you have the child's attention and cooperation, you can start by lightly percussing in a systematic manner all four quadrants of the abdomen for a sense of tympany and dullness. Remember to establish a pattern of examination, such as starting on the RUQ or LUQ and following in a circular motion until the entire areas have been assessed. In children, the predominant sound heard is tympany due to the air in the stomach and the intestines. If you are examining an obese child, tympany may be difficult to elicit due to the increase in adipose tissue. Dullness should normally be heard over organs such as the liver, the spleen, a full bladder, or the colon with feces.

After general percussion, percuss the liver span. Stand on the right side of the child and begin at the midclavicular line at the iliac crest. Percuss upward to determine the lower border of the liver. Next, starting over an area of lung resonance and at the midclavicular line, percuss downward to an area of dullness. Normally, the span of a child's liver is not percussed below the costal margin, although an infant's liver may be percussed 1–2 cm below the costal margin.

Continuing to stand at the right side of the patient, reach across the abdomen and percuss upward from the iliac crest along the midaxillary line until dullness is achieved. Follow this with percussion over an area of lung resonance, and percuss downward along a midaxillary line until dullness is ascertained.

In some children, the spleen lies too deeply to be discernable by percussion. During percussion of the spleen, you may hear a tympanic sound that is lower in pitch over the gastric air bubble, which is in the LUQ in the left lower anterior rib cage. In children, splenic enlargement and/or tenderness is due to bacterial or viral infections.

Adolescents

Abdominal percussion of the adolescent is the same as that of the school-age child, following the same pattern until tympanic assessment has been performed over the entire abdomen.

Common Gastrointestinal Disorders

Quality and character of abdominal pain is associated with related conditions, although infants and young children are unable to describe the type of pain they are experiencing. School-age children, when given some examples, such as a feeling of something hot or burning in their stomach, will help with the differential diagnosis. Determining where the pain is located, other than periumbilical, and what makes it feel better or worse (e.g., Does it feel better before or after you eat?) helps narrow the diagnosis.

Characteristics of the quality of abdominal pain and associated conditions follow:

- *BURNING*: Peptic ulcer
- *CRAMPING*: Gastroenteritis
- *COLICKY*: Appendicitis
- *SHARP*: Pancreatitis, obstruction
- *GRADUAL ONSET*: Viral infection
- *SUDDEN ONSET*: Bacterial infection, obstruction

Other common descriptors used are dull, crampy, gnawing, aching, and stabbing.

Conditions perceived in the *RUQ* include:

- Hepatitis
- Right lower lobe pneumonia
- Duodenal ulcer

Conditions perceived in the *RLQ* include:

- Appendicitis
- Salpingitis
- Ovarian cyst
- Ruptured extopic pregnancy
- Renal stone
- Strangulated hernia
- Meckel diverticulum
- Perforated cecum
- Regional ileitis

Conditions perceived in the *LUQ* include:

- Ruptured spleen
- Gastric ulcer

Conditions perceived in the *LLQ* include:

- Salpingitis
- Ovarian cyst
- Ruptured ectopic pregnancy
- Renal stone
- Strangulated hernia
- Ulcerative colitis
- Regional ileitis
- Constipation

Conditions perceived in the *periumbilical region* include:

- Intestinal obstruction
- Early appendicitis
- Gastroenteritis

Common Gastrointestinal Disorders in Children

Infants

INGUINAL HERNIA is a scrotal or inguinal swelling that includes the abdominal contents. It presents as a bulge or swelling in the scrotal sac or the groin, and the size increases based on intra-abdominal pressure from crying or straining. See **Figure 11-16.**

TABLE 11-2   CLUES IN DIAGNOSING ABDOMINAL PAIN

There are all types of rules for telling whether pain in the abdomen has significance. A few of them follow:

- Patients may give a "touch-me-not" warning—that is, to not touch in a particular area; however, these patients may not actually have pain if their faces seem relaxed and unconcerned, even smiling. When you touch they might recoil, but the unconcerned face persists. (Actually, this sign is helpful in other areas of the body, as well as the abdomen.)
- Patients with an organic cause for abdominal pain are generally not hungry. A negative response to the "Do you want something to eat?" question is probable, particularly with appendicitis or intraabdominal infection.
- Ask the patient to point a finger to the location of the pain. If it is not directed to the navel but goes immediately to a fixed point, there is a great likelihood that this has significant physical importance. The farther from the navel the pain, the more likely it will be organic in origin (Apley rule). If the finger goes to the navel and the patient seems otherwise well to you, you should include psychogenic causes in the list of differential diagnoses.
- Patients with nonspecific abdominal pain may keep their eyes closed during abdominal palpation, whereas patients with organic disease usually keep their eyes open.

Source: This article was published in *Health & Physical Assessment*, 3rd edition, Barkauskas, Baumann, and Darling-Fisher. Clues in Diagnosing Abdominal Pain, page 547. Copyright Mosby (2002).

TABLE 11-3   QUALITY AND ONSET OF ABDOMINAL PAIN

Characteristic	Possible Related Condition
Burning	Peptic ulcer
Cramping	Biliary colic, gastroenteritis
Colic	Appendicitis with impacted feces; renal stone
Aching	Appendiceal irritation
Knifelike	Pancreatitis
Gradual onset	Infection
Sudden onset	Duodenal ulcer, acute pancreatitis, obstruction, perforation

Source: This article was published in *Health & Physical Assessment*, 3rd edition, Barkauskas, Baumann, and Darling-Fisher. Clues in Diagnosing Abdominal Pain, page 547. Copyright Mosby (2002).

TABLE 11-4 SOME CAUSES OF PAIN PERCEIVED IN ANATOMIC REGIONS

Right Upper Quadrant	Periumbilical	Left Upper Quadrant
Duodenal ulcer	Intestinal obstruction	Ruptured spleen
Hepatitis	Acute pancreatitis	Gastric ulcer
Hepatomegaly	Early appendicitis	Aortic aneurysm
Pneumonia	Mesenteric thrombosis	Perforated colon
Cholecystitis	Aortic aneurysm	Pneumonia
	Diverticulitis	
Right Lower Quadrant		**Left Lower Quadrant**
Appendicitis		Sigmoid diverticulitis
Salpingitis		Salpingitis
Ovarian cyst		Ovarian cyst
Ruptured ectopic pregnancy		Ruptured ectopic
pregnancy		
Renal/ureteral stone		Renal/ureteral stone
Strangulated hernia		Strangulated hernia
Meckel diverticulitis		Perforated colon
Regional ileitis		Regional ileitis
Perforated cecum		Ulcerative colitis

Source: This article was published in *Health & Physical Assessment*, 3rd edition, Barkauskas, Baumann, and Darling-Fisher. Clues in Diagnosing Abdominal Pain, page 547. Copyright Mosby (2002).

UMBILICAL HERNIA is a weakness or imperfect closure of the umbilical ring. It presents as a soft swelling in the umbilical area that can be easily reduced by pushing the bowel back through the fibrous ring. It is a common condition in infants and occurs more frequently in black children (Stoll, 2007). See **Figure 11-17**.

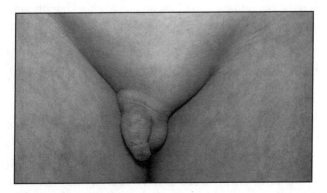

Figure 11-16 Inguinal Hernia on Left

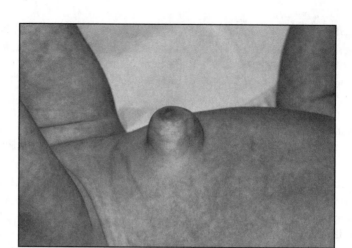

Figure 11-17 Umbilical Hernia (See Color Plate)

HYDROCELE is a collection of peritoneal fluid in the scrotal sac. It is similar in presentation to an inguinal hernia, although it does not change in size or shape in association with straining or crying. It is not reducible and can be easily transilluminated.

GASTROESOPHAGEAL REFLUX is return of gastric contents into the lower esophagus through the lower esophageal sphincter. See **Figure 11-18**. It occurs as the result of relaxation of the lower esophageal sphincter. It is one of the most common GI disorders in children (Suwandhi, Ton, & Schwarz, 2006). Anatomically, the infant is more prone to reflux because of the short, narrow esophagus, which allows for easy reflux of the stomach contents into the esophagus. In addition, the infant's lower esophageal sphincter is shorter and positioned slightly above the diaphragm, making it a less effective barrier to gastric contents than it is in the older child.

GASTROESOPHAGEAL REFLUX DISEASE is considered a more pathologic process of gastroesophageal reflux. The presenting symptoms are infants with poor weight gain, recurrent vomiting, generalized irritability, refusal to feed, arching, and respiratory symptoms such as wheezing (Gold & Gremse, 2006). These symptoms are accompanied by reflux of stomach contents into the lower esophagus.

COLIC is seen in children younger than 3 months of age and presents with recurrent episodes of unexplained crying. The infant often draws the legs up toward the abdomen, in association with loud persistent crying. The

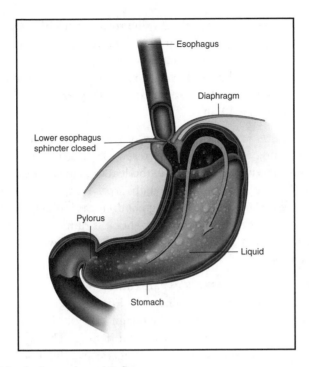

Esophagus

Diaphragm

Lower esophagus
sphincter closed

Pylorus

Liquid

Stomach

Figure 11-18 Gastroesophageal Reflux

etiology of colic is unknown, although excessive air swallowing, improper feeding techniques, food allergies, infant behaviors, and parental factors have all been considered as contributing. The "rule of 3" (Schmitt, 1986) is still used as a definition: Colic is present if crying occurs during the first 3 months, lasts longer than 3 hours per day, occurs more than 3 days per week, and continues for at least 3 weeks.

Toddlers and School-Age Children

ANAL FISSURE is a small linear tear in the anal mucosa. It is generally due to the passage of hard, large stool. Presentation is crying in association with bowel movements, bright red streaks of blood in the stool or diaper, and withholding of stool. Small tears in the anal mucosa will be visible on examination.

CONSTIPATION is defined as the difficult passage of stool or infrequent passage of hard stool. It is associated with straining and abdominal pain.

Constipation is common in toddlers due to toilet training practices and autonomy struggles of this age group. A child who is constipated will present with hard, small stools that may by be passed in regular intervals or large masses of stool passed every couple of days. Abdominal pain or distention as well as loss of appetite may also be present. A palpable fecal mass is often felt in the LLQ.

GASTROENTERITIS is an inflammatory process of the stomach and intestines whose etiology can be viral, bacterial, or parasitic. It presents with vomiting and diarrhea. Rotovirus is the leading cause of gastroenteritis in children. The concern is decreased absorptive capacity due to inflammation; as a result, infants and young children can quickly become dehydrated and are at risk for hypovolemic shock if fluid and electrolytes are not replaced. Children are often hospitalized due to dehydration secondary to gastroenteritis.

INTESTINAL PARASITE INFECTIONS are caused by a variety of organisms. One of the most common is the pinworm, *Enterobius vermicularis*, which is white, threadlike, and 1 cm long (see **Figure 11-19**). The pinworm resides in the colon and rectum, and causes rectal itching. The eggs come from contaminated fomites such as the anus, fingers, and the mouth. They survive in bedding, clothing, and house dust for approximately 2 weeks. The eggs are easily transmitted within families, schools, and day-care settings. Diagnosis is frequently based on the tape test (Leder & Weller, 2010).

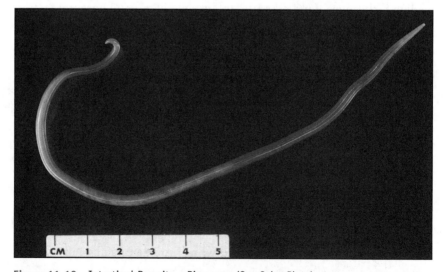

Figure 11-19 Intestinal Parasite—Pinworms (See Color Plate)

RECURRENT ABDOMINAL PAIN is most commonly seen in school-age children. It presents with a history of periumbilical pain without constitutional symptoms of fever, vomiting, or diarrhea. It may be accompanied by school avoidance, and children rarely have nighttime pain. The physical examination is generally normal. Research has evidenced that children with recurrent abdominal pain feel controlled by their parents and have little sense of independence. Treatment is focused on the release of stress within the family setting. Research by the AAP on this topic refers to recurrent abdominal pain as "functional abdominal pain" and indicates that there is no evidence that emotional or behavioral symptoms predict the clinical course or that families of children with chronic abdominal pain differ in broad areas of family functioning.

Adolescents

APPENDICITIS is inflammation of the vermiform appendix. It is the most common cause for abdominal surgery in children. Presenting symptoms can be vague and poorly localized. Pain generally starts in the periumbilical area gradually migrating to the RLQ. Following the initial symptoms of pain,

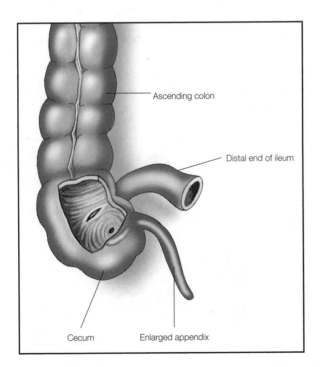

Figure 11-20 Appendicitis

anorexia, and nausea with or without vomiting may occur. The most reliable information is the sequence of the symptom of pain followed by anorexia and nausea. Constipation or diarrhea may be additional symptoms. Misdiagnosis places the child at risk for perforation, abscess, and infection.

INFLAMMATORY BOWEL DISEASE includes two distinct chronic disorders, ulcerative colitis and Crohn's disease. These disorders are similar in their symptomatology and present primarily during adolescence.

- *ULCERATIVE COLITIS* is a chronic inflammation of the large intestine characterized by bloody diarrhea, weight loss, abdominal pain, leukocytosis, and fever. The inflammatory process is limited to the mucosa of the large intestine. This disorder occurs primarily in adolescents.

- *CROHN DISEASE* is a chronic inflammatory disease that is immune mediated. It can affect any portion of the intestinal tract from the mouth to the anus. It is commonly localized to the ileum and the cecum, as well as to the colon.

Both disorders present with abdominal pain, weight loss, diarrhea, growth failure, and hematochezia (bloody diarrhea).

PEPTIC ULCER DISEASE is erosion of the mucosal tissue in the upper part of the stomach or lower end of the esophagus. Commonly presenting symptoms include vomiting and poor appetite, and periumbilical or epigastric pain that is intermittent and accompanied by the classic history that the pain is relieved by eating.

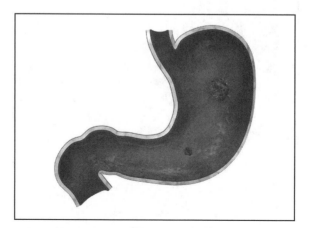

Figure 11-21   Gastric Ulcer

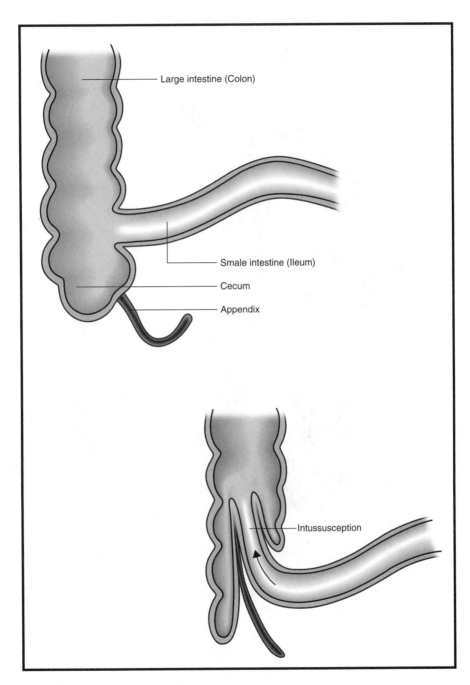

Figure 11-22 Normal Bowel/Intussusception

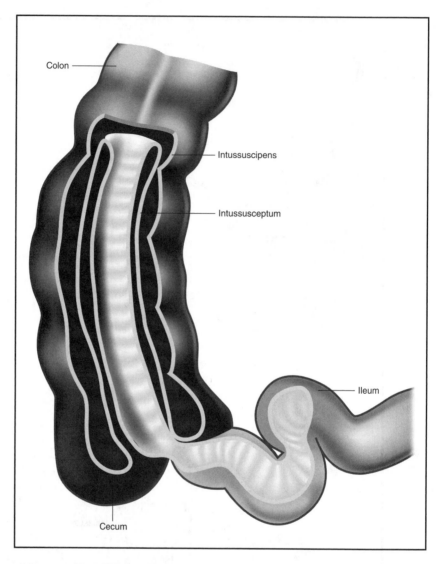

Figure 11-23 Intussusception

> ### Red Flags

Necrotizing enterocolitis is a life-threatening condition seen primarily in the newborn. Symptomatology is abdominal distention, vomiting, lethargy, respiratory distress, hepatomegaly, anorexia, jaundice, feeding intolerance, and decreased bowel sounds. Prompt intervention is crucial to prevent perforation.

Meckel diverticulum is a blind sac protruding from the wall of the ileum. It presents within the first 2 years of life with painless rectal bleeding. The bleeding occurs because the tip of the pouch hanging from the ileum contains ectopic gastric mucosa rather than ileal mucosa. The gastric mucosa secretes acid, which causes irritation and ulceration, eventually leading to lower GI bleed. The rectal bleeding tends to be excessive. Referral for surgical consultation is necessary.

Intussusception is the telescoping of one section of the bowel into the lumen of the adjacent segment. When one section of the intestine invaginates into another section, compression of the walls of the intestine compromise blood flow, leading to inflammation, edema, bleeding, and complete bowel obstruction. The child presents with four classic symptoms: colic, intermittent abdominal pain, vomiting, and currant jelly-like stools. Referral for nonsurgical hydrostatic reduction with barium or surgical consultation is necessary.

Hirschsprung disease is also called congenital aganglionic megacolon. It is the lack of motility of the bowel caused by the absence of parasympathetic ganglion cells in the large intestine. Lack of parasympathetic stimulation prevents peristalsis and ultimately causes feces to accumulate proximal to the defect, which eventually leads to bowel obstruction. It presents in the newborn period by failure to pass meconium within the first 24–48 hours. The majority of patients with Hirschsprung disease are diagnosed in the neonatal period due to failure to pass meconium. The child presents with abdominal distention, bile-stained vomitus, inadequate weight gain, palpable stool throughout the abdomen, but with an empty rectal ampulla. Referral for surgical consultation is necessary.

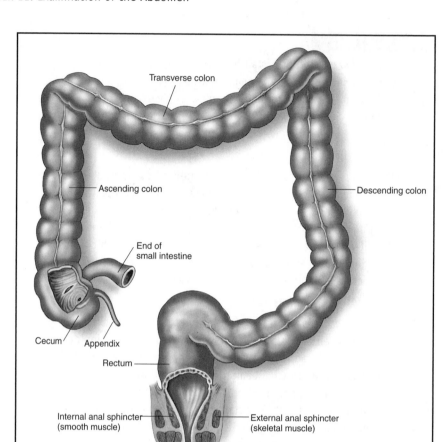

Figure 11-24 Normal Sigmoid Colon and Rectum

Write-Up of the Abdominal Exam

EXAMPLE FOR INFANTS: Abdomen is protuberant with visible pulsations. Umbilicus reveals a small umbilical hernia that is easily reducible. Positive for bowel sounds in all four quadrants. Light and deep palpation without tenderness, distension, or rigidity. Liver palpated 1–2 cm below the right costal margin. Spleen nonpalpable.

EXAMPLE FOR TODDLERS, SCHOOL-AGE CHILDREN, AND ADOLESCENTS: Abdomen is without scars or visible pulsations. Positive for bowel sounds heard in all four quadrants. Light and deep palpation without tenderness, distension, or rigidity. Percussion sounds tympanic in all four quadrants, without hepatosplenomegaly.

Case Study: Boy Presenting with Abdominal Pain

Teddy is a 7-year-old boy who is brought to your office with a chief complaint of intermittent episodes of abdominal pain for the past 6 months. In talking to Teddy, he describes the pain as "sometimes sharp and sometimes dull." It usually lasts about 20–30 minutes and goes away by itself when he lies down. Teddy states that he has to come in from playing when he gets the stomach pains and that he has no warning that they are coming. He indicates that the pain is periumbilical in location without radiation. On further questioning, Teddy reports a soft bowel movement daily and no urinary symptoms such as frequency or dysuria. He denies vomiting or diarrhea with the stomach pain, and has no fever or headache. The pain generally occurs about 2–3 times per week at various times of the day with no specific pattern. It does not wake him at night.

Teddy's past medical history is unremarkable, with no allergies, surgeries, or hospitalizations. Immunizations are up to date. He is an A student in school and has many friends. His family life is stable, with mother, father, and a sibling at home.

His physical examination is entirely normal:

- *HEAD AND NECK*: Unremarkable
- *LUNGS*: Clear without adventitious sounds
- *CARDIAC*: Normal sinus rhythm, normal pulses

- *ABDOMEN*: Soft and nontender with active bowel sounds and no organomegaly, no masses
- *RECTAL*: Normal, stool guaiac negative
- *NEUROLOGIC*: Cranial nerves intact, deep tendon reflexes equal and symmetrical; normal muscle tone and mass; no cerebellar signs

Questions

1. What does your initial evaluation include in order to rule out organic disease?
2. What findings in your history support your diagnosis of recurrent abdominal pain?
3. What is your overall goal of treatment for children with recurrent abdominal pain?

Answers

1. The initial evaluation should include a complete blood count with differential, erythrocyte sedimentation rate, urinalysis, urine culture in females, and guaiac. If there are positive findings further testing may include radiographic studies, throat culture, and liver function tests.
2. The findings that support recurrent abdominal pain are vague, paroxysmal episodes of dull pain located in the periumbilical or suprapubic regions. It is defined by its chronic nature and lacks association with constitutional signs of illness
3. The goal of treatment in recurrent abdominal pain is to avoid attention to and secondary gain that may be derived from these symptoms. The use of medications is discouraged, and the emphasis on normality and independence is encouraged.

References

Gold, D. L. & Gremse, D. A. (2006). Gastroesophageal reflux disease in children. *42*(4), 384–391.

Jarvis, C. (2008). *Physical examination and health assessment* (5th ed.). St. Louis, MO: Elsevier.

Kosloske, A. M., Love, C. L., Rohrer, J. E., Goldthorn, J. F., & Lacey, S. R. (2004) The diagnosis of appendicitis in children: Outcomes of a strategy based on pediatric surgical evaluation. *Pediatrics, 113,* 29–34.

Leder, K. & Weller, P. (2010). *Enterobiasis and trichuriasis.* http://www.uptodate.com

Merritt, L. (2005). Part I: Understanding the embryology and genetics of cleft lip and palate. *Advanced Neonatal Care, 5.*

Seidel, H. M., Ball, J. W., Danes, J.E., Benedict, G. W., (2007). *Mosby's guide to physical examination* (6th ed.). Philadelphia: Mosby.

Schmitt B. D. (1986). Colic: Excessive crying in newborns. *Pediatrics, 77,* 641–648.

Stoll, B. J. (2007). The umbilicus. In R. M. Kliegman, R. Behrman, H. B. Jensen & B. F. Stanton, (Eds.). *Nelson textbook of pediatrics* (18th ed.). Philadelphia: Saunders.

Suwandhi, E., Ton, M. N., & Schwarz, S. M. (2006). Gastroesophageal reflux in infancy and childhood. *Pediatric Annals, 35*(4), 259–266.

Resources

Ball, J., Bindler, R., & Cowen, K. (2010). *Child health nursing* (2nd ed.). Upper Saddle River, NJ: Pearson.

Bickley, L. (2003). *Bates' guide to physical examination and history taking* (8th ed.). New York: Lippincott Williams & Wilkins.

Burns, C., Dunn, A., Brady, M., Starr, N., & Blosser, C. (2004). *Pediatric primary care: A handbook for nurse practitioners* (3rd ed.). St. Louis, MO: Saunders.

Estes, M. (2006). *Health assessment and physical examination* (3rd ed.). Albany, NY: Delmar Publishers.

Hansen, M. (1998). *Pathophysiology: Foundations of disease and clinical intervention*. Philadelphia: Saunders.

Marieb, E. (1995). *Human anatomy and physiology* (3rd ed.). Redwood City, CA: Benjamin/Cummings Publishing Company.

Potts, N., & Mandleco, B. (2007). *Pediatraic nursing* (2nd ed.). Victoria, Australia: Thomson, Delmar Learning.

Tortora, G. J., & Grabvowski, S. R. (2003). *Principles of anatomy and physiology* (10th ed.). New York: Wiley.

Examination of the Musculoskeletal System

Anatomy and Physiology

The musculoskeletal system consists of supporting structures that facilitate movement, including the bones, muscles, joints, and tendons.

Bones

There are more bones in the child's skeleton than in the adult's. These additional bones, such as in the hip and back, fuse by adulthood, yielding 206 total bones in the adult human skeleton. The skeleton has two principal divisions: The axial skeleton is based on the longitudinal axis and consists of the facial bones, skull, hyoid bone, ribs, sternum, and vertebrae. The appendicular skeleton consists of the bones of the upper and lower extremities as well as the pelvis, scapula, and clavicle.

Bones are further classified according to their size and shape. There are several types: long, short, flat, and irregular. The long bones include the fibula, tibia, femur, humerus, and ulna; the majority of growth in these bones occurs during childhood. The short bones include those in the wrist and ankle. The flat bones are the skull, sternum, and ribs. The irregular bones have irregular complex shapes and sizes and include the pelvis bones, scapula, and vertebrae.

Development of the Musculoskeletal System

Bone formation is ongoing, particularly during childhood. It begins in the second month of gestation and primary ossification is complete by birth. Secondary ossification continues during childhood, as bones grow in thickness by appositional growth and long bones lengthen by interstitial growth of the epiphyseal plates. Bones stop growing in the length near the end of adolescents, although may continue to thicken into the early 20's. During

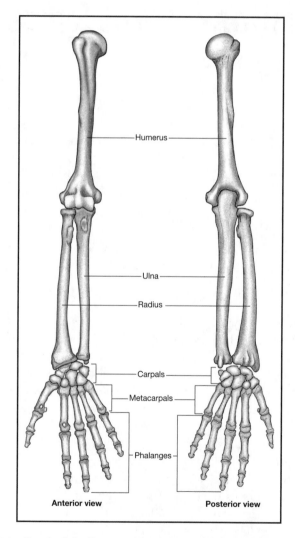

Figure 12-1(a)   Bones of the Upper and Lower Extremities: Arms

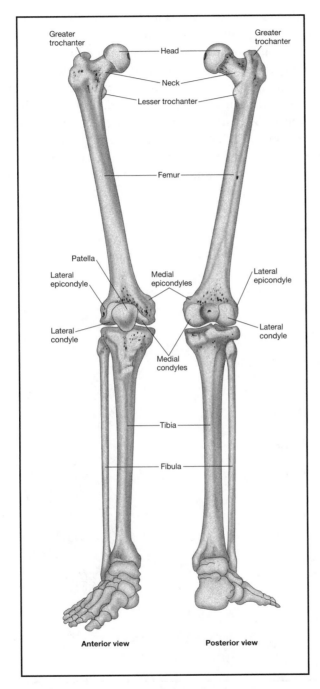

Figure 12-1(b)   Bones of the Upper and Lower Extremities: Legs

this period, the clavicles and the skull bones are the first to ossify. The long bones and spine follow in the process of ossification. The bones of the embryo are composed of hyaline cartilage and fibrous membranes. As growth continues, the membranes eventually become the flat bones such as those in the skull, and the cartilages become the long bones. Ossification of the long bones starts in the diaphysis and the epiphyses and progresses gradually through the continual deposition of bony matrix. Bone is continually being reabsorbed as well as built up. In this process, calcium is being supplied to the extracellular fluids. The dissolution or reabsorption of bone is caused by the osteoclasts, which secrete an enzyme that dissolves the protein matrix, which in turn releases calcium and phosphorus into the blood.

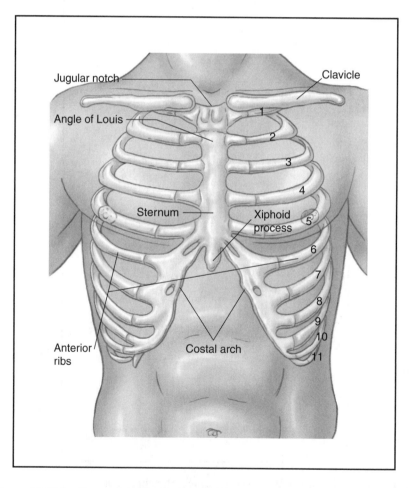

Figure 12-2(a)   Bones of the Trunk, Anterior View

The formation, growth, repair, and metabolism of bone involves calcium, phosphorus, hormones, and vitamins. In a brief overview, vitamin D accelerates the absorption of calcium and phosphate from the gastrointestinal tract. The parathyroid hormone then stimulates the breakdown or reapportion of bone, and the thyroid hormone, calcitonin, inhibits resorption. These hormones are antagonists, maintaining normal levels of calcium in the blood, as well as promoting proper bone formation.

In childhood, bone growth is based on hormonal regulation. Growth hormone is released by the anterior pituitary gland, which in turn stimulates growth of the epiphyseal plate cartilage. Thyroid hormone (T_3 and T_4) modulates the activity of growth hormone, ensuring that proper

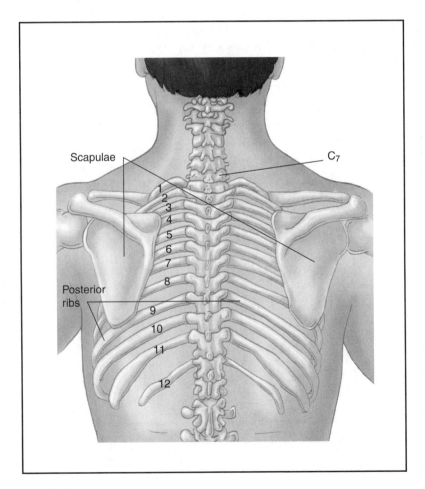

Figure 12-2(b)   Bones of the Trunk, Posterior View

proportions are released for adequate growth. As the child reaches puberty, male and female sex hormones are released (testosterone and estrogen). These hormones produce the growth spurt seen in adolescence, and they also account for the masculinization and/or feminization of specific parts of the musculoskeletal system. These hormones are also responsible for closure of the epiphyseal plate, which ends longitudinal bone growth. See **Figure 12-3, Figure 12-4,** and **Figure 12-5** for examples of epiphyseal plate.

Because this book is solely focused on the growth and development of the child, understanding how children attain longitudinal growth is an important consideration. The epiphyseal plate is a layer of hyaline cartilage in the metaphysis of a growing bone, and the diaphysis, or shaft of the long bone, increases in length through activity of the epiphyseal plate. As a long bone grows, chondrocytes (cartilage cells) form tall columns. The cells at the top of these columns (on the epiphyseal side) divide, increasing the thickness of the epiphyseal plate, and gradually push the epiphysis away from the diaphysis (shaft of the long bone), which subsequently causes the long bone to increase in length. As Marieb (2006)

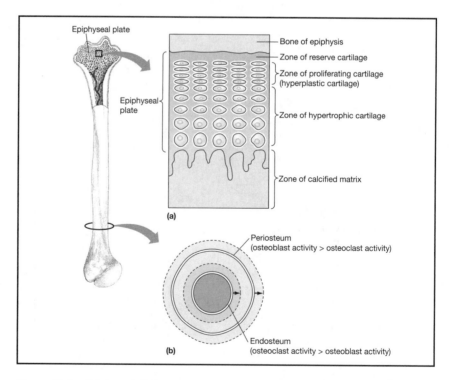

Figure 12-3   Epiphyseal Plate

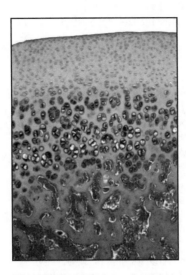

Figure 12-4   Epiphyseal Plate (See Color Plate)

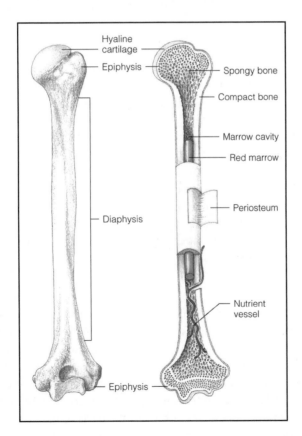

Figure 12-5(a)   Epiphyseal Plate

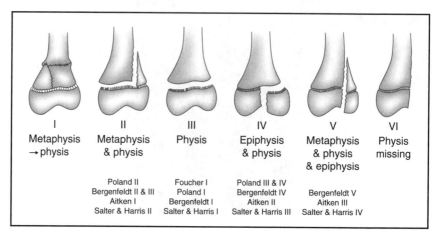

Figure 12-5(b) Peterson Classification of Physical Injuries

Source: With kind permission from Springer Science+Business Media: Journal of Pediatric Orthopaedics, Physeal Fractures: Part 3. Classification, 14, 1994, 439–44, and Peterson, Hamlet.

explains, "During childhood and into adolescence, the epiphyseal plate maintains a constant thickness because the rate of cartilage growth on its epiphyseal face is balanced by its replacement with bone tissue on its diaphyseal side." As a child reaches the end of adolescence, there is decreased division of the cartilage cells of the epiphyseal plates, causing the plate to become thinner and thinner until the entire space is replaced by bone tissue. Gradually, bone growth ends and the epiphysis and diaphysis fuse. While the growth plate is open during childhood, fractures in this area may damage the epiphysis, which can cause progressive angulation or shortening of the limb. Generally, closure of the epiphyseal plate occurs around 18 years of age in females and 21 years of age in males (Marieb, 1995, p. 166).

Muscles

There are basically two types of muscles: Skeletal, or striated, muscles are voluntary and under conscious control. Muscles that involve the biceps, triceps, deltoid, gluteus maximus, and other muscle groups are skeletal. Smooth muscles found in the hollow of visceral organs such as the stomach, bladder, and respiratory system have no striations and do not contract or relax at will; they are, therefore, involuntary. Cardiac muscle is a special striated involuntary muscle. It constitutes the mass of the heart and ensures the heart's constant contraction and relaxation.

Muscles have four basic functions: allow movement, maintain posture, stabilize joints, and generate heat. The skeletal muscles are responsible for maintaining movement and are responsible for quick responses, such as jumping out of the path of a car or pulling your hand back from something hot. Muscles that maintain posture allow sitting, walking, bending over, and lying down, to name a few functions. Stabilizing joints allow one to swing a tennis racket or a golf club, throw a ball, take a step, or bring a fork to one's mouth. As muscles contract, they generate heat, which is important in maintaining normal body temperature.

To better understand the musculoskeletal system, this chapter will focus on the skeletal muscles that are composed of bundles of muscle fibers, or fasciculi. These skeletal muscles are attached to bone by tendons, which are strong connective tissue. Aponeuroses are flat, sheetlike tendons that attach muscles to other muscles or to bones. Ligaments are dense connective tissues that bind bones together at joints. They contain more elastic fibers than tendons and provide support for various movements. It is important to remember that muscles do not increase in number, but rather in length and circumference, as the child grows. Muscle fibers reach maximum diameter in girls at around 10 years of age, and in boys at 14 years. Muscle strength continues to increase until 25 to 30 years of age (Chamley, Carson, & Randall, 2005; Ball, Binder, & Cowen, 2010). Ligaments and tendons are stronger than bone until puberty.

Joints

Joints, or articulations of two bones, serve two fundamental functions: They hold the skeleton together, and they allow mobility needed for everyday activities. Joints are classified based on the material binding the joint together and whether a joint cavity is present, which allows for movement at the joint. They are classified as synovial or nonsynovial. Fibrous (nonsynovial) joints, also called synarthrotic joints, are immovable and no joint cavity is present; an example is the sutures of the skull where the bone edges interlock so that the joint is immovable. Cartilaginous (nonsynovial) joint implies that the articulating bones are united by cartilage. These joints, like the fibrous joints, do not have a joint cavity. They are only slightly moveable. Examples include the vertebrae and the pubic bones and symphysis, where there is slight movement during pregnancy.

Synovial joints, which are the majority of joints in the body, are composed of articulating bones separated by a fluid-containing cavity that allows sliding of opposing surfaces, which in turn permits a sliding movement. In these joints, there is a substantial freedom of movement such

(a)

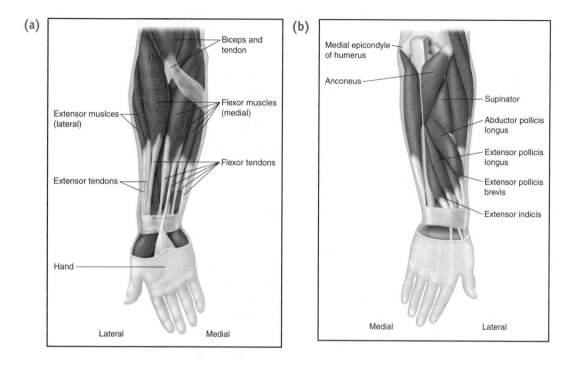

Biceps and tendon

Flexor muscles (medial)

Extensor muslces (lateral)

Flexor tendons

Extensor tendons

Hand

Lateral   Medial

(b)

Medial epicondyle of humerus

Anconeus

Supinator

Abductor pollicis longus

Extensor pollicis longus

Extensor pollicis brevis

Extensor indicis

Medial   Lateral

(c)

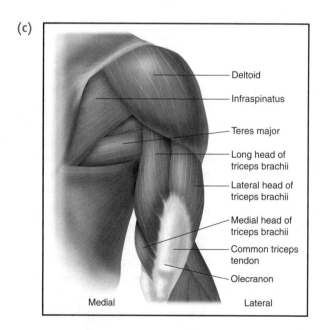

Deltoid

Infraspinatus

Teres major

Long head of triceps brachii

Lateral head of triceps brachii

Medial head of triceps brachii

Common triceps tendon

Olecranon

Medial   Lateral

Figure 12-6   Muscles of the Upper Extremities: (a) Anterior Arm; (b) Posterior Arm; (c) Upper Arm

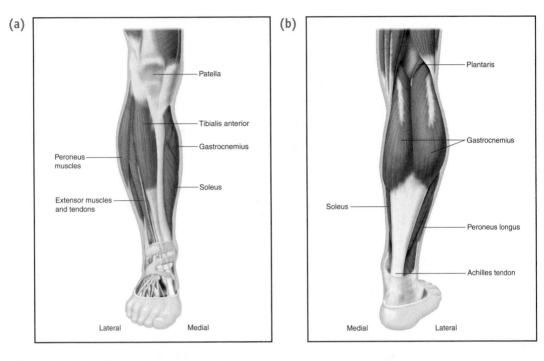

Figure 12-7   Muscles of the Lower Extremities

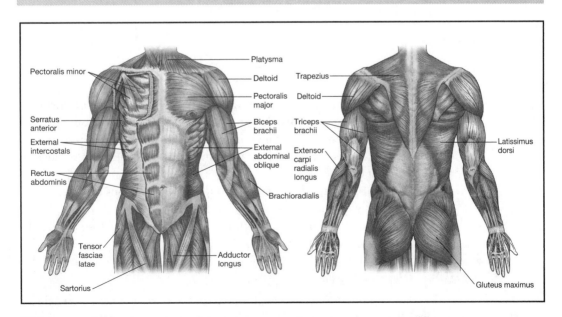

Figure 12-8   Superficial Muscles of the Trunk, Anterior and Posterior View. Adult Images Used to Demonstrate Specific Muscle Groups.

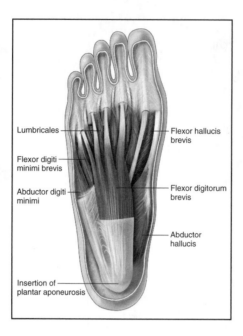

Figure 12-9 Front View of Foot Muscles

as in the shoulder, elbow, knee, and hip. The synovial joints have five distinguishing features:

1. Articular cartilage, or hyaline, covers the opposing bone surfaces. This cartilage is avascular and receives nourishment from synovial fluid that circulates during joint movement, which serves as a cushion for the bones and provides a smooth surface to facilitate movement.
2. A joint cavity is present.
3. An articular capsule, which is a tough, flexible fibrous capsule, is continuous with the periostea of the articulating bones.
4. A synovial membrane, which is loose connective tissue, covers the internal joint surfaces.
5. Synovial fluid, which is a slippery fluid, occupies all free spaces within the joint capsule.

In conjunction with the synovial joints are the bursae, which are enclosed sacs filled with synovial fluid. The bursae reduce friction between adjacent structures during joint activity such as the prepatellar bursa of the knee or

(a)

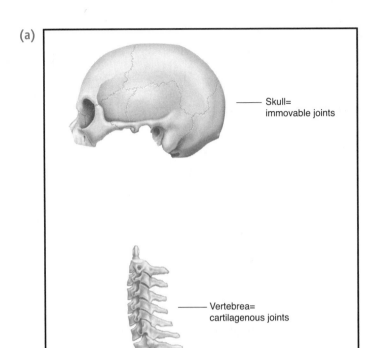

Skull=
immovable joints

Vertebrea=
cartilagenous joints

(b)

Ribs and vertebrea=
semi-mobile joints

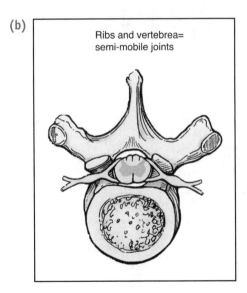

Figure 12-10 Types of Joints Found in the Human Body: (a) Skull and Vertebrae;
(b) Ribs and Vertebrae

(c)

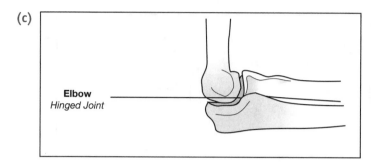

Elbow
Hinged Joint

(d)

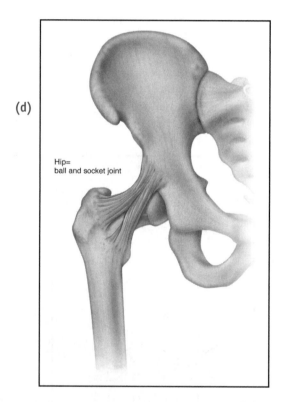

Hip=
ball and socket joint

Figure 12-10 Types of Joints Found in the Human Body: (c) Elbow; (d) Hip Joint

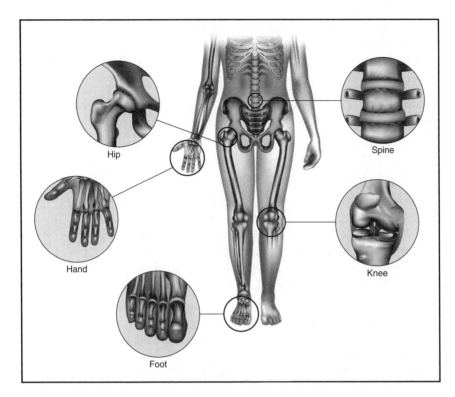

Figure 12-11   Human Joints

the subacromial bursa of the shoulder. Synovial joints are further classified into six major categories:

- *PLANE JOINTS* allow for only short slipping or gliding movements; they include the intercarpal and intertarsal joints and the joints between the vertebrae.
- *HINGE JOINTS* allow motion along a single plane, similar to that of a mechanical hinge; such motions include the bending and straightening of the elbow and interphalangeal joints.
- *PIVOT JOINTS* allow movement in a uniaxial rotation of one bone around its own long axis, such as the movement of the head from side to side.
- *CONDYLOID JOINTS* permit all angular motions, including flexion and extention, abduction and adduction, and circumduction, such as the wrist and the metacarpophalangeal joints (knuckles).

- *SADDLE JOINTS* are shaped like a saddle and allow freedom of movement; an example is the carpometacarpal joints of the thumb.
- *BALL-AND-SOCKET JOINTS* allow movement in all axes and planes; examples include the shoulder and hip.

Muscles and tendons of the skeletal system enable body parts to move in various positions. Following are movements carried out by the skeletal muscles (Jarvis, 2008, p. 599):

- *FLEXION*: Bending a limb at a joint
- *EXTENSION*: Straightening a limb at a joint
- *ABDUCTION*: Moving a limb away from the midline of the body
- *ADDUCTION*: Moving a limb toward the midline of the body
- *PRONATION*: Turning the forearm so that the palm is down
- *SUPINATION*: Turning the forearm so that the palm is up
- *CIRCUMDUCTION*: Moving the arm in a circle around the shoulder
- *INVERSION*: Moving the sole of the foot inward at the ankle
- *EVERSION*: Moving the sole of the foot outward at the ankle
- *ROTATION*: Moving the head around a central axis
- *PROTRACTION*: Moving a body part forward and parallel to the ground, such as jutting out your jaw.
- *RETRACTION*: Moving a body part backward and parallel to the ground, such as retracting your jaw back to its original position.
- *ELEVATION*: Raising a body part
- *DEPRESSION*: Lowering a body part

The temporomandibular joint (TMJ) is the articulation of the mandible and the temporal bone, and is the most active joint in the body. This joint is formed by the two bones of the zygomatic arch and the fossa of the mandible. The TMJ allows the jaw to open and close as in chewing and speaking. There are three motions: hinge action to open and close the jaw, gliding action for protrusion and retraction, and gliding for side-to-side movement of the lower jaw (Jarvis, 2008, p. 600).

The Spine

The spine is composed of 33 vertical connecting vertebrae; it is the central supporting structure of the trunk. The spine extends from the base of the skull to its anchoring point in the pelvis and is shaped in an S curve to distribute body weight. The cervical and lumbar areas have a concave curve, whereas the thoracic and sacrococcygeal spine have convex curves, all of which help to distribute upper body weight to the pelvis and lower extremities, as well as to cushion the concussive impact of walking or running.

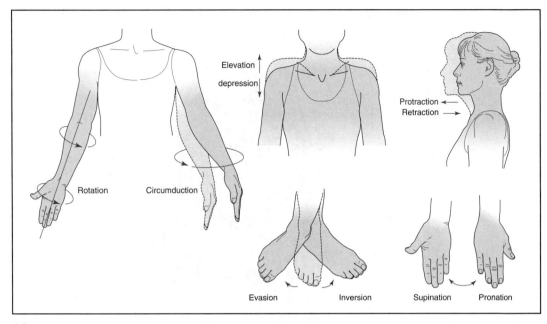

(a)

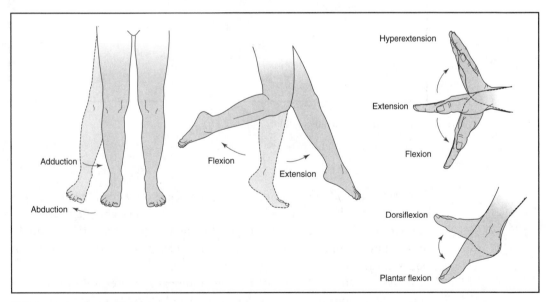

(b)

Figure 12-12   (a) (b) Muscle Movements

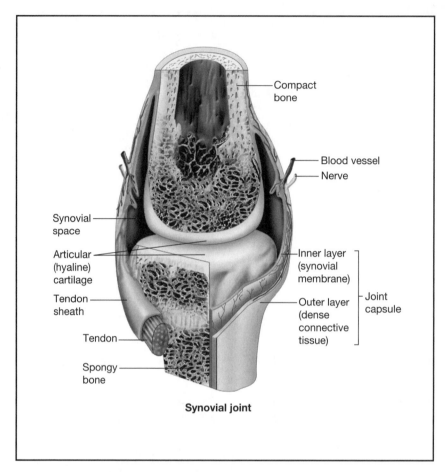

Figure 12-12(c) Synovial Joint

The vertebral column also provides attachment points for the ribs and the muscles of the back. The spine is composed of 7 cervical, 12 thoracic, 5 lumbar, 5 sacral, and 3 to 4 coccygeal vertebrae. (Remembering common meal times—7 am, 12 pm, and 5 pm—may help you recall the number of bones in these areas of the spine [Marieb, 1995].)

In assessment of the spine, surface landmarks are helpful in orienting you to the various levels. These levels are based on an older adolescent and will vary slightly depending upon the age of the child.

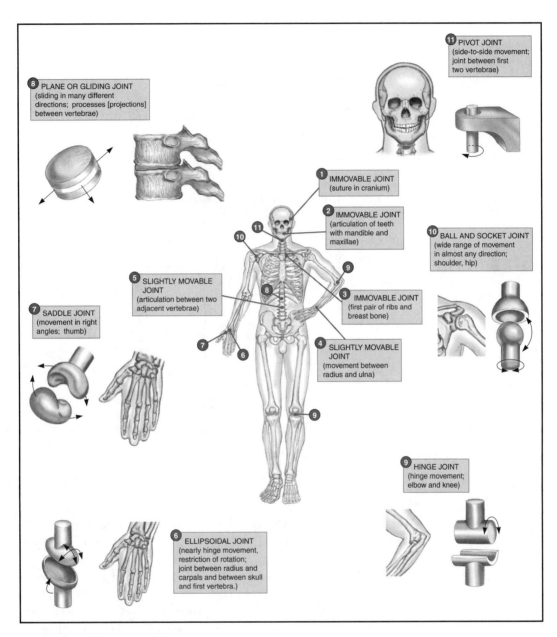

Figure 12-12(d)   Types of Joints

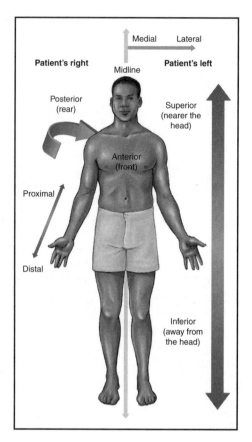

Figure 12-12(e) Anatomic Terms

- The spinous processes C7 and T1 are prominent at the base of the neck.
- The inferior angle of the scapula normally is at the level of the interspace between T7 and T8.
- An imaginary line connecting the highest point on each iliac crest crosses L4.
- An imaginary line joining the two symmetric dimples that overlie the posterior superior iliac spine crosses the sacrum and may be observed in the adolescent.

When viewing the vertebral column from the side, observe the four curves (double S shape). The cervical and lumbar curvatures are concave posteriorly, and the thoracic and sacral curvatures are convex posteriorly (**Figure 12-14**). These curves are important because they increase the spine's

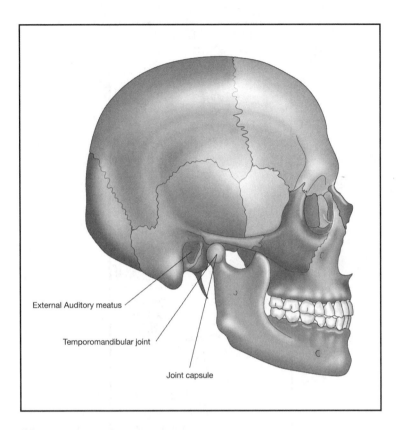

Figure 12-13 The Temporomandibular Joint

resilience and flexibility, allowing flexion (bending forward) and extension (bending backward) and abduction and rotation. All of the vertebrae enclose an opening called the vertebral foramen, which forms the vertebral canal through which the spinal cord passes. The vertebral arch is formed by pedicles, which are short bony cylinders that project from the sides of the vertebral body and form openings through which the spinal nerves can pass. The spinous process is a single midline projection that one palpates in assessment of the vertebral column. The transverse process and the spinous process are attachment sites for the muscles that move the spinal column. Because the spinal cord and spinal nerve roots are close to the vertebral casing, they are often susceptible to disc herniation and impingement from trauma.

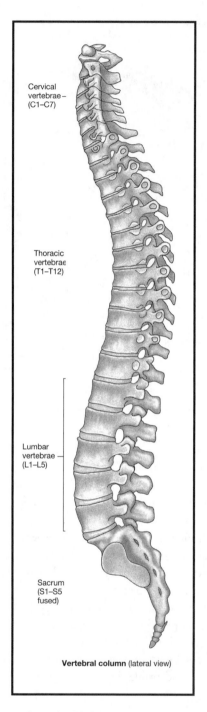

Cervical vertebrae (C1–C7)

Thoracic vertebrae (T1–T12)

Lumbar vertebrae (L1–L5)

Sacrum (S1–S5 fused)

Vertebral column (lateral view)

Figure 12-14 Structures of Vertebral Joints

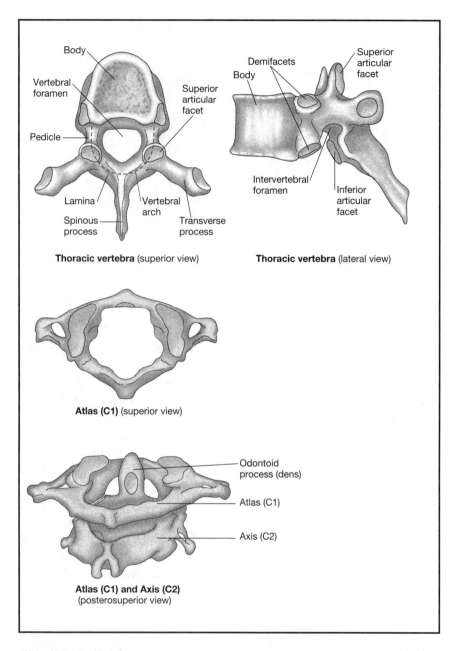

Figure 12-15   Vertebra

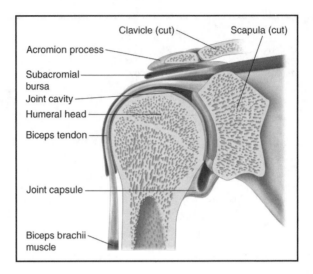

Figure 12-16 Shoulder Joint

Between the vertebral bodies are moveable joints composed of elastic cartilaginous plates. Within each disc is the core, or nucleus pulposus, composed of a soft mucoid center. These cartilaginous plates between the discs act as a cushion or shock absorber and allow for movements of the spine such as bending or flexing. When the spine moves, the discs allow for compression and expansion, with one side compensating for the other. When compression of the disc becomes too great, it can rupture, causing the nucleus pulposus to herniate outside of the vertebral column. This results in pain by causing compression on the associated spinal nerves.

The principal muscle groups that work in conjunction with the spine, starting at the cervical area, include the sternocleidomastoid and trapezius, which provide for neck extension, flexion, and rotation. The lumbar muscles include the psoas muscles; the abdominal muscles, including the obliques and rectus abdominis; and the intrinsic muscles of the back, which provide for extension, rotation, and bending.

The Shoulder

The shoulder, or glenohumeral joint, consists of two bones, the anterior clavicle and the posterior scapula. Anteriorly, the medial end of each clavicle joins the sternum, and the distal ends of the clavicles meet the scapulae laterally. Articulation at the shoulder includes the humerus and glenoid fossa of the scapula. The capsule surrounding and protecting the joint is composed of the acromion and coracoid processes, which make up the rotator cuff of the shoulder (**Figure 12-17**). The shoulder is an example of a ball-and-socket joint stabilized by the clavicle and acromion that allows shoulder movement with a wide range of motion on many axes.

In examination of the shoulder, the bones have palpable landmarks to help guide your assessment. After identification of the manubrium, sternoclavicular joint, and clavicle, palpate the clavicle laterally. From behind, follow the bony spine of the scapula laterally and upward as it becomes the acromion or the bony prominence at the top of the shoulder. Palpating down and outward from the acromion process is the greater tubercle of the humerus, another bony prominence. From here, palpate medially until you feel a large bony prominence, which is the coracoid process of the scapula.

In summary, within the shoulder joint there are three different points of articulation: the glenohumeral joint, which is articulation of the head of the humerus with the glenoid fossa of the scapula; the sternoclavicular joint, which is articulation with the clavicle, which is part of the concave hollow in the upper sternum; and the acromioclavicular joint, which is articulation of the clavicle with the acromion process of the scapula. These landmarks may be difficult to palpate due to their deep location within the shoulder capsule.

The principal muscle groups attached at the shoulder include the scapulohumeral group. These include muscles inserting directly on the humerus, also know as the "SITS muscles of the rotator cuff" (Bickley,

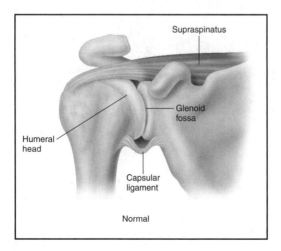

Figure 12-17   Rotator Cuff Muscles: Anterior Normal

2003, p. 470): the supraspinatus, which runs above the glenohumeral joint and inserts on the greater tubercle; the infraspinatus and the teres minor, which cross the glenohumeral joint posteriorly and insert on the greater tubercle; and the subscapularis, which crosses the joint anteriorly and inserts on the lesser tubercle. Two other groups of muscles include the axioscapular group, which attaches the trunk to the scapula and rotates the scapula, and the axiohumeral group, which attaches the trunk to the humerus and produces internal rotation of the shoulder. In addition, the muscles of the upper arm—the biceps and triceps—connect the scapula to the bones of the forearm and are also involved in movement of the shoulder.

The Elbow

The elbow forms the articulation of three bones, the humerus, radius, and ulna.

The ligaments of the radius and ulna protect the joint of the three contiguous surfaces that are enclosed in a single synovial cavity. The olecranon

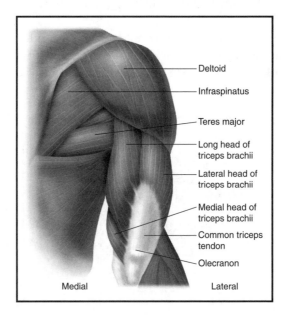

Figure 12-18 Muscles of the Arm in an Adult

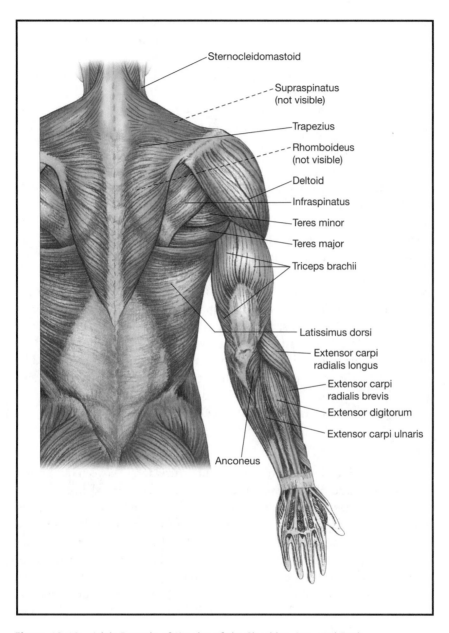

Figure 12-19 Adult Example of Muscles of the Shoulder, Arm, and Back

bursa is situated between the olecranon process and the skin. The elbow is an example of a hinge joint with the radius and ulna articulating to permit pronation and supination of the hand and forearm.

The muscle groups traversing the elbow include the biceps and the brachioradialis. The ulnar nerve runs posteriorly between the medial epicondyle and the olecranon process and is responsible for the painful tingling sensation you feel when you hit your "funny bone" (Marieb, 1995, p. 205).

The Wrist

The wrist, or radiocarpal joint, forms the articulation of the distal radius and the eight small carpal bones. The wrist is a condyloid joint that allows movement in two planes—flexion and extension as well as side-to-side deviation. Articulations in the hand are between the middle carpals and metacarpals, metacarpals and proximal phalanges, and the middle and distal phalanges. The joints of the metacarpophalangeal joints are condyloid joints and are enclosed in synovial sheaths. Further description of the hand joints includes the metacarpophalangeal (MCP) joints, proximal interphalangeal (PIP) joints, and the distal interphalangeal (DIP) joints.

The muscle groups associated with wrist flexion include two carpal muscles that provide supination and pronation. The thumb is controlled by three muscles that provide flexion, abduction, and opposition. Movements in the digits are dependent upon action of the flexor and extensor tendons of muscles in the forearm and wrist (Bickley, 2003, p. 474).

The Hip

The hip is a ball-and-socket joint and forms articulation between the acetabulum and the head of the femur. The anterior iliac crest and the acetabulum surround the capsule, providing stability, strength, and leverage for movement. During childhood, the pelvic girdle, or coxal bone, is made up of three separate bones: the ilium, ischium, and pubis. By adulthood, these bones become fused and are referred to as the acetabulum, although their names are retained in order to refer to specific regions. The ilium is the large, flaring bone that forms the major portion of the coxal bone. The ischium forms the posterior inferior part of the hip bone, and the pubis forms the anterior portion of the coxal bone.

There are marked differences between the male and female pelvis. The female pelvis is wider, shallower, lighter, and rounder than the male pelvis; it is reflective of modifications necessary for childbearing. In the male, the pelvis bones are heavier and thicker, and the pelvis itself is narrower, longer, and less movable.

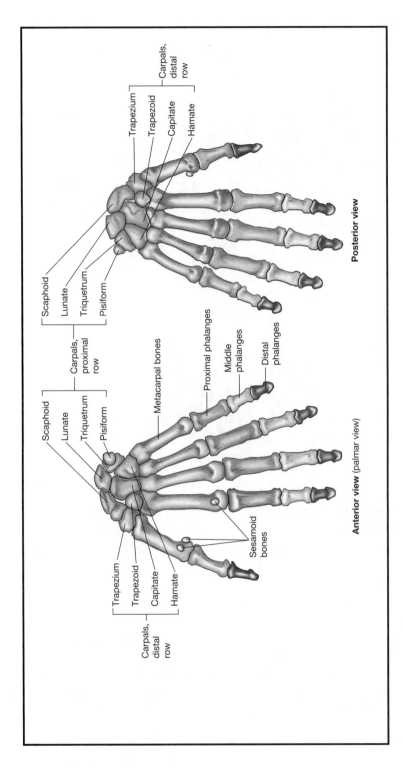

Figure 12-20(a) Hand/Wrist

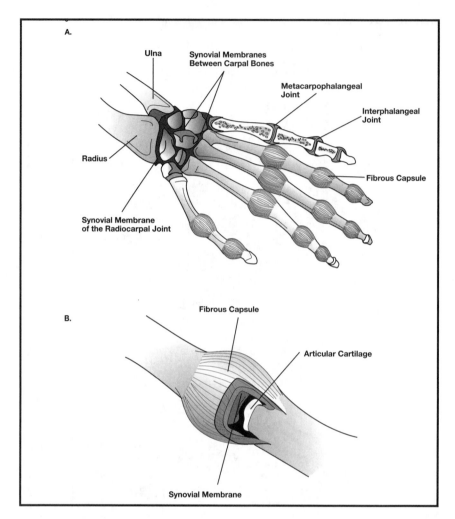

Figure 12-20(b)   Hand/Wrist

In examination of the hip, there are bony landmarks that will help guide your assessment. These landmarks are variable depending upon the age of the child. The iliac crest is located at the anterior aspect of the hip at the level of L4. From here, palpate downward to locate the iliac tubercle, which is the widest point of the iliac crest. Continue downward to the anterior superior iliac spine. With your thumbs on the anterior superior spine, move your fingers downward to the greater trochanter of the femur. From here,

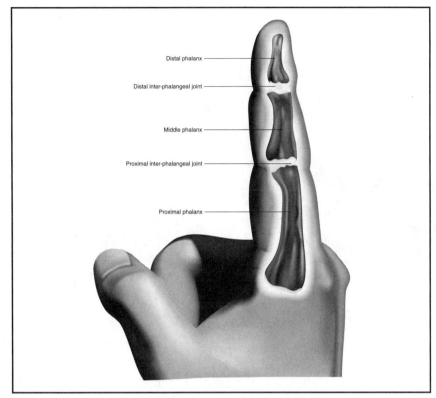

Distal phalanx

Distal inter-phalangeal joint

Middle phalanx

Proximal inter-phalangeal joint

Proximal phalanx

Figure 12-21

Source: Medical Multimedia Group LLC, www.eOrthopod.com

move your thumbs medially to the public symphysis, which is at the same level as the greater trochanter. To assess the posterior aspect of the hip, locate the posterior superior iliac spine, which is underneath the dimples just above the buttocks. Place your thumb and index finger over the posterior superior iliac spine, and locate the greater trochanter at the level of the gluteal fold. From here, you can place your fingers medially on the ischial tuberosity (Bickley, 2003, p. 478).

Muscle groups associated with the hip include the flexor group, which lies anteriorly. The primary hip flexor is the iliopsoas, which flexes the thigh. The extensor group lies posteriorly and includes the gluteus maximus, which is the primary extensor of the hip. The adductor group is medial and functions to swing the thigh toward the body, whereas the abductor group is lateral and functions to move the thigh away from the body.

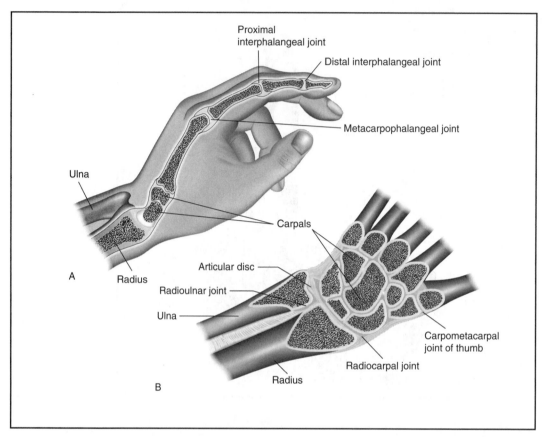

Figure 12-22 Structures of the Wrist and Hand Joints

Source: This article was published in *Physical Examination and Health Assessment,* 5th edition, Jarvis. Fractures of the wrist and hand. Copyright Saunders (2007).

The Knee

The knee is the largest and most complex joint. It involves three bones and forms three articulation surfaces, one between the patella and the distal end of the femur and another between the femoral condyles above and the menisci of the tibia below. It is a hinge joint and provides flexion and extension of the lower leg. This is a unique joint in that it is susceptible to sports injuries because it carries the body's weight. The knee can absorb vertical force but is vulnerable to horizontal blows such as those that occur during football blocking and tackling maneuvers. Lateral blows to the extended knee are most dangerous because they are likely

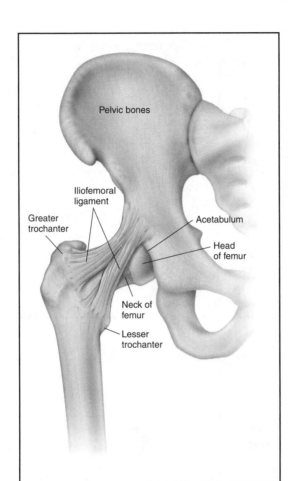

Pelvic bones

Iliofemoral
ligament

Greater
trochanter

Acetabulum

Head
of femur

Neck of
femur

Lesser
trochanter

Figure 12-23   Hip

to tear the medial collateral ligament and the medial meniscus that are attached to it. The knee joint itself is composed of two rounded condyles of the femur that rest on the flat portion of the tibia. The patella slides in a groove on the anterior aspect of the distal femur, the trochlear groove. You can palpate the patella with the knee flexed about 90 degrees. By pressing your thumbs downward along the groove of the tibiofemoral joint, you will be able to feel the edge of the tibial plateau. By following it medially and then laterally, you will be able to palpate the converging femur and tibia. Continue by moving your thumbs upward toward the

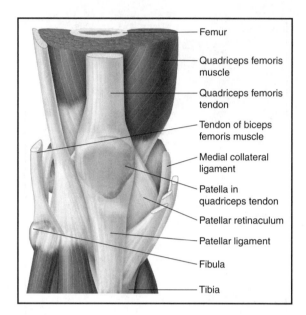

Figure 12-24 Knee

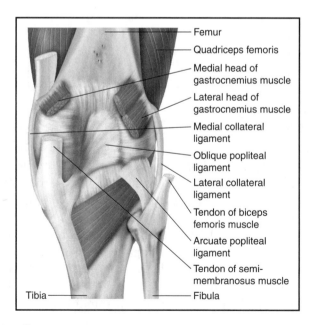

Figure 12-25 Knee

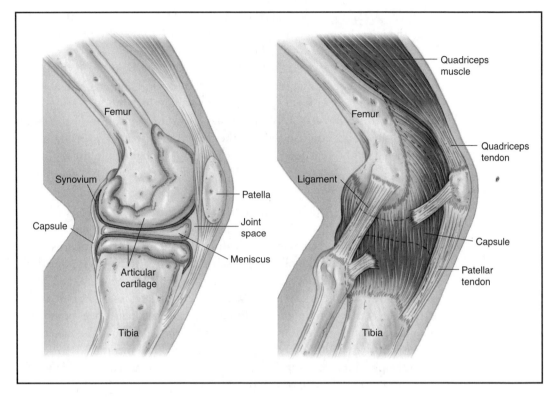

Figure 12-26   Knee

midline to the top of the patella. and follow this line to identify the margins of the joint.

Muscle groups associated with the knee include two important pairs of ligaments: the collateral ligaments and the cruciate ligaments (Bickley, 2003 p. 482):

- The *MEDIAL COLLATERAL LIGAMENT* (MCL) connects the medial condyles of the femur and the tibia. To palpate this region, move your fingers medially and posteriorly along the joint line, then palpate along the ligament from its origin to insertion.
- The *LATERAL COLLATERAL LIGAMENT* (LCL) connects the lateral femoral condyle and the head of the fibula. To palpate this region, cross one of the patient's legs so that the ankle rests on the opposite knee, and find the firm cord that runs from the lateral epicondyle of the femur to the head of the fibula. Medial and lateral stability is provided to the knee by these two collateral ligaments, the MCL and LCL.

- The *ANTERIOR CRUCIATE LIGAMENT* (ACL) crosses obliquely from the lateral femoral condyle to the medial tibia, thereby preventing the tibia from sliding forward on the femur.
- The *POSTERIOR CRUCIATE LIGAMENT* (PCL) crosses from the lateral tibia and lateral meniscus to the medial femoral condyle, thereby preventing the tibia from slipping backward on the femur.
- The *MEDIAL AND LATERAL MENISCI* cushion the action of the femur on the tibia. You can palpate the medial meniscus by pressing on the medial soft tissue depression along the upper edge of the tibial plateau.

The Ankle and Foot

The ankle and foot joint, or tibiotalar joint, forms articulations with the tibia, fibula, and talus. It is a hinge joint that provides flexion (dorsiflexion) and extension (plantar flexion) of the foot. Two important landmarks of the foot include the medial malleolus, which is the bony prominence at the distal end of the tibia, and the lateral malleolus, which is at the distal end of the fibula. Body weight is carried by the two largest tarsals—the talus, which articulates with the tibia and the fibula, and the calcaneus (heel bone). The Achilles tendon of the calf muscles attaches to the calcaneus. The metatarsus consists of five small long bones, the metatarsals. The metatarsals articulate with the proximal phalanges of the toes, and the enlarged head of the first metatarsal forms the ball of the foot (Marieb, 1995, p. 214).

Muscle groups associated with the ankle and foot include the gastrocnemius, which controls the posterior tibial muscle and the toe flexors necessary for plantar flexion, as well as the anterior tibial muscle and the toe extensors necessary for dorsiflexion.

(a)

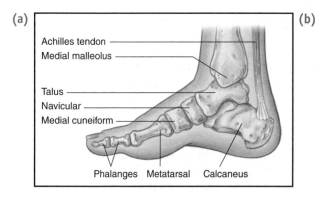

Achilles tendon
Medial malleolus

Talus
Navicular
Medial cuneiform

Phalanges   Metatarsal   Calcaneus

(b)

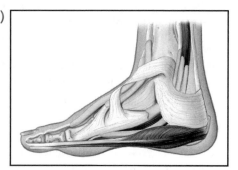

Figure 12-27   Foot

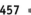

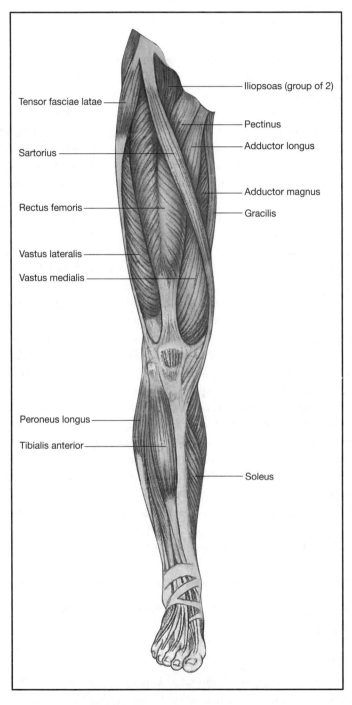

Tensor fasciae latae

Sartorius

Rectus femoris

Vastus lateralis

Vastus medialis

Peroneus longus

Tibialis anterior

Iliopsoas (group of 2)

Pectinus

Adductor longus

Adductor magnus

Gracilis

Soleus

Figure 12-28   Lower Leg Muscles

Differences Between the Child's and the Adult's Musculoskeletal System

There are a number of differences between the bones of the child and those of the adult. Ossification, or bone formation continues after birth through primary and secondary ossification centers such as the fontanels, the fibrous membrane that exists between the cranial bones. The anterior fontanelle does not close until approximately 18 months of age, allowing for growth of the brain and skull. The posterior fontanelle closes earlier, between 2 and 3 months of age. The majority of skull growth occurs by 2 years of age, with the skull reaching full size by 16 years (Chamley, Carson, Randall, 2005; Ball, Binder, & Cowen, 2010, p. 1438).

In children, growth takes place at the epiphyseal plates of long bones, and injuries to this portion of the bone can cause abnormalities in growth. Due to rapid bone growth during this period, fractures heal more quickly than in adulthood. To provide for adequate bone growth and density during childhood, calcium intake is essential. Inadequate calcium and Vitamin D intake during this period can lead to weak and brittle bones in adulthood.

In children, the epiphyseal plate remains open and is not replaced by bone until late adolescence. Because the bones of children are more porous and less dense than those of an adult, they are more likely to buckle, splinter, or fracture. The spinal vertebrae also change in shape as the child grows. In the newborn, the thoracic and sacral regions of the spine are convex, and as the infant develops and gains better head control, the cervical vertebrae become concave. Around the end of the first year when the child learns to stand and walk, the lumbar region becomes concave, distributing the upper body weight to the pelvis and lower extremities. Muscle development and strength increase until the child reaches the mid 20s. Prior to puberty, both ligaments and tendons are stronger than bone. Gradually, as the child reaches puberty and hormonal release occurs, cartilage is replaced by bone. This new bone is stronger than the ligaments or tendons; consequently, trauma to the long bones now more frequently results in injuries to ligaments and tendons rather than fractures.

Assessment Considerations: Subjective Information

The following sections present considerations for the assessment of the musculoskeletal system.

Infants and Toddlers

- Was the baby premature and what was the birth weight? A baby born premature with a low birth weight may be at risk for cerebral palsy and muscle tone disorders.

- Was the baby breech? Developmental dysplasia of the hip (DDH) is associated with breech presentation.
- Was there a history of ETOH (ethyl alcohol) abuse during pregnancy?
- Did the mother have a difficult delivery? Did the baby come headfirst? Were forceps used? A difficult delivery may increase the risk for fracture, such as fracture of the clavicle or brachial plexus..
- Did the baby need resuscitation or ventilator support at birth? If the baby was anoxic at birth, muscle tone disorders may be noted when monitoring development.
- Were abnormal fingers or toes noted at birth, including polydactyly (extra fingers) or syndactyly (webbed fingers or toes)?
- Were there any defects noted along the spinal column? Tufts of hair or dimples? These findings can be associated with spina bifida occulta or other defects of the spinal cord that can cause neurologic dysfunction.
- Were the baby's motor milestones, such as sitting and walking, achieved at the appropriate chronologic age of development?
- Were the baby's hips checked for signs of dislocation such as an audible click heard with the Ortolani or Barlow test?
- Was there concern regarding leg length discrepancy or thigh crease asymmetry, which can be associated with developmental hip dysplasia?
- Are any bony deformities evident, such as unusual shape of the toes or foot (e.g., clubfoot)?
- Has the baby had any broken bones or dislocations? How did they occur?
- Is extreme bowing or unilateral bowing of the legs evident? This finding can be associated with pathologic causes such as rickets or tibia vara.
- Are there concerns regarding in-toeing or out-toeing of the feet, knock knee, or bow legs? These are often developmental findings and generally resolve without intervention. .

School-Age Children and Adolescents

- Is there a history of subluxation of the elbow or nursemaid's elbow due to a tugging or swinging injury?
- Does the child have a history of joint or bone deformity, such as swelling, inflammation, contracture, joint stiffness, or unusual positioning?
- Is the child experiencing altered function, such as weakness, limp, or decreased range of motion?
- Is there an altered gait pattern such as toe walking, in-toeing, or out-toeing?
- Does the child complain of back pain? Factors that may contribute to back pain can be the type of shoes worn (e.g., platform shoes), use of a backpack, and the amount of weight in the backpack.
- Has the child been screened for scoliosis?

- Is the child involved in sports? If so, which sport and how many times per week? If relevant consider asking about pitch count for baseball or softball.
- Is there special equipment or training needed for the sport?
- Does the child work with a trainer such as working on weight lifting?
- Is the child on a special diet, such as vegetarian or vegan?
- Does the child get an adequate amount of calcium and Vitamin D?
- Does the child take herbal supplements?

Family History

- Is there a family history of orthopedic problems?
- Is there a family history of scoliosis or developmental dysplasia of the hip (DDH)?
- Is there a family history of genetic disorders such as osteogenesis imperfecta, dwarfing syndrome, neurofibromatosis, Marfans, or Ehlers Danlow syndrome?
- Is there a family history of juvenile rheumatoid arthritis?

Review of Systems

In review of the musculoskeletal system, determine if there is a history of generalized weakness. Question if there is concern about clumsiness, frequent falling or tripping, or abnormal gait. Does the child have a history of persistent or chronic pain, such as joint pain or increased pain with movement? Is there concern of swelling of joints, warm or painful joints, or limitation of range of motion of joints? Does the child complain of back pain or have a history of scoliosis? Is there complaint of injuries/trauma or previous fractures?

Sports Physical

Schools today require that players have a complete sports physical. The purpose is to screen for potential illnesses or conditions that may restrict or limit the child's activity. It ensures that the child does not have any medical condition that may be aggravated by intense exercise and that the child is physically capable of meeting the demands of the sport. Obtaining a comprehensive history and performing a thorough physical exam is the cornerstone in identification of the majority of problems affecting children participating in athletics.

A detailed history is important and should focus on the hereditary component of cardiovascular disorders, including questions pertinent to a family history. Important considerations include sudden death in a close relative before the age of 50 years, long QT syndrome, and a history of Marfan syndrome or any other cardiovascular disorders. Specific questions pertinent to the child should focus on symptoms related to the cardiovascular system such as shortness of breath, chest pain, dizziness, tiring easily with exercise, and palpitations. History of the following physical findings indicates the need for further evaluation and possibly referral (Green, 2002):

- Early fatigue, dizziness, syncope, chest pain, shortness of breath, or palpitations with exercise
- Family history of sudden death or significant cardiovascular condition
- Physical signs of Marfan syndrome
- Significant head or spinal injury
- Best-corrected vision of less than 20/40 in either eye
- Significant musculoskeletal problem or injury
- History of surgeries or hospitalizations

When performing a preparticipation physical exam, the goals include (Green, 2002):

- Identify conditions that would predispose children to serious injury or death.
- Identify current medical or psychological conditions that could be worsened by exercise.
- Diagnose previously undetected conditions.
- Assess general health and risk-taking behaviors.
- Satisfy school, state, and insurance requirements.
- Assess fitness level and performance parameters (optional).

Timing of the evaluation is approximately 6 weeks prior to the beginning of the athletic season, or preseason practice. This length of time allows for further evaluation, diagnostic testing, and/or rehabilitation or conditioning of specific problems.

Questions to Consider in a Preparticipation Sports History

GENERAL questions include:

- Do you have a history of allergies to medications, foods, and the environment, such as pollens or beestings?
- Are your immunizations up to date? Obtain a record of proof.
- Have you ever become ill from exercising in the heat?

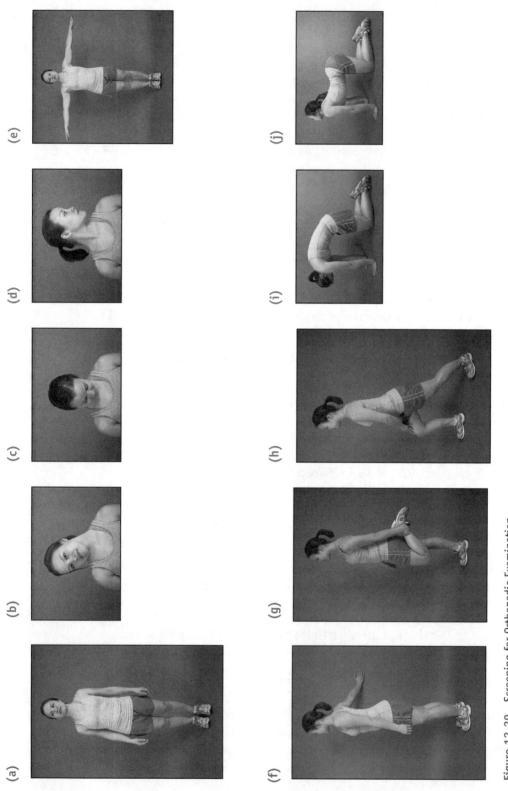

Figure 12-29 Screening for Orthopedic Examination

High School Sports
Physical Evaluation

Name:_____

Sex: M or F   Age:____   DOB: _____   Height_____ Weight:____

Emergency Contact:

Name:_____ Relationship:_____ Phone:_____

Yes or No

1. Do you have any medical   Y   N   10. Do you have severe headaches Y   N
condition or injuries?   Or migraines?

2. Have you ever had
any surgeries?   Y   N   11. Have you ever broken or   Y   N
                                                     fractured any bones?

3. Are you currently
taking any prescriptions or   Y   N   12. Do you have seasonal   Y   N
over-the-counter medications?   Allergies?

4. Are you allergic to any   Y   N   13. Do you feel dizzy during   Y   N
medications?   Or after exercise?

5. Have you ever been   Y   N   14. Have you ever become ill   Y   N
hospitalized?   From the heat?

6. Do you have asthma?   Y   N   15. Do you feel stressed out?   Y   N

7. Do you wear glasses   Y   N   16. Have you ever been knocked   Y   N
or contacts?   Out or blacked out?

8. Has any family member   17. Have you ever had a seizure
died of heart problems   Y   N   or had a family member have   Y   N
before the age of 40?   A seizure?

9. Have you ever been told   Y   N
you have a heard murmur?

Figure 12-30   Preparticipation Physical Evaluation Form: History Questionnaire

- Do you need any special protective or corrective equipment such as hearing aids or a knee brace?
- Do you want to weigh more or less than you do?
- Do you lose weight to meet requirements for your sport?

SKIN-RELATED questions focus on any current skin problems, including rashes, itching, warts, blisters, and fungal infections.

EAR, NOSE, AND THROAT questions focus on any problems with the child's eyes/vision: Have you experienced injury to your eyes during sports? Hearing problems?

RESPIRATORY questions include:

- Do you have difficulty breathing, such as coughing or wheezing, after physical activity?
- Do you have a history of asthma? If so, do you use a metered-dose inhaler? How often?
- Do you smoke? Does anyone in your house smoke?

CARDIOVASCULAR questions include:

- Do you experience dizziness, shortness of breath, or chest pain associated with exercise?
- Do you tire more easily than friends?
- Do you have a history of high blood pressure, high cholesterol, or heart murmur?
- Have you ever been restricted from sports due to cardiovascular problems?

MUSCULOSKELETAL questions include:

- Have you ever had a sprain, strain, or swelling after an injury?
- Have you ever dislocated a joint or fractured a bone

NEUROLOGIC questions include:

- Have you ever been knocked out or experienced loss of consciousness or memory loss?
- Do you have a history of seizures, headaches, or numbness or tingling in your hands or feet?

PSYCHOLOGICAL questions include:

- Do you feel stressed? Is there anything you are worried about and want to talk about?
- Do you have a history of depression or suicide?
- Do you drink alcohol or use drugs? How frequently?

PAST MEDICAL HISTORY questions include:

- Do you have any history of hospitalizations, accidents, or motor vehicle accidents?
- Do you have any history of chronic illness such as diabetes or epilepsy?
- Have you had any changes, illnesses, or accidents since your last physical exam?

MEDICATION-related questions include:

- Do you take any medication on a regular basis?
- Do you use an inhaler?
- Do you take vitamins or dietary supplements? Herbal remedies?
- Do you take any pain medicine for sore muscles and/or headaches?
- Do you take medicine to gain or lose weight or to improve your athletic performance?

FEMALES should be asked the following questions:

- What was your age of menarche?
- Are your menses regular, and what is the duration?
- Do you have intermenstrual bleeding or pain? Perimenstrual symptoms?
- What was the date of your last menstrual period?
- Do you use contraception? What type?

Physical Examination

A complete physical exam includes vital signs, height/weight, BMI, and hearing and vision screen. Routine laboratory screening and radiographs are not necessary in an asymptomatic child.

Determining Eligibility for Participation

Conditions that require further evaluation for participation in sports include:

- *CARDIOVASCULAR*: Hypertension, congenital heart disease, dysrhythmia, mitral valve prolapse, heart murmur
- *NEUROLOGIC*: Cerebral palsy, epilepsy, history of serious head trauma, head injury, craniotomy
- *RESPIRATORY*: Acute respiratory infection, pulmonary compromise such as history of cystic fibrosis
- *EYES*: History of serious eye injury, loss of an eye
- *GENITOURINARY*: Absence of one kidney
- *MUSCULOSKELETAL*: Musculoskeletal disorders
- *SKIN*: Methicillin-resistant staphylococcus aureus, herpes, impetigo, scabies, Molluscum contagiosum

- *GASTROINTESTINAL*: History of mononucleosis with enlarged liver/spleen
- *BEHAVIORAL*: Obesity, anorexia nervosa, bulimia nervosa

Clearance to participate in sports is classified according to three categories:

- *UNRESTRICTED*: There is no limiting abnormality, and the child is approved to participate in all sports.
- *CONDITIONAL CLEARANCE*: Clearance is given, pending further evaluation.
- *NOT CLEARED FOR ALL SPORTS*: This category includes children with potentially life-threatening conditions.

Conditions that need to be considered but may not preclude participation in sports include:

- *ENDOCRINE*: Diabetes mellitus
- *IMMUNOLOGIC*: HIV infection
- *GENITOURINARY*: Absence of one ovary, absent or undescended testicle
- *RESPIRATORY*: Asthma that is well managed
- *HEMATOLOGIC*: Sickle cell disease
- *NEUROLOGIC*: Seizure disorder that is well controlled

Under the Rehabilitation Act of 1973 and the Americans with Disabilities Act of 1990, athletes may have the legal right to participate in a sport despite medical advice.

As a healthcare provider, you should consult with an expert in the field in regard to a child whom you feel should be restricted from participation or excluded from a sport. Consulting an expert reassures both the parents and the child that restriction from a specific sport is the correct course of action. It also provides the healthcare provider with liability protection when making the recommendation (Graham & Uphold, 2003; Green, 2002).

Assessment Considerations: Objective Information

Examination of the musculoskeletal system varies according to age group.

Newborns

Musculoskeletal examination of the newborn is covered in Chapter 4, "Newborn Assessment."

Infants and Toddlers

Examination of the musculoskeletal system of the infant and toddler starts with inspection with the child undressed to the diaper and *supine* on the examining table or in the parent's lap. The actual extent of the assessment should be based on each individual child. A functional screening of a joint by joint evaluation is not necessary on an active, coordinated toddler who demonstrates basic gross and fine motor functioning that is appropriate for his or her age. If the child is actively playing, you can conduct much of the exam by playing with the child and observing him or her at the same time.

Initially, observe for symmetry of the extremities as the infant is kicking and moving about on the table. Note if one side is moving more or is more active than the other side. The child who presents with weakness or specific joint pain, immobility, or signs of joint infection requires a more thorough examination. In the actual assessment, palpation and joint and muscle evaluation is performed by putting the joints through passive range of motion in an infant or a toddler who is too young to follow instructions.

During the first year of life, positioning of the child on the examination table is important to emphasize facilitation of certain movements. For example, at 4–6 months of age, a child in a prone position demonstrates the ability to push up on his or her hands and roll from a prone to a supine position. By 7 months, placing the child in a standing position allows you an opportunity to evaluate the child's ability to bear weight and to assess the muscle strength of the child's legs. At 8 months, placing the child in a sitting position allows you to observe the strength of his or her back, as well as stability in reaching out.

Specific body parts are assessed as follows:

FEET AND ANKLE: Start the exam from a distal point and approach the child slowly by initially playing with the toes, inspecting for color and deformity, and palpating for temperature, tenderness, and limitation in movement, as well as capillary refill, posterior tibial pulse, and doralis pedis pulse. Gradually move to the child's ankle and gently put it through passive range of motion, at the same time assessing muscle strength and noting color, warmth, deformity, and/or any limitation in movement. Movement at the ankle joint is limited to dorsiflexion and plantar flexion.

KNEE: With the child in a supine position, either on the table or on the parent's lap, inspect the knee, assessing color and shape. Gently palpate the knee for warmth and tenderness, and put it through passive range of motion, noting any limitation in movement. The knee joint can be assessed for flexion and extension.

HIP: A hip exam assessing for congenital hip dislocation is covered in detail in Chapter 4; this exam is performed until the child demonstrates independent walking (Durtz, 2010).. In the infant and toddler, the hip is initially inspected for shape, color, and/or any deformity. This is followed with palpation and assessment for tenderness and warmth. Next, put the hip joint through passive range of motion that includes flexion, extension, abduction, adduction, and internal and external rotation.

FINGERS, WRIST, AND ELBOW: As you approach the child's hands and arms, gently inspect the fingers and wrist, assessing for color and deformity. Palpate the fingers and wrist for tenderness, strength, and temperature while putting them through passive range of motion, as well as checking capillary refill and a radial pulse. Movement of the fingers includes primarily flexion and extension. The thumb includes opposition to the tip or base of the little finger as well as flexion. Movement of the wrist includes flexion and extension as well as radial and ulnar deviation. From the wrist, move up to the elbow, inspecting for size, contour, and color. Palpate for tenderness and passive range of motion. Movement of the elbow includes flexion and extension.

SHOULDER: Assessing the child's shoulder should begin with inspection both posteriorly and anteriorly, assessing for contour and symmetry. Then palpate for tenderness and temperature as you put the shoulder through passive range of motion. Movements of the shoulder include forward flexion, backward extension, horizontal flexion and extension, as well as abduction, adduction, and internal and external rotation.

SPINE: Assessment of the spine for the infant can be performed with the child in a prone position or sitting on the table. In an older child, have the child stand up on the table or on the floor. Begin with inspection of the shoulder height, inspecting downward and noting the height and placement of the scapulae. Next, assess the vertebrae. If the child is standing, you can evaluate the hip height for symmetry. If assessing a school-age child, ask the child to bend over to touch the toes, then hyperextend and rotate from side to side. Remember, in a toddler, observing the child playing, bending, and moving about will allow you to observe for range of motion of the hips and spine.

HEAD: Observation of movement of the head while the child is playing allows observation of flexion, extension, and rotation. Playing along with the child and placing toys in various positions encourages the child to reach out, bend toward, rotate, stand up, and sit down, all presenting opportunities to assess active range of motion.

School-Age Children and Adolescents

General assessment starts by observing the child's posture and ease of mobility as the child walks into the room, bends over, sits down, and stands up. Start by having the child change into a hospital gown and sit on the exam table.

Temporomandibular Joint

INSPECTION: With the school-age child and adolescent, you can begin the exam by starting at the head and assessing the TMJ. Initially, inspect the area anterior to the ear in front of the tragus for any redness or rash.

PALPATION: Palpate the TMJ by placing the tips of your index and middle finger in front of each ear, and ask the child to open and close the mouth. You will be able to palpate a depressed area over the joint next to the mandible.

RANGE OF MOTION: When the child opens and closes the mouth, assess for smoothness and movement without crepitation or clicking. Swelling, tenderness, or decreased range of motion may indicate an inflammatory process. Clicking and/or crepitation may be palpated and can be considered a normal finding in some children.

Shoulder

INSPECTION: Inspect the shoulders, assessing the clavicles and placement of the scapulae; note the size and contour of the shoulders, particularly assessing for any asymmetry (one shoulder higher than the other). Note any swelling, deformity, color change in skin, or abnormal positioning. Scoliosis in the child may cause elevation of one shoulder.

PALPATION: Palpate the shoulders, noting any warmth or tenderness. Identify the bony landmarks of the shoulder—the acromion process, the acromioclavicular joint, and the coracoid process—and palpate these areas for pain.

RANGE OF MOTION: Assess range of motion by asking the child to put the shoulder joint through six motions: flexion, extension, abduction, adduction, internal rotation, and external rotation.

- FLEXION AND HYPEREXTENSION: With the child's arms at the sides and elbows extended, move both arms forward and up in wide vertical arcs, then move them back.
- ABDUCTION AND ADDUCTION: With the child's arms at the sides and elbows extended, raise both arms in wide arcs above the child's head.
- EXTERNAL ROTATION: Touch both of the child's hands behind the head with elbows flexed and rotated posteriorly.
- INTERNAL ROTATION: Rotate the child's arms internally behind the back, and place the back of the hands as high as possible toward the scapulae.
- STRENGTH: To assess shoulder strength, ask the child to shrug the shoulders against your resistance. You expect the shoulders to rise symmetrically. This procedure also assesses the integrity of cranial nerve XI, the spinal accessory.

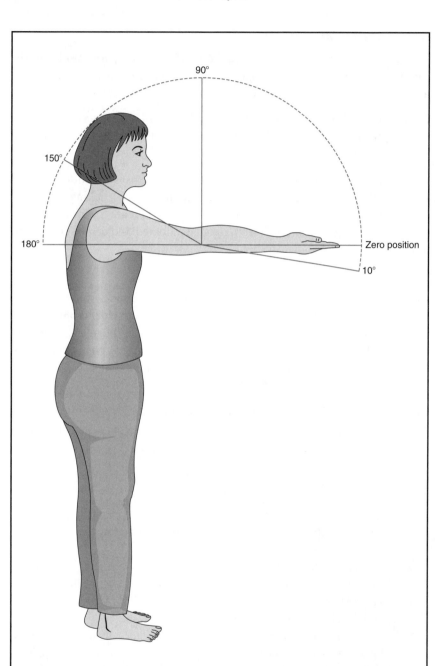

Figure 12-31 Range of Motion

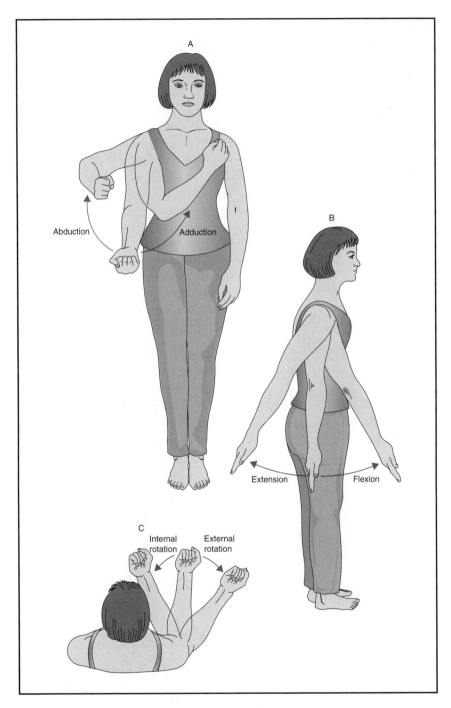

Figure 12-32 Range of Motion at the Shoulder

Elbow

INSPECTION: With the child in a sitting position, inspect the contour of the elbow in both flexed and extended positions. Inspect for any redness, swelling, and contour.

PALPATION: Palpate the elbow by supporting it with your opposite hand. Flex the child's elbow about 70 degrees; with your thumb and index finger, palpate the contours of the elbow, identifying the medial and lateral epicondyles and the olecranon process of the ulna. Palpate the olecranon process for tenderness. See **Figure 12-34.**

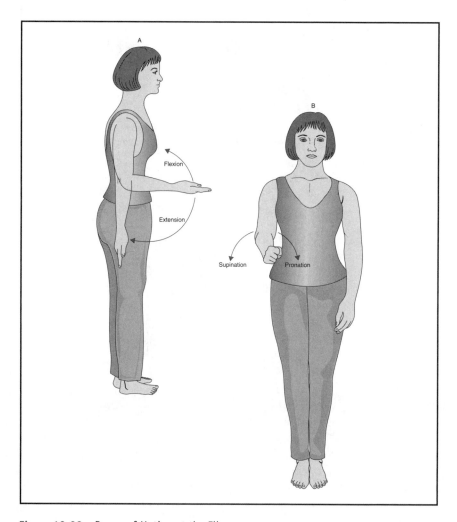

Figure 12-33   Range of Motion at the Elbow

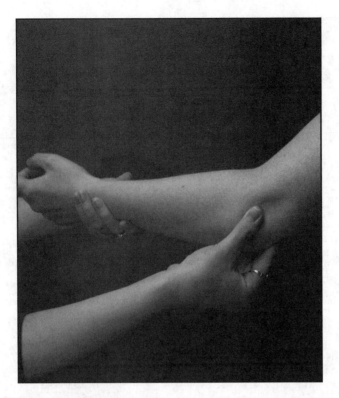

Figure 12-34 Palpate the Elbow

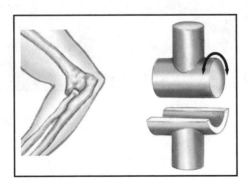

Figure 12-35(a) Knee Joints

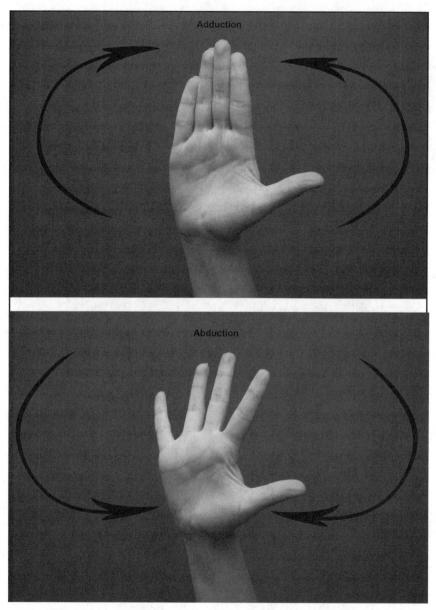

Figure 12-35(b) Range of Motion at the Finger Joints

RANGE OF MOTION: To assess range of motion, ask the child to flex and extend the elbow.

Wrist and Hand

INSPECTION: With the child in a sitting position, inspect the hands and wrists on both the dorsal and palmar sides, noting contour, color, and positioning. Inspect for swelling and shape of fingers.

PALPATION: Palpate each joint in the wrist and in the hand, particularly if assessing for tenderness secondary to trauma from a fall or sports. Palpate the metacarpophalangeal joints as well as the interphalangeal joints. There should be no swelling or tenderness.

RANGE OF MOTION: To assess for range of motion, ask the child to bend the hand upward at the wrist and then downward at the wrist. Bend the fingers up and down, spread the fingers apart, and touch the thumb to each finger and to the base of the little finger.

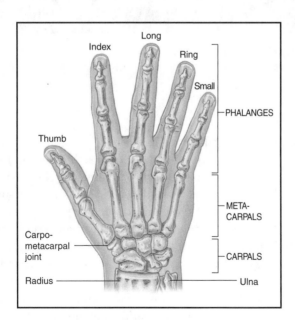

Figure 12-35(c)   Anatomy of the Wrist and Fingers

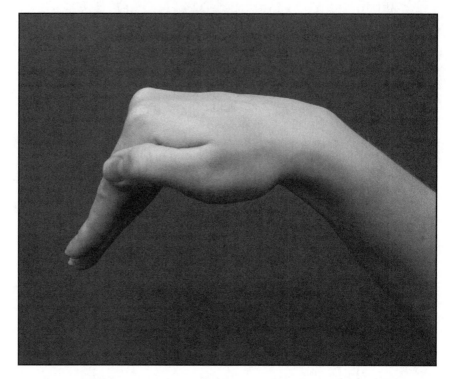

Figure 12-35(d) Normal Range of Findings

Cervical Spine

INSPECTION: With the child standing, inspect the spine; note the spinous processes, including the major landmark of vertebrae C7 and T1 that are usually most prominent. Next inspect for symmetric shoulders, scapulae, and iliac crest heights. The curves of the cervical and lumbar spines should be concave, and the curve of the thoracic spine should be convex. Be sure the knees and feet are in alignment with the head and trunk and pointing forward. Children often tend to stand with a bend or angle in their hip or knee, which will give a false impression of the cervical spine and scapulae.

Screening for *scoliosis* is most important during the preadolescent growth spurt. Several types of scoliosis may present during childhood. The majority of cases of scoliosis are idiopathic, accounting for approximately 75% of cases, most of which are seen in girls.

To screen for scoliosis, the child must be in his or her underwear so that the entire back is visible. Start with the child standing upright and the feet pointing forward. Start at the top and inspect for symmetry of the shoulders. Next, ask the child to bend over in the "forward bend test," or the *Adams bend test*. Seat yourself behind the standing child and ask the child to stand with the feet shoulder-width apart and bend forward slowly to touch the toes. The child's back should remain symmetrical with a straight vertical spine while standing and while bending forward. The posterior ribs should be symmetrical, and there should be equal elevation of the shoulders, scapulae, and iliac crests. In this position, inspect and palpate the spinous processes starting at the cervical spine and progressing to the sacral area. When using a scoliometer, place it on the thoracic vertebrae in the midspinal line. Measure the angle of the trunk rotation, and a reading on the scoliometer of greater than or equal to a 7 degree curve should be evaluated further (Green, 2002, p. 697). On overall inspection, you are inspecting for uneven shoulders, one scapula that appears more prominent than the other, an uneven waist, one hip higher than the other, limb length discrepancy, back pain, and difficulty breathing.

RANGE OF MOTION: To assess the thoracic and lumbar range of motion, have the child in a standing position and perform the following maneuvers:

- *FLEXION*: Bend forward at the waist and touch the toes.
- *HYPEREXTENSION*: Bend backward at the waist as far as possible.

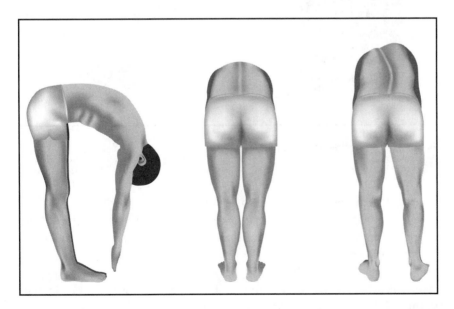

Figure 12-36   Scoliosis

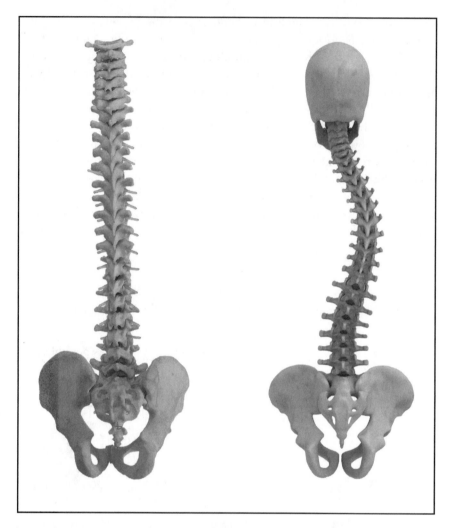

Figure 12-37 Normal Spine vs. Deformity from Scoliosis

- *BILATERAL BENDING*: Bend to each side as far as possible.
- *ROTATION OF THE UPPER TRUNK FORWARD AND BACKWARD*: Rotate the upper trunk from the waist in a circular motion, front to side to back to side.

PALPATION: With the child standing, assess the spinous processes by palpating each vertebra. Palpate the paravertebral muscles for tenderness. Muscles that are in spasm will feel firm and knotted. Tenderness may be noted secondary to trauma and increased physical activity.

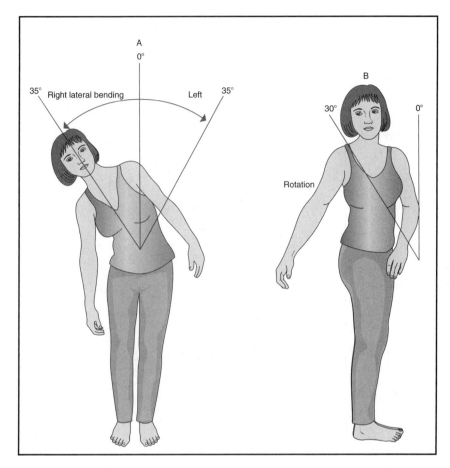

Figure 12-38 Normal Range of Findings

Hip

INSPECTION: Inspection of the hip starts as the child walks into the office and you observe the child's gait, noting whether the child has in-toeing, out-toeing, or tibial torsion; is walking on the toes; or has a limp. Note whether the child exhibits a normal gait with a smooth continuous rhythm.

PALPATION: With the child supine on the exam table, initially identify landmarks such as the iliac tubercle and the anterior superior iliac spine. Ask the child to place the heel of the leg being examined on the opposite knee. Then palpate along the inguinal ligament for tenderness. Repeat this maneuver on the opposite side.

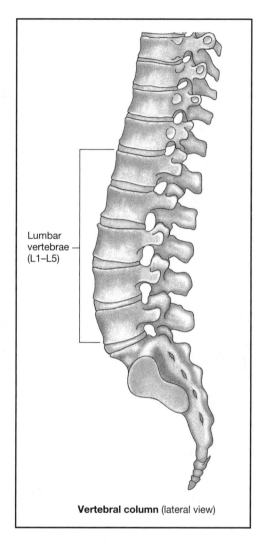

Lumbar
vertebrae
(L1–L5)

Vertebral column (lateral view)

Figure 12-39 Anatomy of the Lumbar Spine

RANGE OF MOTION: Ask the child to perform the following maneuvers (on both sides):

- *FLEXION:* While the child is supine, raise the leg with the knee extended above the body.
- *ADDUCTION AND ABDUCTION:* While the child is supine, move the leg laterally and medially with the knee straight.

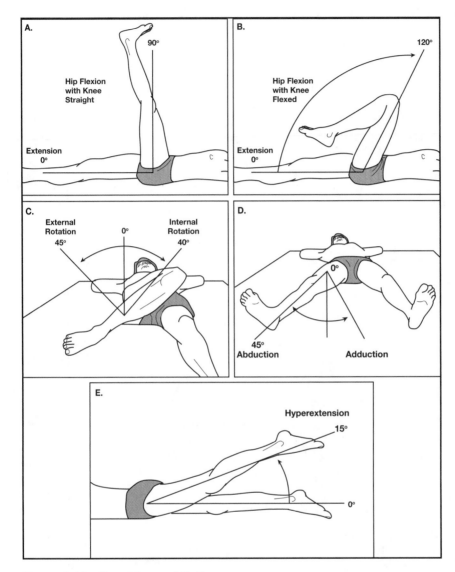

Figure 12-40 Normal Range of Findings

Source: Jarvis.

- *INTERNAL ROTATION:* While the child is supine, flex the knee and rotate the leg inward toward the other leg.
- *EXTERNAL ROTATION:* While the child is supine, place the lateral aspect of the foot on the knee of the other leg, and move the flexed knee toward the table.

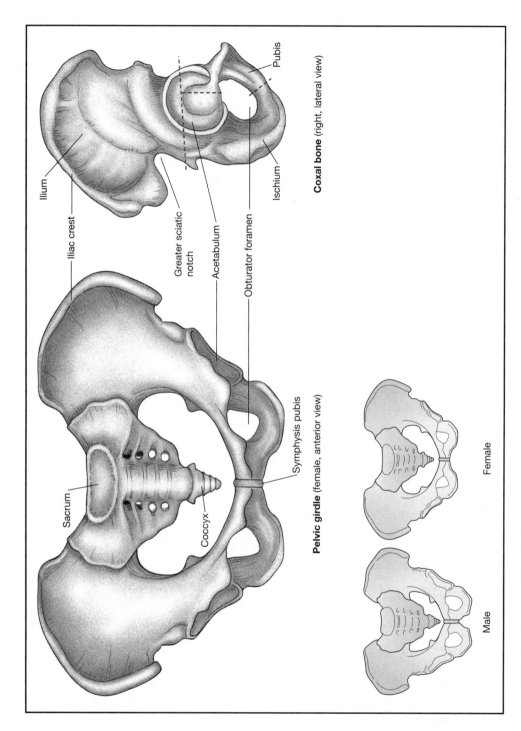

Figure 12-41 Anatomy of the Hip Joint

- *HYPEREXTENSION*: With the child standing or prone, move the straightened leg behind the body.

To evaluate the strength of the hip muscles, the child should be in a supine position with the hip flexed and the knee flexed and in extension. Apply opposing force as you evaluate hip muscle strength. Remember to adjust the force applied depending upon the age of the child. This maneuver would primarily be performed on an adolescent.

Knee

INSPECTION: With the child in a sitting position, inspect the knee both in flexion and extension, noting the contour, any redness, swelling, or deformity.

PALPATION: With the child's knees flexed, place your thumbs on both sides of the patella and palpate the knee both in flexion and extension, noting any tenderness or crepitus. If the child is complaining of tenderness in the knee, assess for bogginess and/or fluid:

- *BULGE SIGN*: The bulge sign indicates fluid in the suprapatellar pouch. Effusion occurs as fluid flows across the joint of the knee. To perform this test, firmly place your thumb and fingers on the lower portion of the thigh and palpate downward toward the knee, assessing the supra- patellar pouch for bogginess or sponginess. The tissue should feel firm

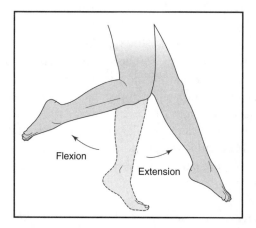

Figure 12-42 Range of Motion at the Knee Joint: Flexion and Hyperextension

(a) 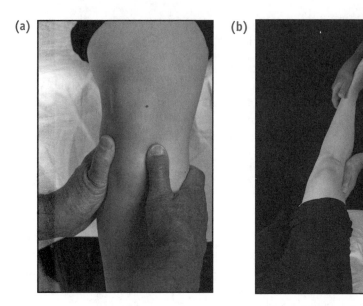 (b)

Figure 12-43 Another Technique for Testing the Collateral Ligaments: (a) Ballottement, (b) Extension

and without edema. If swelling is observed, determine if it is swelling due to soft tissue injury or increased fluid in the joint. Firmly stroke the medial aspect of the knee upward to displace any fluid. With a positive bulge sign, you will observe the fluid move from one side of the joint to the other (Jarvis, 2008, p. 624).

- *BALLOTTEMENT*: If there is concern about a larger amount of fluid on the knee, ballottement of the patella is performed. Use your hand to compress the suprapatellar pouch; as you do so, ballote (push) the patella against the femur. If there is a large effusion, you will observe fluid returning to the suprapatellar pouch or moving into the knee joint. With your other hand, sharply push the patella against the femur. If no fluid is present, the patella will remain snug against the femur (Jarvis, 2008, p. 625).

RANGE OF MOTION: To assess range of motion of the knee, with the child in a standing position, ask the child to bend or flex one knee at a time and then extend each knee to determine if there is limitation in movement. This procedure can be performed in a supine position by flexing the hips and then performing flexion and extension of the knee.

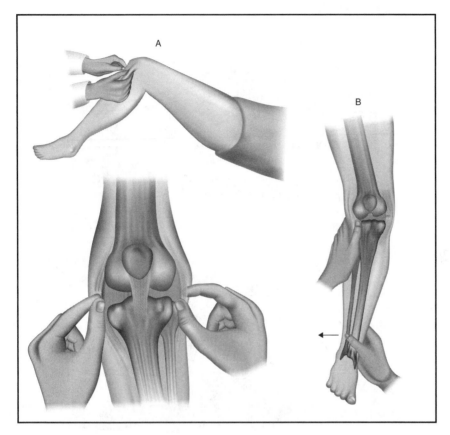

Figure 12-44   Technique for Testing for a Knee Joint Effusion

Source: This article was published in *Textbook of Physical Diagnosis: History and Examination,* 5th edition, Swartz. Technique for testing the collateral ligaments. Copyright Saunders (2005).

Ankle and Foot

INSPECTION: With the child sitting on the exam table, inspect the ankle and feet in a nonweight-bearing position as well as standing and walking. Inspect the feet and toes, noting contour of the joints and any skin alterations such as calluses. The toes should lie flat and point straight ahead. Inspect for flat feet, high arch, hammer toes, and bunions. On inspection of the ankle, the internal and external malleoli are smooth bony prominences with even coloring.

PALPATION: For palpation, support the child's ankle by grasping the heel with your fingers as you palpate the joint spaces on the foot. There should be no edema, tenderness, or swelling. Palpate the metatarsophalangeal joints on the plantar surface of the foot for tenderness and/or inflammation.

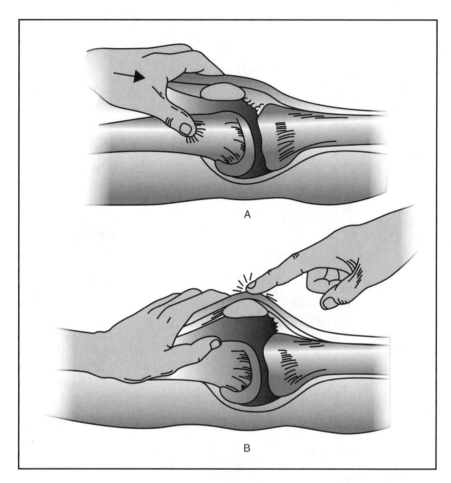

Figure 12-45 Assessment of Bulge Sign in Knee

RANGE OF MOTION: For plantar flexion, ask the child to point the toes toward the floor. For dorsi flexion, ask the child to point the toes toward his or her nose. Turn the sole of the child's foot outward (eversion), then inward (inversion). Follow this by flexing and straightening the child's toes.

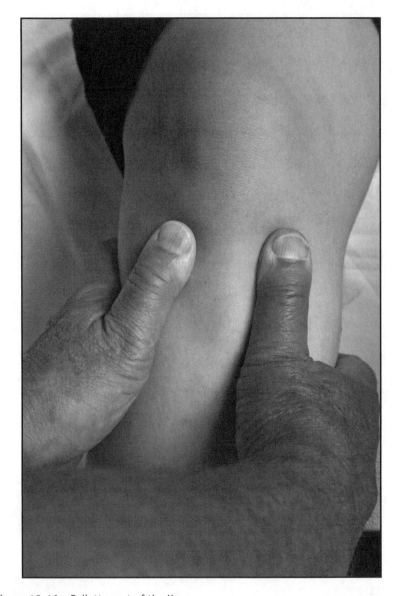

Figure 12-46 Ballottement of the Knee

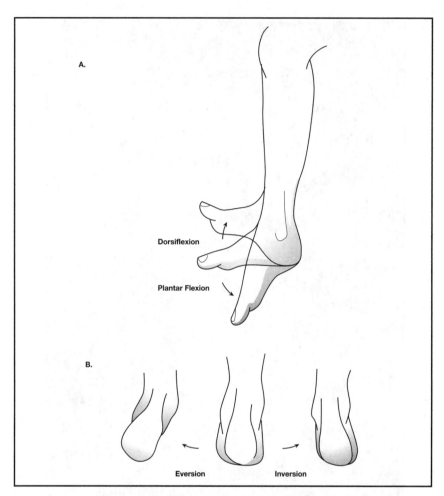

Figure 12-47 Range of Motion at the Ankle and Foot Joints

Common Musculoskeletal Disorders

Infants

BRACHIAL PLEXUS INJURIES: These injuries are characterized by traumatic stretch or traction injuries that occur when innervation to the child's arm is disrupted during labor and delivery, resulting in paralysis. This presentation is dependent upon the location of the nerve and muscle involved. Children born with brachial plexus injuries are referred to an orthopedist for further evaluation.

Toddlers, School-Age Children, and Adolescents

COSTOCHONDRITIS: This is a benign disorder characterized by sharp pain localized at the costosternal junction where the sternum, ribs, and costal cartilage connect. This disorder presents with acute chest pain of short duration. The major finding on palpation is localized tenderness at one or more constochrondral joints. Management includes mild analgesia or anti-inflammatories.

LEGG-CALVÉ-PERTHES DISEASE: This condition is idiopathic osteonecrosis of the femoral head in children. It is characterized by inadequate blood supply to the capital femoral epiphysis, leading to necrosis and deformity of the femoral head. It is primarily seen in young school-age boys. This disorder presents with decreased range of motion, pain, and stiffness. Children are referred to an orthopedic surgeon for further evaluation.

SLIPPED CAPITAL FEMORAL EPIPHYSIS: This condition is characterized by the gradual dislocation of the femoral head from its neck and shaft at the upper epiphyseal plate level (**Figure 12-49**). This displacement involves weakening of the growth plate and surrounding structures, placing the adolescent at risk for avascular necrosis. This disorder presents with hip and/or knee pain, a limp, and marked limitation of range of motion. Patients are referred to an orthopedic surgeon for further evaluation.

OSGOOD-SCHLATTER DISEASE: This is an example of an overuse injury due to the weak link at the bone–tendon junction (**Figure 12-50**). It results from microscopic avulsion fractures at the insertion of the patellar tendon

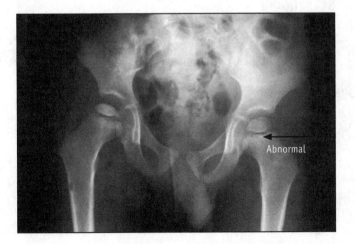

Figure 12-48   Legg-Calve-Perthes Disease

when the child is physically active and the weak secondary ossification center of the proximal tibia is developing. This condition most frequently occurs during adolescence (Green, 2002, p. 581).

GENU VARUM (BOWLEGS): This is an angular deformity at the knee with the tibia medially deviated in relation to the femur. This disorder may be familial and a normal variation of development. Pathologic genu varum is less common and due to rickets, osteogenesis imperfecta, or dyschondroplasia.

GENU VALGUM (KNOCK-KNEES): This is alignment of the knee with the tibia laterally deviated in relation to the femur (**Figure 12-51**). This disorder may be familial and/or a normal variation of development. Extreme or unilateral genu valgum may be associated with underlying bone disease.

INTOEING: This is often due to inward rotation of the femur or tibia. The most common finding is femoral anteversion or increased internal torsion of the femur.

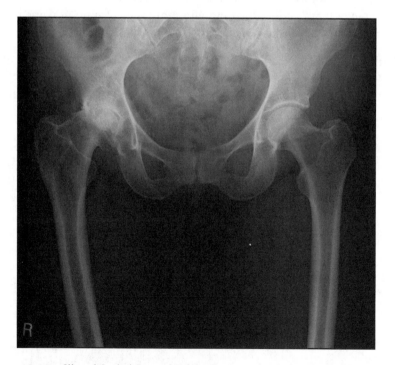

Figure 12-49   Slipped Capital Femoral Epiphysis

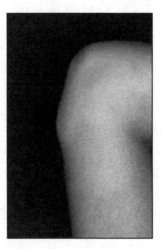

Figure 12-50   Osgood-Schlatter Disease

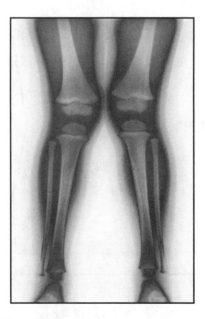

Figure 12-51   Genu Valgum Knocked Knee

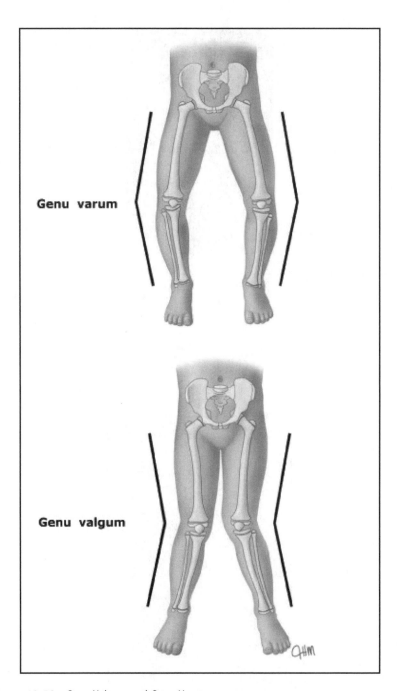

Figure 12-52 Genu Valgum and Geno Varum

TIBIAL TORSION: This is a common problem described as twisting of the long bone along its long axis. It is the most common cause of intoeing and is generally observed around 2 years of age. It is generally a benign condition, although it should be referred if it causes functional problems.

OUTTOEING: This is excessive rotation of the femur (femur retroversion) and the tibia (external tibial torsion). It is a common deviation of normal development and generally observed around 2 years of age. Both intoeing and outtoeing are benign conditions although should be referred if they cause functional problems.

OSTEOCHONDRITIS DISSECANS (OCD): This is a condition in which a segment of articular cartilage and the underlying subchondral bone gradually separate from the surrounding osteocartilaginous tissue (Hergenroeder, 2004). The condition primarily affects boys between 9 and 18 years of age and presents with vague pain with activity. As the process progresses there may be intermittent swelling and locking of the knee.

GROWING PAINS: This leg pain is described as mild to moderate, intermittent in character, and more noticeable in the evening or at night following a day of increased activity or sports. Exam should focus on identifying any infection, masses, inflammation, lymphadenopathy, abnormal joint movement, instability, or neurologic deficits. Growing pains are a benign self-limiting disorder that may occur intermittently for several months.

TRANSIENT SYNOVITIS: This disorder is characterized by pain, limitation of motion in the hip, and occasionally a low-grade fever. Some studies show it follows an upper respiratory infection. Management is use of nonsteroidal anti-inflammatory drugs and a return to full activity as tolerated. To rule out other disorders, a comprehensive examination of the hips and knees should be performed as described next (Whitelaw & Schikler, 2010).

- *HIP EXAMINATION*:
  - ➤ During the physical examination, hold the hip in flexion with slight abduction and external rotation.
  - ➤ Examination of the individual with transient synovitis usually reveals mild restriction of motion, especially to abduction and internal rotation, although one-third of patients with transient synovitis demonstrate no limitation of motion.
  - ➤ The hip may be painful even with passive movement.
  - ➤ The hip may be tender to palpation.
  - ➤ The most sensitive test for transient synovitis is the log roll, in which the patient lies supine and the examiner gently rolls the involved

limb from side to side. This procedure may detect involuntary muscle guarding of one side when compared to the other side.

- *KNEE EXAMINATION*: The knee of the individual with transient synovitis may have decreased range of motion only as it includes hip motion. Any effusion or joint abnormality within the knee should suggest another disease process.

FRACTURES: These are common injuries in active children due to the plasticity of a child's bone. In children, bones heal faster because of the thicker and stronger fibrous periosteum that covers the surface of the bone. This fibrous membrane has a rich supply of blood vessels that supply oxygen and nutrients to the osteoblasts, thus increasing the rate of healing and remodeling. Common fractures in children include the *greenstick fracture*, which involves a bend on one side of the bone and a partial fracture on the other side (like breaking a green stick) (**Figure 12-53**). Another common fracture is a *Torus fracture*, or buckle fracture, which occurs if one side of the bone bends, raising a little buckle, without fracturing the other side.

JUVENILE IDIOPATHIC ARTHRITIS: This disorder includes autoimmune inflammatory diseases that affect joints and connective tissues. Diagnosis is based on history, physical examination, and criteria established by the

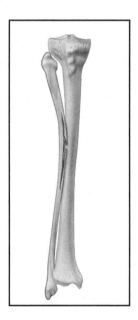

Figure 12-53 Greenstick Fracture

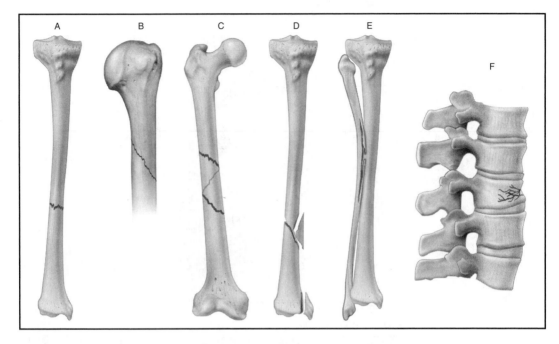

Figure 12-54 Typical Fractures: a. Transverse, b. Oblique, c. Spiral, d. Comminuted, e. Greenstick, f. Compression fracture

American College of Rheumatology, which include onset before 16 years of age, arthritis of at least 6 weeks' duration involving joint swelling or effusion, and two of the following: warmth, pain on motion, or limited range of motion (Edgerton & DuPlessis, 2000, p. 859; Potts, 2007). There are no specific laboratory tests for juvenile idiopathic arthritis because tests reflecting inflammation are nonspecific and can reflect other conditions causing inflammation.

SCOLIOSIS: This is defined as a lateral curvature of the spine. The highest risk for curve progression is during a growth spurt in puberty. Spinal deformities also include kyphosis (humpback), which is a convex curvature at the thoracic level of the spine, and lordosis, which is a concave curvature of the lumbar spine (**Figure 12-56**). Treatment is dependent upon the severity of the curvature and the age of the child. Standard assessment is based on evaluation with a scoliometer with a reading of greater or equal to 7 degree curve requiring referral. Treatment options include monitoring, bracing, and surgery.

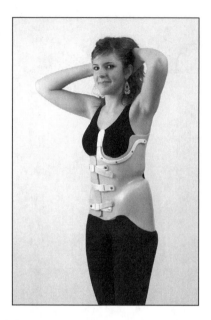

Figure 12-55 Scoliosis Brace

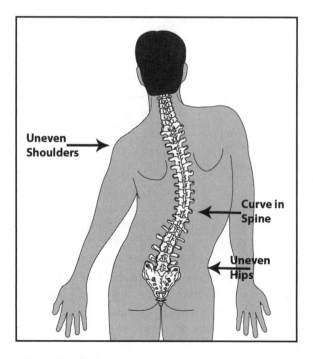

Figure 12-56 Signs of Scoliosis

TOE WALKING: This can be a variation of normal in children, referred to as idiopathic toe walking, particularly noted when a child begins to walk. If it persists past 18 months, pathologic causes should be ruled out such as cerebral palsy, muscular dystrophy, occult hydrocephalus (upper motor neuron signs), and intraspinal abnormality (cavus feet, unilateral involvement). A detailed birth history is critical.

NURSE MAID'S ELBOW: This is also known as subluxation of the radial head and is the most common elbow injury in children less than 5 years of age. It is associated with increased laxity of the ligaments, and occurs from tugging on a child's arm or lifting the child by grabbing the hand. "The mechanism of injury is a pull on the forearm when the elbow is extended and the forearm is pronated" (Green, 2002, p. 594). The child will favor that side by holding the arm by their side with the elbow slightly flexed and the forearm pronated. Treatment is to reduce the sublimation by placing your thumb over the radial head and supinate the forearm. A snap will be appreciated as the ligaments slip back into normal position and the radial head reduces in size.

> ## Red Flags

Osteomyelitis: This condition is characterized by infection of a bone with localized swelling, erythema, and tenderness over the involved area; fever may be present. Infection can initiate in the bone or spread to the bone secondary to trauma. This is a serious condition that requires aggressive treatment to prevent spread of infection.

Developmental dysplasia of the hip: This condition is characterized by abnormal development of the hip joint. Several disorders are included: dysplasia, subluxation, or complete dislocation of the femoral head out of the acetabulum. This disorder presents with positive Ortolani or Barlow sign. It is seen in infants during the first 3 months of life and requires immediate referral to an orthopedic surgeon for further evaluation and treatment.

Talipes equinovarus (clubfoot): This condition is present at birth and requires immediate referral to an orthopedist (**Figure 12-57**). It may have a genetic basis, be idiopathic, or be associated with spina bifida or neuromuscular disorders.

Torticollis: This is a condition that typically develops by two to four weeks of age and presents with the child who prefers to hold the head tilted to one side with limited range of motion. Involvement of children who have congenital muscular torticollis may have associated musculoskeletal anomalies, including hip

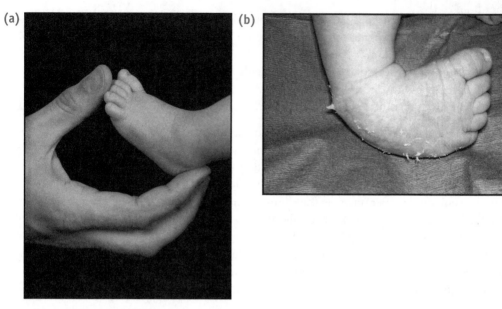

Figure 12-57 Normal vs. Congenital Clubfoot

dysplasia, metatarsus, adductus, talipes equinovarus and C1 and C2 sublixation (Macias, 2009).

Septic arthritis: This is caused by bacterial infection in the synovial fluid and is a medical emergency in order to prevent damage to the joint.

Gower's sign: This is a medical sign classically seen in muscular dystrophy that describes a child that has to use his or hands and arms to 'walk up' his own body from a squatting position. This is due to weakness of the proximal muscles, primarily those of the lower limbs. Observation of this behavior requires referral to a specialist.

Write-Up of the Musculoskeletal Exam

INFANTS: Feet/hands appear normal, no abnormalities of digits/toes, hips: negative Ortalani, and Barlow, equal leg lengths, thigh creases symmetric; spine straight-no tufts/dimples, full range of motion (ROM) of all extremities, no swelling, or erythema of joints.

TODDLER: Full ROM of all extremities, no swelling, erythema, or deformities of joints, wide stance gait to waddle gait, normal lumbar lordosis in spine, reasonable strength of upper and lower muscle groups with symmetrical appearance.

SCHOOL-AGE AND ADOLESCENT: Temporomandibular joint without click or crepitation, neck full ROM, vertebral column without deformity or curvature in both upright and bending position, no tenderness, full extension, lateral bending, and rotation, iliac crests of equal height and shoulders equal height. Arms and legs symmetric, full ROM, without pain. Muscle strength able to maintain flexion against resistance. Gait smooth with symmetric arm swing.

Case Study: Girl with Hip Pain

Kelly, a 6 year old came to your office with a chief complaint of severe pain in her right hip and leg for the past 24 hours. Her father states" that she refuses to walk and insists that I carry her." He further tells you that Kelly woke up experiencing severe pain in her right hip and upper leg, which she describes as "aching." She rated her pain as a 9 on a visual analog scale of 1–10 (with 1 being the lowest and 10 the highest). Kelly denied any recent changes in weight and appetite and denied having fatigue or chills. Her medical history was noncontributory, except for an upper respiratory infection approximately 9 days ago that resolved spontaneously without antibiotics.

On examination, you observe the following:

- Kelly was alert, tearful, but cooperative upon examination.
- Vital Signs: within normal limits (WNL)
- Height & Weight: 75%
- Integument, Head, Eyes, Ears, Nose, Throat (HEENT), Resp, Card, Abd: all WNL
- Musculoskeletal: right hip revealed the hip held in flexion, abduction, and external rotation
- Left hip: full range of motion
- Knees: full range of motion for flexion and extension
- Ankles: full range of motion with dorsiflexion, plantar flexion, and inversion and eversion.

Questions
1. What is the differential diagnosis of a painful limp in children?
2. What laboratory and or radiographic tests would you order for this child?
3. What is your diagnosis?
4. What management would you recommend for Kelly?

Answers

1. The differential diagnosis of a painful limp includes trauma, slipped capital femoral epiphysis, toxic synovitis, osteomyelitis, and septic arthritis.
2. Laboratory tests that are indicated are complete blood count and erythrocyte sedimentation rate (or c-reactive protein) to rule out systemic disease or infection. Hip radiographs may be useful in determining the etiology of the pain. In some cases where it is difficult to determine toxic from septic arthritis, aspiration of the hip joint may be necessary.
3. The diagnosis is transient synovitis, which is an acute inflammation of the hip.
4. The symptoms of transient synovitis are generally self-limiting and resolve within 3-5 days. Management includes bed rest, anti inflammatories and or analgesics and restricting activity as necessary. Follow-up with the primary care provider is necessary to ensure symptoms are resolving.

References

Ball, J., Bindler, R., & Cowen, K. (2010). *Child health nursing* (2nd ed.). Upper Saddle River, NJ: Pearson.

Bickley, L. (2003). *Bates' guide to physical examination and history taking* (8th ed.). New York: Lippincott Williams & Wilkins.

Chamley, C. A., Carson, P. Randall, D. & Sandwell, M. (2005). Developmental anatomy and physiology of children, St. Louis, MO: Elsevier. Taken from Ball, Bindler, Cowen, *Child Health Nursing*, 2010, Pearson.

Durtz, J. (2010). The pediatric physical examination: Back, extremities, nervous system, skin, lymph nodes. Retrieved from http://www.uptodate.com/

Edgerton, E., & DuPlessis, H. (2000). Juvenile rheumatoid arthritis. In C. Berkowitz (Ed.), *Pediatrics: A primary care approach* (2nd ed.; pp. 549–552). Philadelphia: Saunders.

Graham, M. V., & Uphold, C. R. (2003). *Clinical guidelines in child health* (3rd ed.). Gainesville, FL: Barmarrae Books.

Green, W. B. (2002). *Essentials of musculoskeletal care* (2nd ed.). Rosemont, IL: American Academy of Orthopaedic Surgeons.

Hergenroeder, A.C. (2004). Causes of knee pain in the young athlete. Retrieved from http://www.uptodate.com

Jarvis, C. (2008). *Physical examination and health assessment* (5th ed.). St. Louis, MO: Elsevier.

Macias, C. & Vanthaya, G. (2009). Congenital muscular torticollis. Retrieved from http://www.UpToDate.com

Marieb, E. (1995). *Human anatomy and physiology* (3rd ed.). Redwood City, CA: Benjamin/Cummings Publishing Company.

Potts, N., & Mandleco, B. (2007). *Pediatraic nursing* (2nd ed.). Victoria, Australia: Thomson, Delmar Learning.

Whitelaw, C. C., & Schikler, K. N. (2002). Transient synovitis. In: Myones BL (ed). eMedicine: Pediatrics.

Resources

Burns, C., Dunn, A., Brady, M., Starr, N., & Blosser, C. (2004). *Pediatric primary care: A handbook for nurse practitioners* (3rd ed.). St. Louis, MO: Saunders.

Estes, M. (2006). *Health assessment and physical examination* (3rd ed.). Albany, NY: Delmar Publishers.

Hansen, M. (1998). *Pathophysiology: Foundations of disease and clinical intervention*. Philadelphia: Saunders.

Mayo Clinic. (n.d.). Scoliosis. Retrieved July 16, 2010, from www.mayoclinic.org/scoliosis/diasgnosis.html

Seidel, H. M., Ball, J. W., Dains, J. E., & Benedict, G. W. (1999). *Mosby's guide to physical examination* (4th ed.). St. Louis, MO: Mosby.

Slcheri, S.A. (2010). Clinical features: Evaluation and diagnosis of adolescent idiopathic scolosis. Retrieved from http://www.UpToDate.com

Tortora, G. J., & Grabvowski, S. R. (2003). *Principles of anatomy and physiology* (10th ed.). New York: Wiley.

Examination of the Central Nervous System

Anatomy and Physiology

The nervous system is the primary communicating center for the body. It is divided into two main parts: the central nervous system (CNS), which includes the brain and spinal cord, and the peripheral nervous system, which is outside of the CNS and includes 12 pairs of cranial nerves, 31 pairs of spinal nerves, and all of their branches.

The brain is protected by the skull, the meninges, and cerebrospinal fluid, which act as a cushion. It is further protected from harmful substances in the blood by the blood–brain barrier.

The meninges are composed of three layers of connective tissue that cover and protect the CNS: the dura mater, arachnoid mater, and pia mater.

- The *DURA MATER* is the thick, tough, outermost layer.
- The *ARACHNOID MATER* is the middle layer that forms a loose covering over the brain. Beneath the arachnoid mater is the sub-arachnoid space where cerebrospinal fluid is circulated.
- The *PIA MATER* is a thin, vascular layer composed of delicate connective tissue that covers convolutions of the brain.

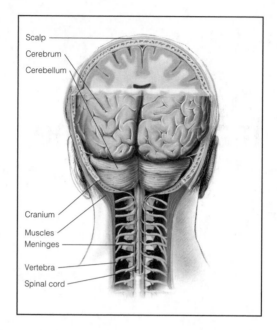

Figure 13-1(a)   Brain and Spinal Cord

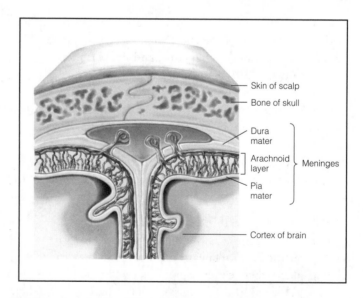

Figure 13-1(b)   Cross Sectional View of Brain and Meningeal Layers

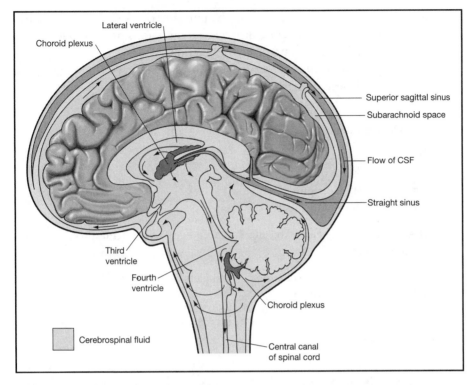

Figure 13-1(c) Sagittal View of the Brain

Meningitis, or inflammation of the meninges, is a serious brain infection, either bacterial or viral, that can spread into tissue of the CNS. Encephalitis is an acute infection of the CNS that involves inflammation of the brain itself.

The peripheral nervous system carries impulses to the brain and away from the brain. It carries impulses to the brain from the skin and skeletal muscles via the *sensory*, or *afferent*, division. The *motor*, or *efferent*, division transmits impulses away from the CNS to muscles and glands, resulting in a motor response or glandular secretion. This efferent part of the CNS is further divided into the autonomic nervous system, which consists of two branches—the *sympathetic* and *parasympathetic*. The sympathetic nervous system sends impulses from the CNS to visceral effectors such as cardiac muscle, smooth muscle, and glandular epithelium. This system is beyond conscious control and is therefore viewed as involuntary. It is a catabolic system that responds to the "fight-or-flight response" by shunting blood to the heart and muscles, and dilating the pupils in times of stress. The parasympathetic nervous system conserves energy and is an anabolic system that slows the heart rate and digestive functions.

The following outline describes the differences between sympathetic functions and parasympathetic functions.

The sympathetic nervous system affects body structures as follows:

EYE: Dilates the pupil

GLANDS:
- *LACRIMAL*: No significant effect
- *SALIVARY*: No significant effect
- *SWEAT*: Stimulates secretion

HEART: Increases heart rate, increases myocardial contractility, increases blood pressure

BLOOD VESSELS: Dilates cardiac and skeletal blood vessels, constricts skin and digestive blood vessels

LUNGS: Increases respiratory rate, increases respiratory depth, promotes bronchial dilation

GASTROINTESTINAL TRACT: Inhibits motility, decreases gastric secretions, increases glycogenolysis, decreases insulin production, promotes sphincter contraction

ADRENAL GLAND: Stimulates secretion of adrenaline

GENITOURINARY TRACT: Decreases urine output, decreases renal blood flow

The parasympathetic nervous system affects body structures as follows:

EYE: Contracts the pupil and contracts the ciliary muscle for accommodation

GLANDS:
- *LACRIMAL*: Stimulates secretion
- *SALIVARY*: Stimulates secretion
- *SWEAT*: No significant effect

HEART: Decreases heart rate, decreases myocardial contractility

BLOOD VESSELS: No significant effect

LUNGS: Constricts bronchial tubes, stimulates bronchial gland secretion

GASTROINTESTINAL TRACT: stimulates motility, increases gastric secretion, promotes sphincter dilation

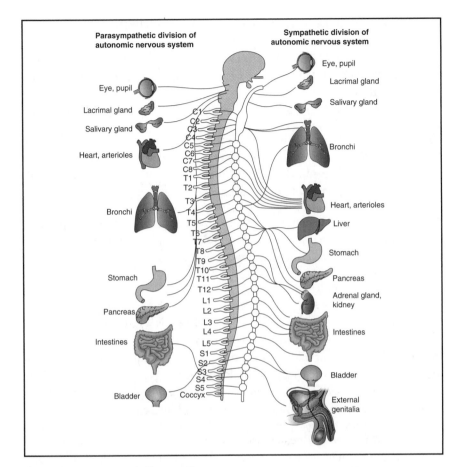

Figure 13-2 Autonomic Nervous System

Source: This article was published in *Pathophysiology: Foundations of Disease and Clinical Intervention,* 1st edition, Hansen. Autonomic nervous system, page 624. Copyright Saunders (1998).

ADRENAL GLAND: No significant effect

GENITOURINARY TRACT: No significant effect

Anatomic Components of the CNS

The *CEREBRUM* controls a human's highest functioning, which includes memory, reasoning, sensation, communication, intellectual processing, and voluntary movements, all associated with conscious behavior. The cerebrum is divided into the left and right hemispheres, and each hemisphere is divided into four lobes—the *frontal, parietal, temporal,* and *occipital.*

- The *FRONTAL LOBE* is the site of behavior, intellectual function, personality, and emotion.
- The *PARIETAL LOBE* is the primary site for the somatic sensory area.
- The *TEMPORAL LOBE* is the site for hearing, memory, and speech perception.
- The *OCCIPITAL LOBE* is the primary site for vision and visual perception.

The *BROCA AREA*, which mediates motor speech, is located within the frontal lobe. When there is damage to this area, expressive aphasia results. The child can understand language spoken to him or her but cannot speak or produce appropriate sounds in response.

The *WERNICKE AREA* is another speech area associated with language comprehension. It is located in the temporal lobe. A lesion in this area results in receptive aphasia. The child hears what is said but is not able to interpret the meaning of the words.

The *CEREBRAL CORTEX* is referred to as the gray matter of the brain because of its color. The interior part of the brain is white due to the myelin sheath that insulates the axon of the nerves. The gray matter is composed of neurons made up of axons and dendrites. On the surface are *gyri*, which are elevated ridges of tissue; grooves between the gyri are called *sulci*. The two hemispheres are connected internally by the *corpus callosum*, a body of white matter composed of axons that extend into each hemisphere.

The *BASAL GANGLIA* are located deep within the cerebral cortex and function as the extrapyramidal system that receives input from the cerebral cortex and relays impulses that regulate initiation and termination of movements.

The *CEREBELLUM* is a cauliflower-shaped structure located under the occipital lobe. It processes motor coordination such as skeletal muscle contraction needed for activities such as swimming, riding a bicycle, or playing the piano. Cerebellar activity occurs subconsciously in control of voluntary movements, equilibrium, and muscle tone.

The *DIENCEPHALON* is located at the midline of the brain above the brainstem. It is composed of the thalamus, hypothalamus, optic tracts and optic chiasma, infundibulum, third ventricle, mammillary bodies, posterior pituitary gland, and pineal gland.

The *BRAINSTEM* is the pathway between the cerebrum and the spinal cord. It is composed of the midbrain, pons, and medulla oblongata. The reticular activating system is located in the brainstem and mediates control of respiratory, cardiovascular, and vegetative functions. The midbrain, which sits

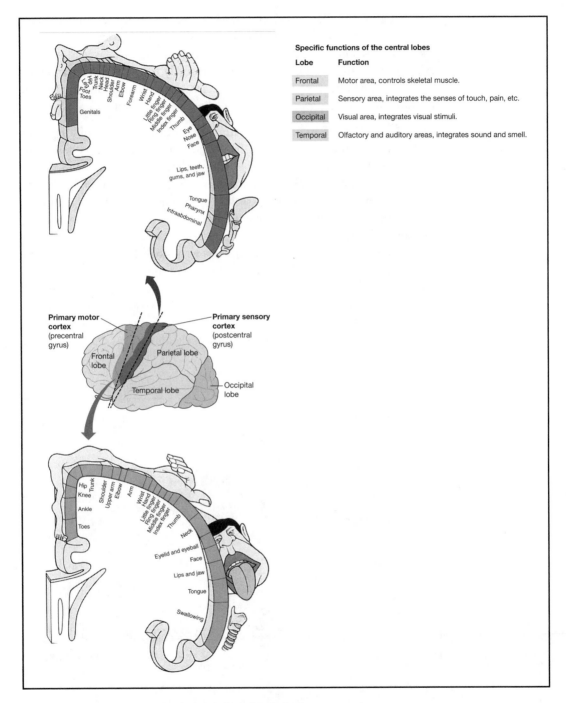

Specific functions of the central lobes

Lobe	Function
Frontal	Motor area, controls skeletal muscle.
Parietal	Sensory area, integrates the senses of touch, pain, etc.
Occipital	Visual area, integrates visual stimuli.
Temporal	Olfactory and auditory areas, integrates sound and smell.

Figure 13-3   Homunculus—Cortical Mapping of Body Surfaces

directly below the diencephalon, houses the nuclei of the 12 cranial nerves in locations between the midbrain, pons, and medulla oblongata. The pons sits below the midbrain and contains the ascending and descending fiber tracts. The medulla oblongata is located directly below the pons and contains ascending and descending fiber tracts, which control vital autonomic functions such as respiration, heart rate, and gastrointestinal function.

The *SPINAL CORD* is basically a continuation of the medulla oblongata at the area of the foramen magnum. It functions as the main relay center for the ascending and descending fiber tracts. The descending tracts (pyramidal and extrapyramidal) carry motor impulses away from the brain. The ascending tracts (dorsal columns or spinothalamic) carry sensory impulses to the brain. Anatomy of the spinal cord, when viewed from a cross-section, resembles a butterfly, with gray matter in the center composed of axons and dendrites and unmyelinated fibers. It is surrounded by white matter, the myelinated nerve fibers. The posterior portion of this butterfly is referred to as the dorsal horn, and the anterior portion is the ventral horn. The dorsal horn contains afferent (sensory) neurons that receive and transmit sensory signals from the afferent fibers in the spinal cord. The ventral horn contains efferent (motor) neurons, which innervate skeletal muscles, carrying signals

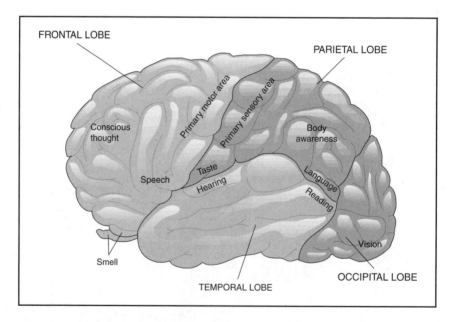

Figure 13-4(a)   Cerebral Cortex

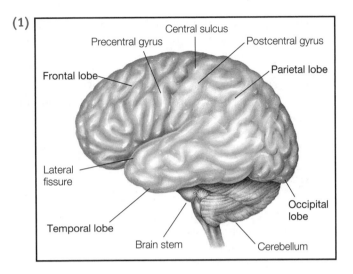

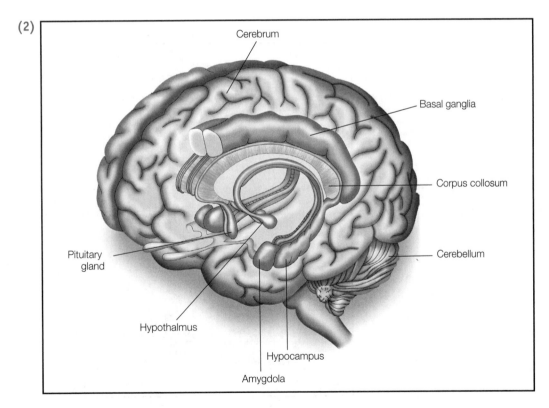

Figure 13-4(b) Anatomy of the Brain

from the brain and the spinal cord. It serves as a relay center between the basal ganglia and the cerebellum. See **Figure 13-5**.

The *CRANIAL NERVES* are composed of 12 peripheral nerves, each possessing motor or sensory function. The cranial nerves and their nuclei arise from the brainstem. The following is a description of the cranial nerves and their functions:

- *OLFACTORY (CRANIAL NERVE [CN] I)*: Smell
- *OPTIC (CN II)*: Visual acuity, visual fields (assessed by fundoscopic examination)
- *OCULOMOTOR (CN III)*: Cardinal fields of gaze, equal ocular movement (EOM), eyelid elevation, pupil reaction (assessed by doll's eyes phenomenon test)
- *TROCHLEAR (CN IV)*: EOM
- *TRIGEMINAL (CN V)*:
  - ➤ Motor: Strength of temporalis and masseter muscles

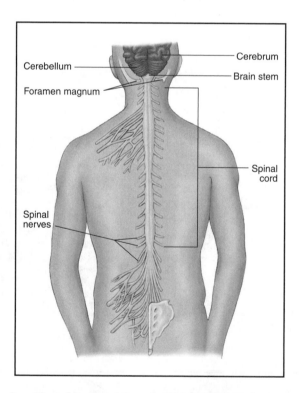

Figure 13-5 Base View of Brain and Cross-Section of Spinal Cord

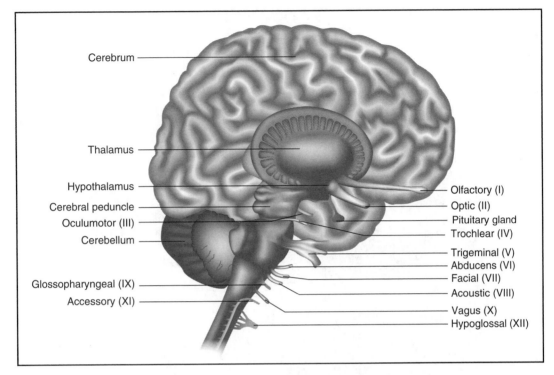

Figure 13-6(a)   Structures of the Diencephalon and Location of the Cranial Nerve Roots

Source: This article was published in *Advanced Neurological and Neurosurgical Nursing*, Rudy. Structures of the diencephalon and location of the cranial nerve roots, page 760. Copyright Mosby (1984).

> ➤ Sensory: Light touch, superficial pain and temperature to face, corneal reflex
- *ABDUCENS (CN VI)*: EOM
- *FACIAL (CN VII)*:
  > ➤ Motor: Facial movements
  > ➤ Sensory: Taste in the anterior two-thirds of the tongue
  > ➤ Parasympathetic: Tears and saliva secretion
- *ACOUSTIC (CN VIII)*:
  > ➤ Cochlear: Gross hearing (assessed by Weber and Rinne tests)
  > ➤ Vestibular: Vertigo, equilibrium, nystagmus
- *GLOSSOPHARYNGEAL AND VAGUS (CN IX AND X)*:
  > ➤ Motor: Soft palate and uvula movement, gag reflex, swallowing, guttural and palatal sounds as the child says 'ahhh'
  > ➤ Sensory: Taste in the posterior one-third of the tongue

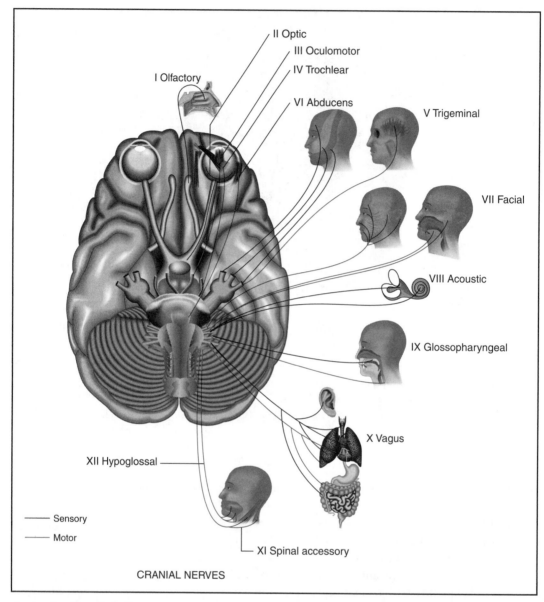

Figure 13-6(b) Cranial Nerves

Source: This article was published in *Physical Examination and Health Assessment,* 5th edition, Jarvis. Cranial nerves. Copyright Saunders (2007).

- *SPINAL ACCESSORY (CN XI)*: Movement of sternocleidomastoid and trapeziums muscles
- *HYPOGLOSSAL (CN XII)*: Tongue movement, lingual sounds

A mnemonic for remembering the names of the cranial nerves is, "**O**n **O**ld **O**lympus' **T**owering **T**ops, **A** **F**inn **A**nd **G**erman **V**iewed **S**ome **H**ops," in which the first letter of each word represents, in order, the cranial nerves (olfactory, optic, oculomotor, trochlear, trigeminal, abducens, facial, acoustic, glossopharyngeal, vagus, spinal accessory, hypoglossal).

Motor and Sensory Pathways of the CNS

Motor Pathways

The CNS is composed of three motor pathways: the corticospinal (or pyramidal) tract, the extrapyramidal tract, and the cerebellum.

The *pyramidal tract* is so named because of the pyramidal shape of the cells located in the motor cortex. The motor nerve fibers originate in the motor cortex in the cerebrum and migrate through the midbrain, pons, and medulla. At the level of the medulla, they cross over, or decussate, to the opposite side and travel down the lateral column of the spinal cord, called the anterior corticospinal tract. Fibers from this tract synapse in the anterior horn at all levels before they leave the spinal cord. Motor neurons that synapse above the anterior horn or above the corticospinal tract are referred to as the upper motor neurons and are located totally in the CNS. Motor neurons that synapse in the anterior horn connect with the corticospinal tract and innervate skeletal muscles that are responsible for voluntary and purposeful movements.

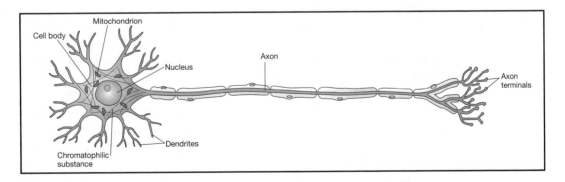

Figure 13-7   Neuron

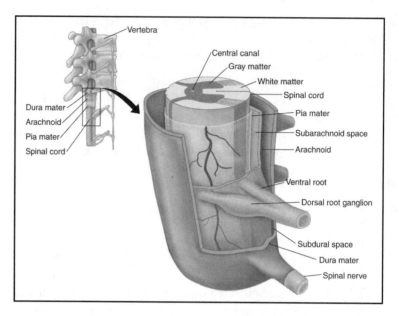

Figure 13-8 Spinal Cord and Protective Layer

The *extrapyramidal tract* includes all of the motor neurons located in the motor cortex, basal ganglia, brainstem, and spinal cord that are outside of the pyramidal tract. This more primitive or lower motor tract is referred to as the *extra*pyramidal tract because it is outside of the pyramidal tract. This tract is responsible for maintaining muscle tone and gross automatic movements such as running and walking.

Understanding of the upper and lower motor neurons is complex. To help clarify, the upper motor neurons are completely located within the cerebrum or the CNS. These neurons send impulses from motor areas of the cerebral cortex to the lower motor neurons in the anterior horn cells of the spinal cord. An example of an upper motor neuron disease in children is cerebral palsy, in which there is damage such as anoxia to the upper motor neurons often located along the motor strip. Damage to this area results in various types of spasticity, affecting motor control from walking to talking.

The lower motor neurons are located within the anterior gray matter of the spinal cord and are the direct pathway to innervations of muscles. These neurons are part of the peripheral nervous system. Examples are cranial nerves and spinal nerves. Diseases associated with lower motor

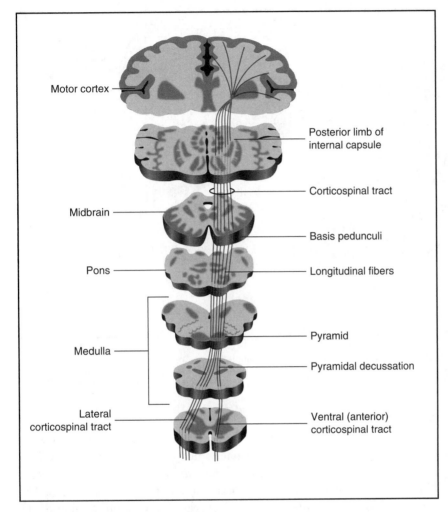

Figure 13-9   Tracts of the Spinal Cord

Source: This article was published in *Mosby's Guide to Physical Examination*, 6th edition, Seidel, Ball, Dains, and Benedict. Tracts of the spinal cord, page 762. Copyright Elsevier (2006).

neurons are spinal cord lesions and poliomyelitis. Damage to this area can affect the respiratory center, which ultimately leaves the child dependent upon a respirator.

The *cerebellar system* receives impulses on a subconscious level regarding body position and equilibrium, and coordination of movement. The cerebellum integrates information from the cortex as it is relayed to lower motor neurons in the spinal cord.

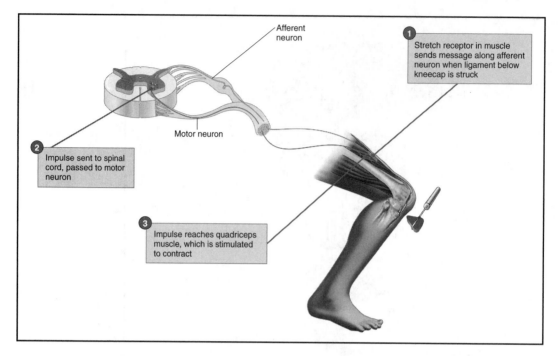

Afferent neuron

1 Stretch receptor in muscle sends message along afferent neuron when ligament below kneecap is struck

Motor neuron

2 Impulse sent to spinal cord, passed to motor neuron

3 Impulse reaches quadriceps muscle, which is stimulated to contract

Figure 13-10 Cross Sectional View of Spinal Cord Showing Simple Reflex Arc

Sensory Pathways

The sensory pathways include the spinothalamic tracts and the posterior column, which are part of the peripheral nervous system (PNS). The PNS consists of afferent fibers that carry messages to the CNS and efferent fibers that send messages into the periphery, or outside of the CNS. The process starts with the afferent nerve fiber receiving an impulse, entering the spinal cord through the dorsal roots. Once in the spinal cord, the impulse travels up the spinothalamic tracts, where it decussates to the opposite side. There, the impulse travels up the spinothalamic tract to the CNS. Impulses such as temperature are transmitted via this tract to the sensory area of the cerebral cortex.

The posterior column carries sensory sensations of vibration, position sense, and touch sensation up to the medulla where it synapses. It is at this point that the neurons decussate to the opposite side of the medulla, and the impulse is transmitted to the sensory cortex of the CNS.

When assessing deep tendon reflexes, activation of the reflex arc, such as the patellar reflex, involves a monosynaptic reflex involving two neurons—one afferent and one efferent (Estes, 2006, p. 649). By using a reflex hammer and tapping a tendon, you are actually stretching the muscle spindles, which in turn stimulates the sensory afferent nerve. The sensory afferent fibers then carry the message from the receptor through to the dorsal root of the spinal cord. The impulse synapses with the motor neuron in the anterior horn. The motor efferent fibers then leave via the ventral root of the horn and travel to the muscle, ultimately stimulating a muscle contraction (Jarvis, 2008, p. 660).

There are four types of reflexes:

- Deep tendon reflexes such as the patellar
- Superficial reflexes such as the corneal
- Visceral reflexes such as pupillary constriction or accommodation in response to light
- Pathologic reflexes such as the Babinski

Dermal segmentation is cutaneous distribution of the spinal nerves. It comes into clinical application when assessing, for example, a child with herpes zoster (shingles). A dermatome is a circumscribed area of skin that is innervated through a particular spinal nerve. Many times, there is overlap of the spinal nerves so that if one is severed, another one can take over and transmit the necessary signal.

- Thumb, middle finger, and fifth finger: spinal nerves C6, C7, and C8
- Axilla spinal nerve: T1
- Nipple spinal nerve: T4
- Umbilicus spinal nerve: T10
- Groin spinal nerve: L1
- Knee dermatome: L4

Development of the CNS

During development of the brain and spinal cord, the neural plate evolves into the neural groove and neural folds, and closure of the neural tube is completed by 28 days of gestation. Closure of this tube at the appropriate time in utero is important because insult during development such as trauma, teratogens, or infection can result in neural tube defects such a myelodysplasia or spina bifida.

Between 2 and 4 months of gestation, neuronal proliferation occurs, which is followed by migration at 3 to 5 months. By the fifth month of gestation, the gyri formation starts, with the major fissures being formed at this time. Neuronal organization and myelination starts in the third trimester and are the major processes that account for maturation and brain growth. By 36 weeks of gestation, neuronal proliferation, which includes

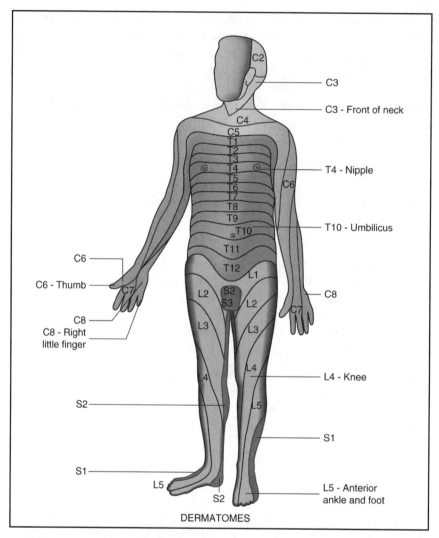

Figure 13-11 Dermatomes

Source: This article was published in *Physical Examination and Health Assessment*, 5th edition, Jarvis. Dermatomes, page 622. Copyright Saunders (2007).

development of dendritic and axonal processes and their connections, is nearly complete.

The next step in the developmental process in brain maturation is myelination. It begins early in the third trimester, with rapid development occurring in the first 2 years of life. This process follows a specific time course and pattern, which is reflected in the acquisition of neurodevelopmental milestones. Myelination occurs early for motor-sensory roots, special senses, and the brainstem, which are necessary for reflex behavior and survival.

The corticospinal tract starts to myelinate at 36 weeks of gestation and is completed by 2 years of age. Myelination of the corticospinal tract begins at the proximal portion of the axon, and the shortest axons are the first to myelinate. Next, the axons for the upper extremities and the trunk myelinate. The axons for the lower extremities, which are the longest axons, are the last to myelinate, with the process being completed by 24 months of age. This myelination pattern correlates with the progressive head-to-toe acquisition of developmental milestones.

At birth, the child's brain and spinal cord are not fully matured. The bones of the skull are not fused and are separated by fontanelles, which are connective bands of tissue that allow for delivery through the birth canal, as well as continued growth of the brain. The anterior fontanelle does not completely fuse until approximately 18 to 24 months of age.

One of the major differences between the spinal cord of the child and that of the adult is found in the facets of the vertebral bodies: In children, they are not vertically aligned, as they are in adults, but are wedge shaped, which allows for more movement in cases of injury. Adult characteristics of the spinal cord are not fully attained until the child is 8 to 9 years of age, when the vertebral bodies lose their wedge shape and the facets become more vertically aligned (Dogan et al., as cited in Ball, Binder, Cowen, 2010).

Because myelination is not complete in the neonate, primitive reflexes are present in the newborn and infant. This developmental process occurs in a cephalocaudal direction as myelination progresses and integration of the primitive reflexes occurs. This is demonstrated through the acquisition of increasing coordination in both fine and gross motor skills.

The following is a list of primitive reflexes and their normal findings (Jarvis, 2008; Ball, 2007).

MORO: Startle the infant with a sudden noise or change in position. The arms extend and the fingers form a C as they spread. The arms slowly move together as in a hug. This is present at birth and starts to decrease by four months of age, disappearing by six months of age.

PALMAR GRASP: Place finger across the infant's palm along the ulnar side noting a tight grasp of the baby's fingers. This is present at birth and disappears around three to four months of age.

PLANTAR GRASP: Place your finger across the foot at the base of the toes. The toes normally curl tightly as if gripping the finger. This is present at

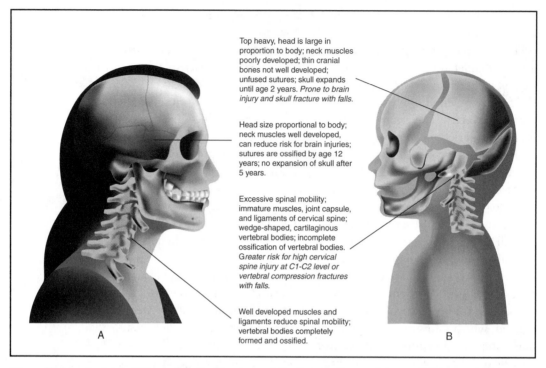

Figure 13-12 Anatomic Difference in the Structures of the Nervous System Between Children and Adults

Source: Ball, Jane W.; Bindler, Ruth C.; Cowen, Kay J., *Child Health Nursing: Partnering With Children and Families*, 2nd ©2010. Printed and Electronically reproduced by permission of Pearson Education, Inc., Upper Saddle River, New Jersey.

birth and disappears at around eight months of age, when the baby is staring to stand.

PLACING: Hold the infant upright under the arms and touch the top or dorsal side of one foot to the underside of the table. The infant normally lifts the foot, as if to step up onto the surface. This presents four to five days after birth and disappears around four to eight weeks of age.

STEPPING: Hold the infant upright under the arms and touch the bottom of the feet on the surface of the table. The feet lift in an alternating pattern as if to walk. This is present at birth and disappears between four and eight weeks of age.

TONIC NECK REFLEX (TNR): Place the infant in a supine position and turn the head to one side with the chin over the shoulder. Note ipsilateral extension of the arm and leg. Repeat by turning the head to the opposite side again noting ipsilateral extension of the arm and leg into a fencing position. This appears about two months of age and decreases by four months of age and then disappears by six months. This reflex must become integrated in order for the baby to turn over.

SUCKING REFLEX: Place a gloved little finger in the infant's mouth. Note the strong suckling reflex. This reflex is present at birth and disappears at ten to twelve months.

ROOTING REFLEX: Brush the infant's check near the mouth. The infant should turn the head toward that side and open the mouth. This appears at birth and disappears at 3–4 months.

BABINSKI REFLEX: Stroke your finger up the lateral edge and across the ball of the infant's foot. The infant's toes should fan out (positive Babinski reflex.) This reflex is presents at birth and disappears (change to adult response by 24 months of age). (Jarvis, 2008; Ball, 2007).

Assessment Considerations: Subjective Information

The following sections present considerations for assessment of the CNS.

Prenatal History

Prenatal history is important, as it may affect the infant's neurologic development.

- Did the mother have any health problems during her pregnancy? Did she have any infections or illnesses, exposure to TORCH viruses (i.e., toxoplasmosis, other viruses, rubella, Cytomegalovirus, and herpes simplex), toxemia, bleeding, history of trauma, persistent vomiting, or excessive weight gain or loss?
- Does the mother have a history of diabetes, hypertension, or other chronic illnesses?
- Did the mother take any medications during her pregnancy, including prenatal vitamins, prescribed medications, herbal remedies, and over-the-counter medications?
- Did the mother take folic acid prior to becoming pregnant?
- Did the mother drink alcohol during her pregnancy? If so, how much? Did she use street drugs? If so, what was the route of administration and the frequency?
- Did the mother smoke cigarettes? If so, how many per day and for how long?

Infants

- What is the baby's birth history, including Apgar scores and gestational age? Was the baby term or premature? What was the birth weight and presentation? Were instruments used? Was there prolonged or precipitated labor? Fetal distress?
- Did the mother receive the baby in the delivery room to hold right after delivery?
- Did the baby breathe immediately? Was there difficulty with the baby's respiratory status? Was oxygen needed? Were resuscitative efforts needed? Was the baby on a ventilator?
- Were there any congenital anomalies or defects?
- Did the baby spend any time in the special care nursery?
- Were mother and baby discharged together from the hospital?
- Did the baby have any problems when he or she came home from the hospital, such as infections, irritability, seizures, or poor coordination with sucking and swallowing?
- Did the baby have a history of neonatal jaundice?
- Did the baby gain weight as expected?
- Was the parent told what to expect in regard to the baby's growth, including height, weight, and head circumference?

Toddlers, School-Age Children, and Adolescents

- Did the child attain developmental milestones at the appropriate age, such as smiling, head control, eye contact, sitting, crawling, and walking?
- How is this child's development in comparison to siblings or playmates?
- At what age did the child start to speak, put two words together, and speak in sentences?
- Does the child have a history of loss of previously attained developmental milestones?
- Did the child receive early intervention services?
- How is the child doing in school? Does the child have any learning problems or difficulty with fine and gross motor skills? If so, has the child had an IEP (individual educational plan)?
- What is the child's behavior like? Does the child have temper tantrums, hyperactivity, or limited attention span? How does the child adjust to new situations? How does the child get along with other children?
- Does the child have a history of migraine headaches, seizures, tics, or other neurologic disorders?

Family History

- Is there a family history of genetic disorders such as Huntington chorea, muscular dystrophy, Tay-Sachs disease, neurofibromatosis, or epilepsy?
- Is there a history of consanguinity?
- Is there a history of learning disorders or mental retardation?
- Is there is history of psychiatric disorders such as bipolar disorder?
- Is there a history of migraine headaches?

Review of Systems

Review of systems pertinent to the CNS can include almost all systems because all bodily systems are controlled by some part of the CNS.

SKIN: Specific neurocutaneous lesions are associated with neurologic disorders such as café au lait spots associated with neurofibromatosis, hypopigmented ash leaf configuration associated with tuberous sclerosis, and Sturge-Weber disease associated with a port-wine stain on the child's face.

HEAD: Consider head circumference and shape, as well as head control in the infant, head injury with loss of consciousness, seizures, headaches, facial asymmetry associated with the trigeminal nerve (CN V). Low-set ears are associated with cognitive impairment.

EYES: Consider new onset of nystagmus, sudden changes in visual acuity or oculomotor movements associated with the oculomotor, trochlear, and abducens nerves (CNs III, IV, VI, respectively). The facial nerve (CN VII) may be affected, with partial to complete facial paralysis, smoothing of the brow, inability to close one eye, flat nasolabial fold, and drooping of the mouth ipsilateral to the lesion. History of a cherry-red spot in the ocular fundus is associated with metabolic neurodegenerative diseases such as Tay-Sachs disease and Niemann-Pick disease, to name just two.

NOSE: Consider loss of smell associated with the olfactory nerve (CN I).

EARS: Consider hearing loss associated with the acoustic or vestibulo-cochlear nerve (CN VIII).

MOUTH AND THROAT: Consider lack of coordination in swallowing and sucking associated with the glossopharyngeal and vagus nerves (CNs IX and X, respectively).

GENITALIA: Consider developmental changes associated with the increase or decrease in stimulation of the pituitary gland.

DEVELOPMENT: Developmental history is particularly important regarding milestones, language, gross motor and fine motor skills, and social and cognitive development. Delay in developmental milestones may be associated with abnormal development of the CNS.

Assessment Considerations: Objective Information

The nervous system has great influence on development; therefore, assessment of the CNS requires a detailed history and comprehensive physical examination. When performing a neurologic exam on a child, the overall goal includes obtaining neurodevelopmental milestones. They are a key component, as they are a reflection of the maturation of the child's nervous system. Subtle indicators of underlying neurologic disease may present with abnormal or unusual patterns of acquisition of developmental milestones. Determining if a neurologic disorder exists, and where in the nervous system it is located, is a major goal when performing a neurologic exam. Examination of the CNS starts with an overall assessment of the child, observing for coordination, alertness, and muscle tone, and noting any clumsiness or weakness.

Cerebral function is tested first, followed by the cranial nerves, motor function, sensory function, and deep tendon reflexes. Much is learned about the child's cerebral function and/or mental status through observation. Observing as the child plays, explores a new environment, and examines and plays with new toys can be very informative about the child's fine and gross motor skills, and ability to process new information. Further evaluation of behavior and cognitive processing is based on the child's judgment, speech and language skills, ability to interact with others, memory and general knowledge base, and school performance. Many neurologic disorders are pervasive in that they affect not only the child's ability to process and learn, but can also affect both motor and sensory pathways, leading to interruption in appropriate stimulation.

In testing the CNS, there are minimally intrusive procedures such as the ear and throat exam, although the neurologic exam takes time and precision with an alertness toward neurologic function and maturational development. To conduct a comprehensive exam, you need full cooperation from the child in order to evaluate the mental status, the cranial nerves, fine and gross motor functioning, cerebellar functioning, and deep tendon reflexes. The child's comfort with the provider and setting allows you to *seize the opportunity* necessary to obtain the best outcomes.

Unique aspects of the neurologic examination in the child are determined by the age of the child. The CNS examination in the infant is based on assessment and integration of infant reflexes, gross and fine motor development, and deep tendon reflexes, as well as integration of developmental milestones. There is much growth during the first year of life, when developmental milestones are attained. The infant's motor system is initially dependent upon the brainstem and the spinal cord; as the cerebral hemispheres mature, development gradually is influenced by the progressing myelination of the cerebral cortex. Awareness of feeding and nap times in conjunction with the child's ability to maintain an alert and responsive state is necessary to elicit age-appropriate responses during the exam. Further neurologic evaluation of the newborn, ages birth to 3 months, is reviewed in Chapter 4.

The following is a review of the cranial nerves specifically adapted to the infant, ages 4 to 12 months (Bickley, 2003, p. 728):

- *CN I* (olfactory): Assessment of smell is generally not performed in the infant.
- *CN II* (visual acuity): The infant should be able to maintain brief eye contact and should track your face in a horizontal and vertical plane. From birth to 2 months of age, the infant follows a moving object with his or her eyes. From 3 to 5 months of age, the infant moves his or her head to track a moving object.
- *CN III* (oculomotor): Assess the infant's optic blink reflex by initially darkening the room, then use a pen light to assess for a blink response.
- *CN IV AND CN VI* (extraocular movements): Assess the infant's ability to track your face as you move it side to side in a horizontal plane and then in a vertical plane. Note that the child moves the head as he or she tracks your face.
- *CN V* (trigeminal): Assess the rooting reflex and observe the infant as he or she takes the bottle or the breast, or sucks the pacifier. You are observing for coordination of the sucking reflex.
- *CN VII* (facial): Observe for symmetry of the face and forehead as the infant cries or smiles.
- *CN VIII* (acoustic): Test the acoustic blink reflex in response to a loud noise. Observe the infant's ability to tract toward the sound of a loud noise.
- *CN IX AND CN X* (glossopharyngeal and vagus): Observe the infant for coordination of sucking and swallowing. Test the gag reflex.
- *CN XI* (spinal accessory): Observe for symmetry of the shoulders.
- *CN XII* (hypoglossal): Observe the infant for coordination of sucking, swallowing, and tongue thrust. (You will observe tongue thrust up until approximately 4 months of age.)

In the assessment of many of the cranial nerves, playing the game Simon Says and asking the child to imitate you, helps to gain the child's cooperation and in turn provides you with a better outcome. The following is an adaptation of the cranial nerve examination for toddlers and early school-age children (adapted from Bowers & Thompson, 1992):

- *CN I*: Not assessed
- *CN II*: Visual fields can be tested, although you may have to immobilize the child's head by placing your finger under the chin. Visual acuity is assessed by using the Snellen, E, or picture chart.
- *CN III, CN IV, AND CN IV*: Use a finger puppet and have the child follow with his or her eyes, immobilizing the child's head by using a finger under the chin. Try to move the object through the six cardinal positions of gaze.
- *CN V*: Note bilateral jaw strength by observing the child chewing a cookie or cracker. Touch the child's forehead and lower face with a cotton ball, and observe for a response.
- *CN VII*: While observing for symmetry, ask the child to smile, make a sad face, and squeeze his or her eyes shut. Ask the child to show his or her teeth. Ask the child to puff up the cheeks.
- *CN VIII*: Shake a bell out of sight of the child and observe the child turn toward the sound. Whisper a known phrase such as "happy birthday" in the child's ear and ask the child to repeat it. Perform audiometric testing.
- *CN IX AND CN X*: Elicit the gag reflex.
- *CN XI AND CN XII*: Ask the child to stick out his or her tongue and move it back and forth. Ask the child to shrug his or her shoulders.

Many of the maneuvers included in the cranial nerve examinations for young children may have to be demonstrated in order for them to be performed correctly.

In addition to assessing the cranial nerves, evaluate for neurologic soft signs in children. Soft signs are defined as minor abnormalities in the neurologic examination of patients with no other features of fixed or transient neurologic disorders. These clinical disabilities are often associated with behavior, coordination, and learning difficulties (Iannetti, Mastrangelo, & Di Netta, 2005).

The following is a cranial nerve examination of the older school-age child and the adolescent, much of which is the same as that of the adult:

- *CN I* (olfactory): This is not routinely tested in children, although it is tested when there is loss of smell from possible head trauma. To test for smell, first assess patency by occluding one nostril at a time and asking the child to sniff. Then, with the child's eyes closed and one nostril occluded at a time, place an item with a familiar odor under the child's nose and ask the child to identify it. Use an aroma that the child is familiar with such as peppermint candy, bubble gum, or toothpaste.

- *CN II* (optic): Test for visual acuity by using the Snellen chart. Test for visual confrontation (or peripheral vision) by asking the child to look into your eyes and ask if the child can see the moving target in the periphery. If the child is cooperative, you may be able to look in the back of the eye to assess the ocular fundus and to determine the color, shape, and size of the optic disc.

- *CN III, CN IV, AND CN VI* (oculomotor, trochlear, abducens): Start by checking pupils for size, equality, and consensual light response. Ask the child to look over your shoulder at a picture on the wall to assess accommodation. Follow by assessing for nystagmus by, moving your finger in both a horizontal and vertical plane. You may observe a few beats of horizontal nystagmus at end gaze, which is within normal. (Nystagmus occurs with disease of the vestibular system or the cerebellum, or a lesion in the brainstem.) Follow this by assessing for extraocular movements. You may need to hold the child's head still by placing your finger under the child's chin as your other hand moves through the six cardinal positions of gaze. (In children, look for strabismus, which may present as exotropia or esotropia.)

- *CN V* (trigeminal): The trigeminal nerve is divided into three branches— *ophthalmic*, *maxillary*, and *mandibular*. The three areas are assessed by motor and/or sensory function.

  ➤ To test *motor function*, ask the child to clench his or her teeth or to bite down, and assess the muscles of mastication by palpating the temporal and masseter muscle. To assess strength, try pushing down on the chin to separate the jaw; you normally cannot do this. (An abnormal finding would be asymmetry or weakness on one side or pain on clenching the teeth.)

  ➤ To test *sensory function*, ask the child to close his or her eyes and, using a cotton ball, test light sensation by touching the forehead, cheek, and chin bilaterally. Ask the child to say "yes" or raise a hand when he or she feels the wisp of cotton. Remember to demonstrate with a test first so that the child knows what to expect. You are testing for lack of sensation or unequal sensation. The corneal reflex is not generally performed on a child. If the child is not blinking on one side or has no sensation in one eye, the corneal reflex is performed. A wisp of cotton is used to assess the corneal reflex. It is important to touch the cornea and not the conjunctiva when performing this test.

- *CN VII* (facial nerve): Have the child smile and then frown, noting smile and frown lines, and assess for asymmetry. Follow by asking the child to squeeze his or her eyes shut while you attemp to open them, then raise the eyebrows. Assess for weakness on one side. Puff up your cheeks and ask the child to imitate you, pushing on the child's cheeks to assess strength and escape of air from both sides equally. Next, ask the child to show you his or her teeth. Overall asymmetry in strength, movement, and sensation is assessed.
- *CN VIII* (acoustic/vestibulocochlear): In children, hearing is tested by using an audiometer to measure pure tones of various frequencies as a function of intensity measured in decibels.
- *CN IX AND CN X* (glossopharyngeal and vagus): This examination is intrusive in children, as you must use a tongue blade to depress the tongue and note pharyngeal movement as the child says "ahhh." You are looking for the uvula to rise midline and the tonsillar pillars to move medially. In children that are tentative about this part of the exam, asking them to open their mouth and hum a tune often accomplishes the same thing without causing them discomfort. In cases of tonsillar or pharyngeal abscess, the uvula may be deviated to the benign or normal side. This finding generally requires immediate referral.
- *CN XI* (spinal accessory): Ask the child to shrug his or her shoulders while you assess strength and size of the sternomastoid and trapezius muscles by resistance to the shoulder shrug. Next, ask the child to turn his or her head to one side while resisting your pressure to that side of the face. Repeat the same maneuver to the other side of the face.
- *CN XII* (hypoglossal): This assessment is easily performed by asking the child to stick out his or her tongue and wiggle it back and forth. You are looking for fasciculation and/or deviation to one side when the tongue is initially extended. Both of these findings are associated with lower motor neuron disease such as polio.

Examination of the Motor System

When inspecting the muscles and the motor system, children are generally cooperative. Start by asking them to show you how strong they are as you use resistance techniques to assess different muscle groups. Begin with the upper body, including the arms, fingers, and wrists, and move down to the legs, ankles, feet, and toes. Muscles are tested in groups for bulk, contour, and symmetry, as well as hypertrophy or atrophy. (Further discussion regarding palpation, range of motion, and muscle strength is included in Chapter 12, "Examination of the Musculoskeletal System.")

Actual assessment of the motor system starts with the assessment of tone when you first observe the child, noting posture, balance, coordination, speech pattern, and movements. Tone or tonus is defined as the expected state of muscle tone, maintained by partial contraction or alternate contraction and relaxation of neighboring muscle fibers in a group of muscles (Seidel, Ball, Dains, Benedict, 2006). It is particularly important when assessing the newborn and the infant.

For example, observation of 3- to 4-month-old infants can reveal much about tone and development as you observe their ability to raise and maintain their head, to kick their feet alternately, and to pull to sit, noting head lag and ability to align their head with their trunk. Observation of toddlers or school-age children as they remove their clothing, and take off their socks and shoes, can demonstrate purposefulness of movements, symmetry, and overall muscle tone. Difficulty in performing any of these maneuvers, such as limited range of motion, pain with motion, tremors, or weakness, may indicate lower motor neuron disease.

Examination of the Sensory System

The sensory system in children is evaluated by having the child identify various sensory stimuli. Sensory stimuli are separated into primary sensory functions and cortical sensory functions. In assessment of primary sensory stimuli, you do not need to test the entire skin surface for every sensation. Particularly in children, routine sensory stimuli include superficial pain, light touch, and vibration. It is most important to explain to the child what you are going to do and what he or she should expect to feel. To assess *superficial pain*, demonstrate by using a sharp point such as a split tongue depressor and gently apply it to the child's skin; then do the same with a dull end. Ask the child to indicate whether he or she feels a sharp or dull sensation when touched. When ready to begin, ask the child to close his or her eyes, and randomly touch the skin, alternating sites and switching between the sharp and dull end of the tongue depressor. To assess for *light sensation*, repeat the procedure using a wisp of cotton and testing in random order the arms, forearms, hands, chest, thighs, and legs. Remember, the face was assessed for sensation when testing the cranial nerves.

Vibration is assessed by using a tuning fork and placing it over a bony prominence at a distal point, such as the bony surface of the great toe or finger. Ask the child to close his or her eyes and then tell you what he or she feels. Compare sides.

Cortical Sensory Stimuli

Cortical sensory function testing includes stereognosis, graphesthesia, two-point discrimination, extinction and point location, and temperature. In children, stereognosis and graphesthesia are assessed, depending upon the age of the child. Two-point discrimination, extinction, and temperature are assessed if there is concern regarding absence of sensation.

Stereognosis is a test to determine the child's ability to recognize objects by feeling them in the palm of the hand with eyes closed. Use objects that children are familiar with, such as a paper clip, key, or marble. Ask the child to close his or her eyes, and place the object in the child's hand. Allow the child to explore it with the fingers of that hand, then ask the child to identify it. Repeat this on the opposite side with a different object. Difficulty identifying objects is often associated with sensory cortex lesions such as stroke, which is uncommon in children.

Graphesthesia is tested by tracing a number in the palm of the child's hand and asking the child to identify it with eyes closed. Most importantly, the child should know how to write numbers. Misleading findings can occur if the child is too young and/or has not mastered numbers.

Cerebellar Function (Including Proprioception, Coordination, and Fine Motor Skills)

When assessing cerebellar function in children, make a game out of the various maneuvers, allowing the child to become fully engaged and in turn producing better outcomes. Demonstrate to the child what you want him or her to do, and ask him or her to repeat the demonstration to verify that they fully understand and can correctly perform the maneuver.

RAPID ALTERNATING MOVEMENTS: With the child sitting on the table, ask the child to pat his or her thighs with both hands, alternating with the palms and back of the hands. Observe for smoothness and rhythmic pace.

FINGER TO FINGER: With the child sitting on the table, ask the child to alternately touch each finger with the thumb on the same hand. Observe how smoothly, quickly, and accurately it is performed.

FINGER TO NOSE: With the child sitting on the table and arms outstretched at the sides, ask the child to touch his or her nose with the index finger, alternating with each side. Observe for speed and accuracy.

HEEL TO SHIN: With the child sitting on the table, ask the child to run the heel of one foot starting at the knee down the shin of the other leg, maintaining a straight line. Observe for smoothness.

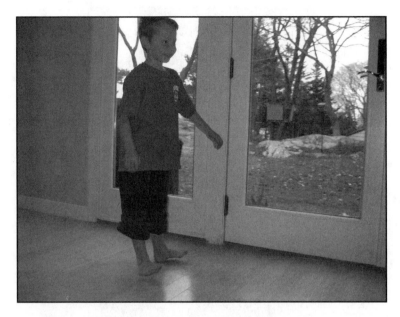

Figure 13-13   Walking on Heels

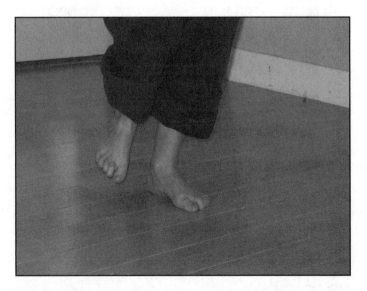

Figure 13-14   Standing on One Foot

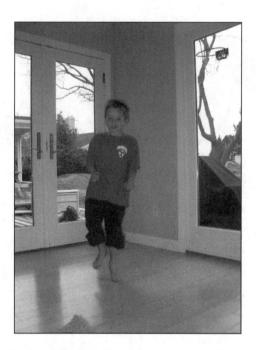

Figure 13-15 Hopping on One Foot

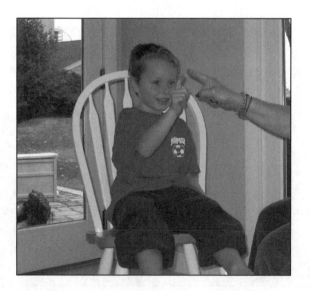

Figure 13-16 Finger to Nose

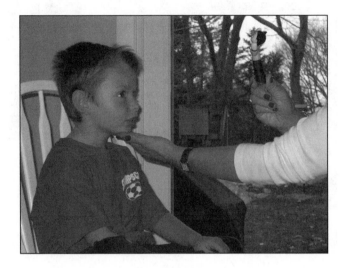

Figure 13-17   Equal Ocular Movements (EOM)

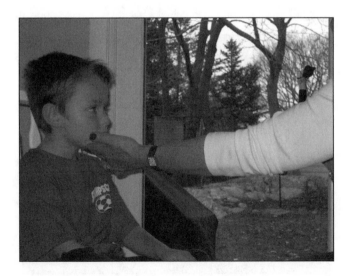

Figure 13-18   Equal Ocular Movements (EOM)

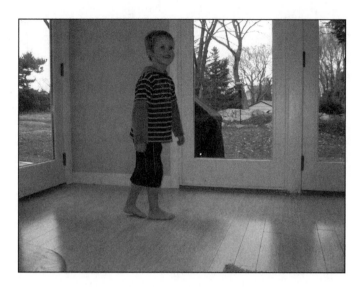

Figure 13-19 Tandem Gait

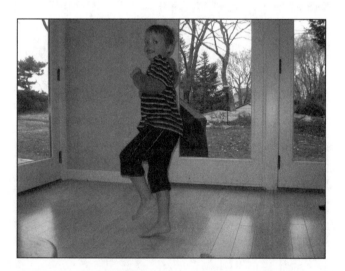

Figure 13-20 Hopping on One Foot

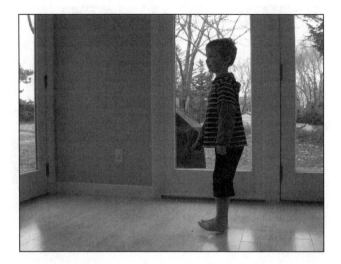

Figure 13-21   Walking on Heels

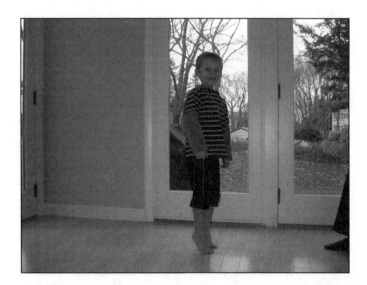

Figure 13-22   Walking on Toes

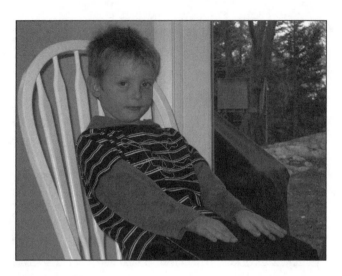

Figure 13-23 Rapid Alternating Movements

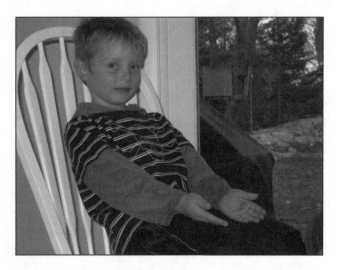

Figure 13-24 Rapid Alternating Movements

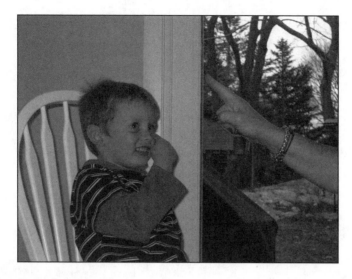

Figure 13-25(a) Finger to Nose

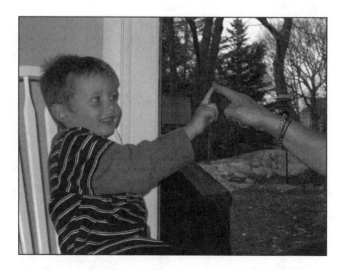

Figure 13-25(b) Finger to Nose

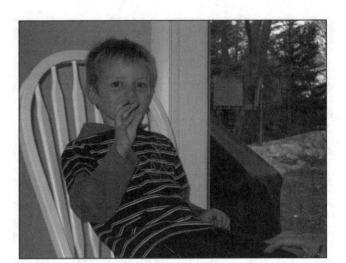

Figure 13-26 Finger to Finger

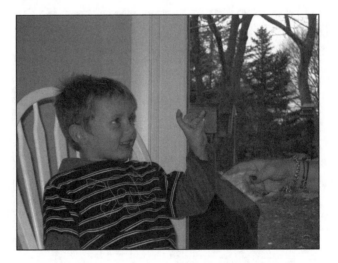

Figure 13-27 Finger to Finger

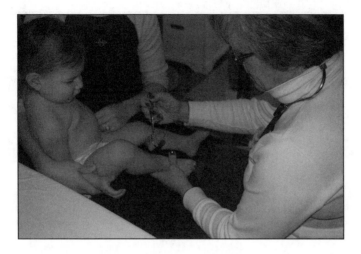

Figure 13-28   Assessing Deep Tendon Reflexes: Patella Reflex

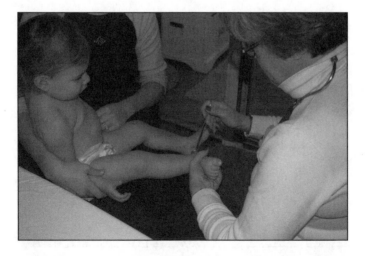

Figure 13-29   Assessing Deep Tendon Reflex: Ankle Jerk or Achilles Reflex

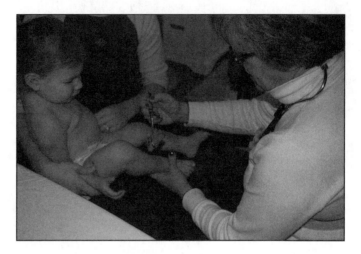

Figure 13-30 Assessing Patella Reflex

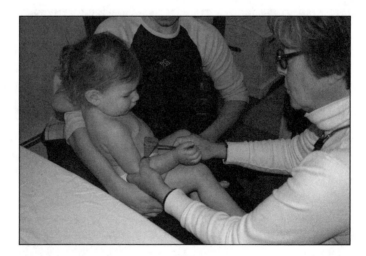

Figure 13-31 Assessing Bicep Reflex

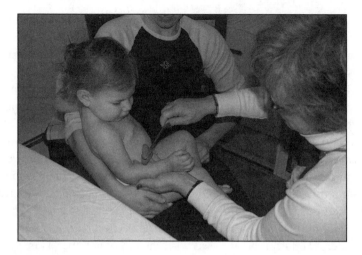

Figure 13-32   Assessing Brachioradialis Reflex

ROMBERG TEST: Ask the child to stand up with feet together and eyes closed. You are assessing for balance, noting whether the child sways or loses balance.

GAIT: Observation of the child as he or she walks into the office starts with assessment of the child's gait, observing if there is a limp, limited weight bearing, abnormal arm swing, or abnormal inward or outward angle of the foot. Ask the child to walk down the hall or across the room to better evaluate gait. Also ask the child to walk across the room on the toes and return on the heels. Next, ask the child to hop on one foot and then hop on the other foot. Ask the child to walk across the room in tandem gait in a straight line with heel to toe.

These maneuvers can be fun for the child by making a game out of them, which in turn may relax the child and reduce the rigidity of the performance. Lack of coordination or inability to smoothly and quickly perform these maneuvers may indicate cerebellar disease such as a vestibular disorder or upper motor neuron disorder (e.g., cerebral palsy).

Deep Tendon Reflexes

In the assessment of deep tendon reflexes (DTRs), the reflex hammer is one of the tools in the doctor's/nurse's play kit, and children may pick up your hammer and imitate tapping with it. Allow children to examine and play with the hammer and to practice tapping on themselves before you actually use it. Demonstrate to them what you are going to do, and emphasize that it will not hurt. In school age-children, DTRs are performed the same as in the adult, starting with the biceps, triceps, brachioradialis, patellar, Achilles, and plantar.

To effectively assess the DTRs, the child should be appropriately positioned and relaxed, and extremities should be loose. You should position the limb so there is slight tension on the tendon to be evaluated. Take the time to palpate the desired tendon prior to actual tapping to ensure that you have the correct location. Hold the reflex hammer loosely between the thumb and index finger so that as you tap the tendon, the hammer can move smoothly but in a controlled direction. It is important not to grip the hammer tightly as though you were hammering nails. Use a rapid, but firm flicking motion of your wrist as you tap the desired tendon. In the infant and toddler, DTRs can be assessed with the reflex hammer as in the older child, although you can also use your index finger in place of the hammer.

DTRs are defined by the reflex arc, which consists of several defined steps along the neural pathways (Bowers & Thompson, 1992):

1. The receptor cells of the tendon are stimulated.
2. The nerve impulse travels along an afferent (sensory) neuron from the receptor cells via the dorsal root and synapses with an anterior horn cell.
3. Following the synapse, the impulse is transmitted to an efferent neuron.
4. This impulse travels along the efferent (motor) neuron via the ventral root until it innervates a skeletal muscle.
5. The skeletal muscle contracts.

DTRs are graded in children the same as in adults, although assessment in infants can be variable due to the immaturity of the corticospinal pathways. Reflexes such as the triceps, brachioradialis, and abdominal reflexes are difficult to elicit before 6 months of age. The anal reflex is present at birth and important to elicit if a spinal cord lesion is suspected (Bickley, 2003, p. 728).

Grading of DTRs can be described as follows:

- *GRADE 0* (absent): No response or visible muscle contraction
- *GRADE 1+* (hyporeflexia): Diminished response, slight or sluggish muscle contraction
- *GRADE 2+* (normal): Average muscle contraction with slight joint movement
- *GRADE 3+* (hyperreflexia): Brisk, slightly hyperactive, with moderate joint movement
- *GRADE 4+* (abnormal): Strong muscle contraction, hyperactive, often associated with one to three beats of clonus

Assessment of clonus, specifically ankle clonus, is performed if the child's reflexes are hyperactive. To test for clonus, hold the child's knee in a partially flexed position and briskly dorsiflex the foot with your other hand, while maintaining the foot in flexion. Clonus is a continuous rhythmic tremor between dorsiflexion and plantar flexion.

The significance of clonus is related to upper motor neuron lesions versus lower motor neuron lesions. The following lists compare the two (Seidel, et al 2006).

UPPER MOTOR NEURON LESIONS:
- Muscle spasticity, possible contractures
- Little or no muscle atrophy
- Hyperreflexia
- Note, damage above the level of the brainstem will affect the opposite side of the body.

LOWER MOTOR NEURON LESIONS:
- Muscle flaccidity
- Loss of muscle tone
- Muscle atrophy
- Hyporeflexia
- Fasciculations
- Changes in muscle supplied by that nerve, usually a muscle on the same side as the lesion

Each tendon reflex is associated with specific spinal segments that include both sensory and motor fibers. Measurement of the reflex response is indicative of the stimulus of the reflex arc at specific spinal levels.

DTRs	Spinal Segments
Biceps	Cervical 5, 6
Brachioradialis	Cervical 5, 6
Triceps	Cervical 6, 7, 8
Patellar	Lumbar 2, 3, 4
Achilles	Sacral 1, 2
Plantar	Lumbar 4, 5; sacral 1, 2

The following is a detailed description of how to elicit DTRs in the toddler, school-age child, and adolescent.

BICEPS REFLEX: Start by flexing the child's arm at the elbow to approximately 45 degrees, then palpate the biceps tendon in the antecubital fossa. Place your thumb over the stretched tendon and strike your thumbnail with the small end of the reflex hammer. You will observe slight flexion of the elbow with contraction of the biceps muscle.

TRICEPS REFLEX: Flex the child's arm at the elbow to 90 degrees and place it along the chest. Palpate the triceps tendon, which is just above the elbow, and strike it directly with the reflex hammer. You will observe slight extension of the forearm. An alternative maneuver to assess the triceps reflex is to extend the upper arm directly from the shoulder, supporting the upper arm with your hand and allowing the forearm to dangle loosely. Tap the triceps tendon directly with the reflex hammer. You will observe minimal sideways movement of the dangling arm.

BRACHIORADIAL REFLEX: Flex the arm at the elbow to approximately 45 degrees, and rest the child's forearm on top of your arm with the child's slightly pronated. Strike the brachioradial tendon directly about 2–3 cm above the radial styloid process or above the wrist. The expected response is slight pronation of the forearm and flexion of the elbow.

PATELLAR REFLEX: This is the reflex that a child will anticipate and possibly exaggerate. As the child is sitting upright on the table with the lower legs dangling, palpate the patellar tendon just below the patella and strike it directly with the reflex hammer. You will observe extension of the leg with contraction of the quadriceps muscle. In some children, you may have to try an additional maneuver by asking them to clasp their fingers together and on the count of three pull hard to separate them. Doing so distracts the child from anticipating the leg extension and allows for full relaxation of the quadriceps muscle, which is necessary for contraction.

ACHILLES REFLEX: With the child sitting on the edge of the exam table and the lower legs dangling, hold the child's foot in dorsiflexion (flex the ankle up to 90 degrees); with your opposite hand, strike the Achilles tendon directly. You will observe plantar flexion of the foot with contraction of the gastrocnemius muscle.

PLANTAR REFLEX (ALSO CALLED THE BABINSKI SIGN): This can be performed with the child in a sitting or supine position. Using the end of the handle of the reflex hammer, lightly stroke the lateral side of the sole of the foot from the heel to across the ball of the foot. A normal response is plantar flexion of the toes. The Babinski sign, which is present in children younger than 2 years of age, is dorsiflexion of the great toe with or without fanning of the other toes. If this response is present in older children, it is an abnormal finding and designated as a positive Babinski, which indicates upper motor neuron disease of the pyramidal tract and requires immediate referral. In some ticklish children, the plantar reflex may be difficult to elicit and the Babinski sign may be observed.

Cutaneous or Superficial Reflexes

These reflexes are responses to scraping of the skin, rather than muscle stretch reflexes, and are graded as present or absent. They are different than muscle stretch reflexes, as the sensory stimulus must travel to the spinal cord and then ascend to the brain as well. Because these reflexes must pass many synaptic reflexes, they can be absent if there is severe lower motor neuron damage or destruction of the sensory pathways from the skin.

ABDOMINAL REFLEX: This is a superficial, or cutaneous, reflex in which the sensory receptors are in the skin rather than in the muscle. Position the child in a supine position. With the handle of the reflex hammer, stroke horizontally and laterally toward the umbilicus. You will observe contraction of the abdominal muscles, with the umbilicus deviating toward the stimulus.

ANAL WINK REFLEX: The anal wink reflex is elicited by gently stroking the perianal skin. It results in puckering of the rectal sphincter due to contraction of the corrugator cutis ani muscle. Both the abdominal reflex and the anal wink may be absent due to spinal cord damage or to disorders that interrupt the pathways between the brain and the spinal cord.

CREMASTERIC REFLEX: This is not typically done in children, although it may be performed in an older adolescent male. Lightly stroke the inner aspect of the thigh with the handle of the reflex hammer. You will observe elevation of the testicle on the stroked side. This reflex may be absent in children with lesions or trauma to the lumbosacral segments of the spinal cord or with lesions of the corticospinal or pyramidal system.

> ### Red Flags

Common disorders of the CNS and red flags (those requiring immediate referral) are sometimes difficult to distinguish in the child and, therefore, will all be included under Red Flags.

Global developmental delay may be indicative of a static encephalopathy often as the result of antenatal or perinatal insult. A question to consider is whether the delay is restricted to a specific area of development such as gross motor skills, and also whether there are signs of developmental regression or a loss of developmental milestones. If these concerns are present, immediate referral to a pediatric neurologist is necessary.

Degenerative disorders:

> ➤ *White matter disease*, such as adrenoleukodystrophy, is a progressive demyelination of the CNS leading to neurologic deterioration, including disturbance of gait and coordination, loss of vision, and loss of hearing, ultimately ending in a vegetative state (Fenichel, 1988, p. 143).

> ➤ *Gray matter diseases*, such as Rett syndrome and Huntington disease, are chronic degenerative diseases of the CNS. Rett syndrome occurs only in girls, with rapid developmental regression and a hallmark sign of hand ringing. Spastic paraparesis and quadriparesis are common endpoints. Huntington disease is transmitted by autosomal-dominant inheritance. Onset is between the ages of 30 and 50 years. Cardinal features are chorea, progressive dementia, and seizures, leading to death (Fenichel, 1988, p. 142).

Nondegenerative disorders:

> ➤ *Cerebral palsy* is a nonprogressive abnormality of the brain that occurs in the prenatal, the perinatal, or postnatal period. It is the most common chronic neurologic disorder of childhood. There are four types of cerebral palsy associated with motor dysfunction: spastic, dyskinetic, ataxic, and mixed. All types are related to the location of the brain insult. Cerebral palsy is thought to be the result of cerebral hypoxia, cerebral ischemia, or an infectious intrauterine insult to the CNS (McKearnan, Kieckhefer, & Engel, 2004). The overall presentation of cerebral palsy includes abnormal muscle tone and lack of coordination with spasticity (Liptak & Accardo, 2004).

> ➤ *Bell's palsy* is defined as an acute process resulting in paralysis or weakening of the trigeminal nerve (facial nerve). It generally presents with drooping on one side of the face, with the eyelid partially or completely closed. Symptoms are often preceded by an upper respiratory infection or exposure to cold temperatures. In children, symptoms resolve within weeks to 6 months without use of steroids.

Epilepsy (seizure disorders) is a chronic disorder characterized by recurrent, unprovoked seizures secondary to a CNS disorder. It presents with abnormal electrical discharges in the brain that cause a variety of involuntary movements and behaviors. The clinical manifestation is dependent upon the type, location, and duration of the seizure, from partial to complex partial seizures, to generalized seizures, to absence seizures. Treatment is variable, depending on the classification of seizure.

Febrile seizures are seizures associated with a fever between 38°C (100.4°F) and 41°C (105.8°F). They are nonfocal generalized tonic-clonic seizures lasting less than 15 minutes. Children with *benign* febrile seizures are developmentally appropriate and neurologically intact.

Headaches: Migraine is the most common cause of recurrent headaches in children. These headaches present with nausea, abdominal pain, vomiting, and pulsating pain; they are relieved by sleep. Often there is a family history of migraine headaches.

Head injury (head trauma) involves damage to brain tissue and its surrounding structures. Closed head injuries result in more diffuse damage and cause multifocal injuries. Open head injuries produce more focal injuries. Primary head injuries cause contusions and hemorrhages within the brain secondary to mechanical forces. Seizures, ischemia, hypotension, and hypoxia can be exhibited with head injuries.

Head growth disorders:

> ➤ *Macrocephaly* is defined as a head circumference more than three standard deviations above the mean for age and sex or one that increases too rapidly.

> ➤ *Hydrocephaly* is defined as a condition with increased volume of cerebrospinal fluid with progressive ventricular dilation. The patient may present with irritability, vomiting, impaired extraocular movements, and excessive rate of head growth.

> ➤ *Microcephaly* is defined as a head circumference three standard deviations below the mean for age and sex or one that is increasing slower than normal. It is often an indicator of delayed brain development, which can lead to delayed developmental milestones and neurologic problems.

> ➤ *Craniosynostosis* is defined as premature closure of the cranial sutures. Bone growth continues in a direction parallel to the prematurely fused suture line, which leads to compensatory overgrowth of normal suture lines and the classic skull

deformities associated with craniosynostosis (Ball, Bindler, & Cowen, 2010, p. 1070).

CNS infections:

> ➤ *Meningitis* is an inflammation of the meninges of the brain commonly caused by viruses or bacteria. Meningitis in infants presents with a bulging fontanelle, irritability, opisthotonic posturing, nausea, vomiting, and difficult consolability. In children school age and older, meningitis presents with nuchal rigidity, headache, vomiting, fever, and irritability, as well as positive Kernig and Brudzinski sign. See Figure 13-39 and Figure 13-40.

Encephalitis is an acute inflammatory process affecting brain tissue. It most commonly presents with viral etiology. With increased vaccines, such as the MMR (mumps, measles, and rubella) and varicella vaccine, encephalitis secondary to childhood illness has decreased dramatically.

Autistic spectrum disorder is one of the most common pervasive developmental disorders. It begins in early childhood and presents with impaired social interactions and communication, with restricted interests, activities, and behaviors (Ball, Bindler, & Cowen, 2010).

Anxiety disorders are common in children as well as in adults. There are a number of disorders such as generalized anxiety disorder, separation anxiety disorder, panic disorder, obsessive-compulsive disorder, social phobia or school phobia, and conversion reaction.

Floppy infant (hypotonic infant) may result from a lesion in various parts of the nervous system, possibly including the cerebrum, spinal cord, peripheral nerve, or myoneural junction. The differential diagnosis for infantile hypotonia is extensive and requires the expertise of a pediatric neurologist.

Meningomyelocele (spina bifida) is a neural tube defect that results in incomplete closure of the vertebral column. As a result, a meningeal sac filled with spinal fluid and containing the spinal cord protrudes through the vertebral defect.

Tourette syndrome is a tic disorder characterized by sudden rapid, recurrent, nonrhythmic, and brief motor movements or vocalizations. It primarily involves the upper body, including blinking of the eyes, coughing, grunting, facial grimacing, and a variety of verbal noises. There is a strong genetic component to this syndrome, with the highest incidence in males. Comorbidities such as obsessive-compulsive disorder and attention deficit hyperactivity disorder (ADHD) often accompany Tourette syndrome.

Write-Up of the CNS Exam

EXAMPLE FOR INFANTS: Positive suck, strong grasp and head control in pull to sit. Patellar and bicep DTRs 2+. Babinski positive bilaterally, no clonus. Cranial nerves: brief eye contact, tracking in both vertical and horizontal plane, positive bilateral red reflex. Symmetrical facies, and startle to loud noise. Positive gag reflex with coordinated suck and swallow.

EXAMPLE FOR SCHOOL-AGE CHILDREN: Patient is alert, oriented, with fluent and clear speech. Attention, naming, repetition, and recall are appropriate. Cranial nerves: pupils are reactive, bilaterally, discs are flat and sharp, extraocular movements are intact, visual fields are full to confrontation. There is no facial asymmetry, palate elevates symmetrically, and tongue is midline. Motor exam: normal tone and bulk. Power is 5/5 throughout. There is no drift, and DTRs are 2+ throughout with downgoing toes bilaterally. Sensory exam: intact to light touch, pinprick, and vibration. Coordination is intact to finger-nose, fine-finger movements and rapid alternating movements. Gait is smooth, coordinated with even toe, heel, and tandem walking.

Case Study: Toddler Presenting with a Febrile Seizure

Jamie is a 20-month-old female who is seen in your office as a follow-up to an emergency room visit 24 hours ago. Jamie's mother reports that she was well until yesterday when she went into Jamie's room after her nap and found her stiff and unconscious in her crib. She also observed that Jamie was very hot. The mother immediately called 9-1-1. When the EMTs arrived, Jamie was alert and responsive and was taken to the local emergency department. A neurologic exam and full septic workup were performed.

On examination, Jamie was febrile, with a temperature of 103°F. She was also found to have a right acute otitis media, which was treated with an antibiotic. She was discharged to home with instructions to follow up with her primary care provider within 24 hours.

Questions

1. What are the criteria to differentiate between simple and complex febrile seizures?
2. What is the appropriate management for this child?
3. What is the differential diagnosis?

Answers

1. Simple febrile seizures are brief, lasting less than 15 minutes; they are generalized without focality, are tonic-clonic in nature, and do not recur within a 24-hour period. Complex febrile seizures last longer than 30 minutes, can recur on the same day, and have focal attributes.
2. Management for this child includes:
   - Protect the airway by placing the child in a side-lying position to prevent aspiration or airway obstruction.
   - Do not put anything in the child's mouth.
   - Reduce the fever with acetaminophen or ibuprofen, using the correct dose.
   - Anticonvulsants are generally not recommended for febrile seizures but may be considered if the child has abnormal neurologic findings or developmental delays, a positive family history of afebrile seizures, or recurrent prolonged simple febrile seizures (Burns, Dunn, Brady, Starr, & Blosser, 2004, p. 693).
3. The differential diagnosis includes meningitis, sepsis, hypoglycemia, trauma, tumor, anoxia, and metabolic or toxic encephalopathy.

References

Ball, J., Bindler, R., & Cowen, K. (2010). *Child health nursing* (2nd ed.). Upper Saddle River, NJ: Pearson.

Ball, J.W., Bindler, R. (2007). *Pediatric nursing: Caring for children*, (4th ed.). New Jersey: Prentice Hall.

Bickley, L. (2003). *Bates' guide to physical examination and history taking* (8th ed.). New York: Lippincott Williams & Wilkins.

Bowers, A. C. Thompson, J. M. (1992). *Clinical manual of health assessment*, (3rd. ed.). Mosby.

Burns, C., Dunn, A., Brady, M., Starr, N., & Blosser, C. (2004). *Pediatric primary care: A handbook for nurse practitioners* (3rd ed.). St. Louis, MO: Saunders.

Dogan, S., Safavi-Abbasi, S., Theodore, N., Horn, E., Rekate, H. L., Sonntag, V. K. (2006). Pediatric subaaxial cervical spine injuries: origins, management and outcome in 51 patients. *Neurosurgical Focus, 20*(2), 1318.

Estes, M. (2006). *Health assessment and physical examination* (3rd ed.). Albany, NY: Delmar Publishers.

Fenichel, G. M. (1988). *Clinical pediatric neurology.* Philadelphia: Saunders.

Iannetti, P., Mastrangelo, M., & Di Netta, S. (2005). Neurological "soft signs" in children and adolescents. *Journal of Pediatric Neurology, 3,* 123–125.

Jarvis, C. (2008). *Physical examination and health assessment* (5th ed.). St. Louis, MO: Elsevier.

Liptak, G. S. & Accardo, P. J. (2004). Health and social outcomes of children with cerebral palsy. *Journal of Pediatraics, 145*(supple), S36–S41.

McKearnan, K.A., Kieckhefer,G.M., Engel, J.M., Jensen, M.P., Kabyal. S. (2004). Pain in children with cerebral palsy. *Journal of Neuroscience Nursing, 36*(5) 252–259. (In Ball, et al)

Seidel, H. M., Ball, J. W., Dains, J. E., Benedict, G. W (2006). *Mosby's guide to physical examination.* Mosby.

Resources

Hansen, M. (1998). *Pathophysiology: Foundations of disease and clinical intervention.* Philadelphia: Saunders.

Marieb, E. (1995). *Human anatomy and physiology* (3rd ed.). Redwood City, CA: Benjamin/Cummings Publishing Company.

Nolan, M. (1996). *Introduction to the neurologic examination.* Philadelphia: F.A. David.

Potts, N., & Mandleco, B. (2007). *Pediatraic nursing* (2nd ed.). Victoria, Australia: Thomson, Delmar Learning.

Tortora, G. J., & Grabvowski, S. R. (2003). *Principles of anatomy and physiology* (10th ed.). New York: Wiley.

Examination of the Male and Female Genitalia

Dianna M. Jones

The Male Reproductive System

Anatomy

The male reproductive system is made up of several parts, includ-ing the testes, which are positioned inside the scrotum; the ducts; and the penis (Jarvis [2009]; Bickley [2003]; and Barkauskas, Stoltenberg-Allen, Baumann, and Darling-Fisher [1998]).

PENIS: The penis is made up of three columns of erectile tissue: the corpus spongiosum and the two corpora cavernosa. The corpus spongiosum contains the urethra. The urethra crosses the corpus spongiosum, and its meatus creates a slitlike opening at the tip of the glans. The penis ends in a cone-shaped structure called the glans penis. The corona is the area on the penis where the shaft and glans meet. The glans is covered by a hoodlike structure, or flap, called the foreskin, or prepuce.

In the male, circumcision refers to the surgical removal of this fore-skin or prepuce. The procedure has been performed for centuries for a variety of reasons including religious, cultural, and medical. Circumcision was initially performed to improve male hygiene and for purification. Today routine circumcision of male infants is a tradition as a religious symbol of Judaism. It is also practiced by followers of Islam and certain aboriginal tribes in Africa and Australia as a rite of passage into manhood. Parents may ask you questions regarding circumcision and when counseling them, it is important to consider the potential medical benefits and risks, as well as the social and religious aspects of this procedure.

It is necessary to understand that the skin of the body of the penis starts to grow over the glans at approximately eight weeks of gestation, eventually covering the entire organ. The purpose of this foreskin is to protect the glans. There is incomplete separation of the foreskin and glans at birth

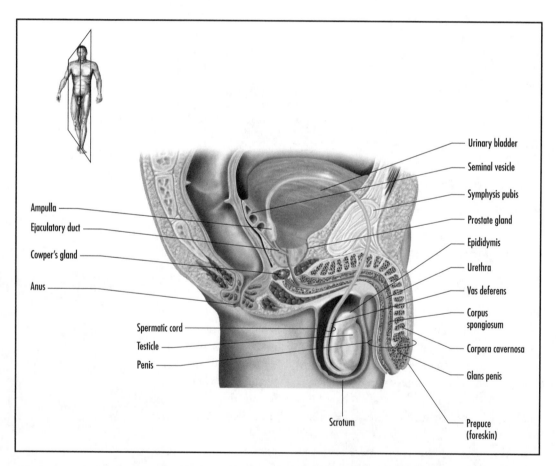

Figure 14-1 Male Genital Structures—Side View

resulting in congenital or physiological phimosis, which is the inability to retract the foreskin or prepuce over the glans. This foreskin becomes easily retracted from the glans over time and 50 percent are easily retractable by three years of age (Shoemaker, 2010).

SCROTUM: The scrotum is made up of loose, wrinkled skin that is divided by a median septum forming two sacs. Each sac contains one testicle.

TESTES: The testes are ovoid structures, which produce sperm and the hormone testosterone. Testosterone initiates the pubertal growth of the male genitalia, prostate, and seminal vesicles. It is also responsible for the development of male secondary sex characteristics, including facial and body hair,

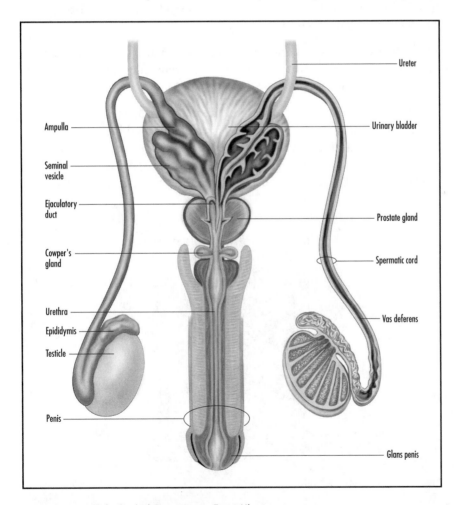

Figure 14-2   Male Genital Structures—Front View

enlarged larynx (causing a deeper voice), and muscle development. The testes are ovoid in shape and have a rubbery consistency. The size varies, measuring approximately 3.5–5.5 cm in length and 2.5 cm in diameter in an adult male. The left testis lies slightly lower than the right. The epididymis is a structure that is the key storage site for sperm. It is coiled and curves over the top outer and posterior surface of each testis. The vas deferens is the lower structure of the epididymis. It is a muscular, cordlike duct that continues down from the tail of the epididymis. The duct and other vessels form the spermatic cord. These vessels include the arteries, veins, lymphatics, and nerves. The spermatic cord passes through the inguinal canal into the abdomen and pelvis. The vas deferens then continues posterior and downward behind the bladder. It connects with the duct of the seminal vesicle to form the ejaculatory duct. The duct then empties into the urethra.

LYMPHATICS: The lymphatics of both the penis and the scrotal surfaces drain into the inguinal lymph nodes and the lymphatics of the testes drain into the abdomen.

INGUINAL AREA: The groin, or inguinal area, is located at the juncture of the thigh and the lower abdominal wall. The inguinal canal is a narrow tunnel that lies above and just parallel to the inguinal ligament. It is a potential space and a common area for hernias. Another potential space for hernias is the femoral canal. The femoral canal lies beneath the inguinal ligament.

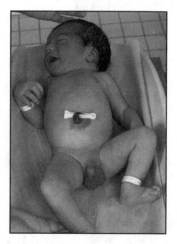

Figure 14-3 Scrotum of Infant

Assessment Considerations: Subjective Information

Consideration pertinent to the male genitalia (Jarvis, 2008):

Infants and Children
- Is the child experiencing any burning or pain with urination?
- Does the child cry or hold his genitals?
- Are there any problems with the child's genitals, such as redness, swelling, lesions, or discolorations?
- Does the child have any history of hernias, hydrocele, undescended testes, or swelling in the scrotum when crying or coughing?

Patients Older Than 2 Years of Age
Ask the parent questions related to toilet training. Has the child started toilet training? Where are they in the process? What steps is the parent taking to facilitate the process?

Patients Older Than 5 Years of Age
At this age, bed-wetting is a concern. Have there been any issues with bed-wetting? How often is this happening? How is the parent handling this?

Preschoolers and Young School-Age Children
Screen for sexual abuse. Ask the child directly if anyone has ever asked to touch his private area or if anyone has ever actually touched his private area. Be sure to let the child know that it is okay to talk about this and that he has not been bad and is not to blame. This is a good time to reiterate that it is not okay for anyone to touch his private area and he should always tell an adult if this happens.

Preadolescents and Adolescents
Approach the adolescent patient in a nonjudgmental manner. Ask questions pertaining to sexual growth and development by phrasing them in a nonjudgmental way such as "when did you first" rather than by asking "do you." It is important to ask questions appropriate for the patient's age. The patient may be apprehensive about discussing these topics with you. Do not be too assertive in your questioning, but offer information on topics such as pubertal development, sexual changes the adolescent may expect, and other more sensitive issues such as nocturnal emissions, sexual activity, contraception, and how STDs are acquired. You may have to explain some of the female physiology, since adolescent boys often to do not understand the relationship of vaginal discharge in the spread of STDs. The adolescent may decline to ask questions often due to their discomfort around this sensitive topic. Always ask if they received sex education in school and if

they have questions on what they learned. Often, discussing this topic while examining the ears or using another distraction can ease any embarrassment. Remember that adolescents often receive much of their sexual information from friends and the media, much of which may be misconstrued or misinformation.

The topics of discussion for the adolescent, such as changes in the genitalia, body and pubic hair growth, change in voice, and muscular growth and development, are based on their age and pubertal development. Always ask the patient if he has discussed these changes with his parents and if he has had sex education at school. At age 12 or 13 you can discuss nocturnal emissions or 'wet dreams,' and the occurrence of random erections at embarrassing times. Assure him that these are normal experiences. When the patient is in his teens, ask if he is dating, if he has a steady girlfriend or boyfriend, or if he has same sex interest. Has he ever had intercourse or engaged in oral sex, and if so, do he and his partner practice safe sex? Assess the patient's knowledge of sexually transmitted diseases such as chlamydia, genital herpes (HSV-2), human papiloma virus, gonorrhea, and HIV. Also screen for sexual abuse at this time. At the end of the exam, ask the adolescent if he has any questions or concerns, and emphasize that what you discuss with him is confidential and you won't tell his parents, unless something he told you is life threatening. Finish by discussing the importance of regularly performing a testicular exam and giving him information on this topic.

The testicular self-examination (TSE) is an important form of health prevention. Although testicular cancer is rare in teenage males, it is the most common cancer in males between the ages of 15 and 35. It is recommended to perform a TSE monthly in order to become familiar with the normal size and shape of the testicles.

The following are basic guidelines with which to instruct your patients:

- It's best to do a TSE during or right after a hot shower or bath. The warmth relaxes the skin of the scrotum making it easier to examine the testicles and feel for anything unusual.
- Use both hands to examine each testicle, one at a time. Place your index and middle fingers underneath the testicle and your thumbs on top. Gently roll the testicle between your thumbs and fingers. It is normal for testicles to be slightly different in size.
- As you feel the testicle, you should be able to feel the epididymis, a cord-like structure on top and in back of the testicle that stores and transports sperm. Do not confuse this with a lump.
- While examining each testicle, feel for any lumps or bumps. They can be pea size or larger and are often painless. Lumps or swellings may

not be cancerous, but should be assessed by a primary care provider as soon as possible.

FAMILY HISTORY: Is there a family history of congenital adrenal hyperplasia, or ambiguous genitalia. Also consider a history of endocrine disorders, genitourinary problems, undescended testes, or testicular malignancy.

REVIEW OF SYSTEMS (ROS): Review problems such as endocrine disorders and genitourinary concerns. Specifically regarding the genitalia consider pain or discharge from the penis, pain, swelling or masses noted in the scrotum, history of hernias, rashes, changes in testicular or penile size. Also consider appearance of pubic hair, history of sexually transmitted diseases, and use of contraception.

Assessment Considerations: Objective Information

All healthcare providers should be well aware of the normal male anatomy before assessing any patient. Understanding what is normal will help you identify if there are any abnormalities. For the older child and adolescent, the genital exam can be very stressful. Be sensitive to this when approaching the patient (Bickley, 2003; Jarvis, 2008).

Newborn Period and Infancy

When examining an infant, the child should be placed in the supine position with the diaper removed. Inspect the penis, scrotum and testes. The penis will be approximately 2–3 cm in length and should appear straight. If there is bowing of the penis, it may be caused by a fibrous band of tissue called chordee. This is associated with hypospadias, which occurs when the uretheral meatus opens on the ventral (under) side of the glands or shaft. In the uncircumcised male the foreskin will appear tight over the glands. Whereas in a circumcised child the glands will appear smooth with the meatus centered at the tip. To assess the glands and meatus the foreskin should be gently retracted, although in the uncircumcised male the foreskin is normally tight for the first 3 months. Use gentle traction to evaluate the degree of foreskin retraction and the meatal location and size (Ball, 2010). If the foreskin is not retractable there may be a phimosis, which is the presence of an abnormal ring of tissue distal to the glands that prevents retraction of the foreskin, which in turn does not allow visualization of the meatus.

Next, inspect the scrotum for size and symmetry and note the presence of rugae. If the scrotum is small without the presence of rugae it is an indication that the testicles are undescended. Palpate the scrotum for the presence of testes, noting that the scrotum should be loose and pendulous, and that the testes are equal in size. If your hands are cold while doing this you may elicit the cremasteric reflex, which is strong in the infant. This reflex pulls the testes up into the inguinal canal from exposure to cold, touch, or emotion. In order to avoid this be sure your hands are warm and palpate from the external inguinal ring down by placing your index finger and thumb over the inguinal canal in the groin and thus preventing the testicles from retracting into the abdomen. The testicles are purposely located outside the body in the scrotum and are suspended by the spermatic cord. The purpose of the scrotum is regulation of the temperature of the testes which expands and contracts in order to facilitate heat transfer. Body temperature can damage sperm and effect male fertility. When a male's testicles get cold, they are automatically pulled up and closer to the body. When the testicles are too warm, the spermatic cord, which is tightened by the cremasteric muscle, relaxes and gets longer, which lowers the testicles into the scrotum to keep them cooler. Assess the scrotum for swelling or edema; an enlarged or asymmetric scrotum may indicate an inguinal hernia or hydrocele. The testes are normally descended and are equal in size. The infant's testes normally measure approximately 10 mm in width and 15 mm in length. Be sure to note if the size changes when the patient cries. This is due to an increase in abdominal pressure. If the scrotal sac appears empty, search for the testicle along the inguinal canal and attempt to milk the testicle down.

Early to Late Childhood
A helpful technique when examining the genitalia of a young boy is placing the child sitting up in a cross-legged position on the table. Inspect the penis and palpate for any abnormalities, paying close attention to the cremasteric reflex. Be sure your hands are warm and start at the inguinal canal. Assess the scrotum and note if the testicles are descended. To assess the cremasteric reflex, simply scratch the medial aspect of the thigh. This will cause the testes to move upward. Be sure to exam the inguinal canal for swelling or tenderness, which may suggest an inguinal hernia. Be sure to gently retract the foreskin to inspect the glands for lesions and hygiene.

INGUINAL HERNIA: In older boys, inguinal hernias present with swelling in the inguinal canal, especially seen with straining.

Adolescence
The adolescent male genitalia exam follows the same procedure as an adult male. There are significant changes that take place during puberty. It is important to be familiar with the sexual maturity rating in boys and the five stages of sexual development. You will want to assign a maturity rating or Tanner staging when examining the patient (**Figure 14-4**). There is much variation in pubertal development of the male genitalia, from enlargement of the testes and scrotum to pubic hair growth. In many males pubic hair

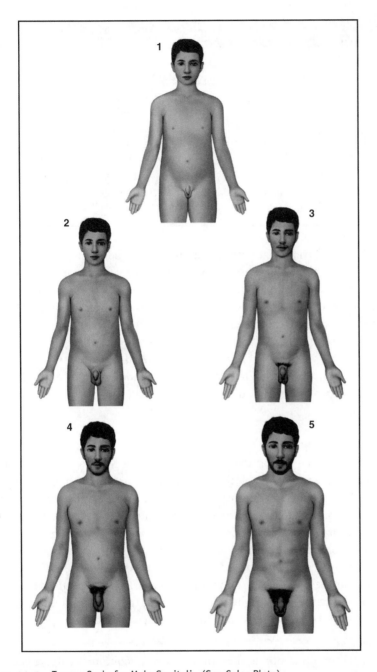

Figure 14-4   Tanner Scale for Male Genitalia (See Color Plate)

Source: Adapted from: Marshall, W.A., and Tanner, J.M. Variations in Pattern of Pubertal Changes in Girls. *Archives of Disease in Childhood*. June 1969, 44(235): 291–303. Marshall, W.A., and Tanner, J.M. Variations in the Pattern of Pubertal Changes in Boys. *Archives of Disease in Childhood*. February 1970, 45(239): 13–23.

TABLE 14–1 TANNER SCALE FOR BOYS		
Tanner Stage	Pubic Hair	Penis/Scrotum
1	None	Childlike
2	Sparse	Scrotum: reddened, thinner, larger. Penis: childlike
3	Darker, begins to curl	Penis length increases. Scrotum continues to enlarge and darken
4	Coarse, less curly than adult	Penis increases in length and circumference
5	Adult	Adult

growth forms a triangular pattern pointing to the abdomen toward the umbilicus. There is also an increase in body hair, from axillary hair to coarse hair on the arms, legs, and chest. There is darkening of the scrotal sac, roughening of the scrotal skin, and increase in penis length and width. The first signs of puberty take place between nine and thirteen years of age. The testicles increase in size first, followed by the growth of pubic hair, and finally, enlargement of the penis in both length and width occurs. It normally takes approximately three years to change from preadolescent to adult anatomy "with a range of 1.8 to 5 years" (Brinkley, 2003).

Penis

Inspection of Palpation

Inspect the penis, noting the skin and assessing for any signs of lesions, which can occur anywhere in the genitalia area. Assess the prepuce, or foreskin. If the patient is uncircumcised retract the foreskin to assess the glands. Note any lesions, such as warts or human papilloma virus (HPV), ulcers, erythema, or signs of inflammation. Inspect the skin at the tip of the penis and note the urethral meatus and its location. Gently compress the tip of the penis with your thumb and index finger. Assess for any discharge or drainage at the opening of the urethral meatus. There should be none. Be sure to retract the foreskin before continuing the examination. Next, palpate the shaft of the penis noting any tenderness or induration.

Scrotum

Inspect the scrotum, noting the skin and scrotal contours. Palpate each testicle and epididymis with your first two fingers and thumb. Hold the scrotum in the palm of your hand and gently feel each testicle. Note the size, shape, and consistency. The testicle is egg-shaped and movable. It feels rubbery with a smooth surface, like a hardboiled egg. The epididymis is on top and behind the testicle; it feels a bit softer. Swelling in the scrotum should be evaluated by translumination. Darken the room and shine a light behind the scrotum through the mass. If it is fluid, the light will appear as a red glow as it illuminates the scrotum. A firm, painless, hard area or enlarged testicle will need further evaluation.

Hernias and Inguinal Lymph Nodes

Inspect and palpate the inguinal and femoral areas. Instruct the patient to strain down or to cough to reveal a hernia. No bulges should be noted. Next, palpate the inguinal canal. To assess the right side, instruct the patient to shift his weight to the left leg. With your index finger, start by following the spermatic cord upward to the inguinal ligament until you feel a triangular slit like opening of the external inguinal ring. Gently admit your finger into the canal and ask the patient to bear down. Normally you will feel no change. Repeat on the left side. Finally, palpate the inguinal lymph nodes horizontally along the groin and the upper inner thigh.

Rectal Exam

The rectal exam is not normally performed as part of the traditional pediatric examination. If an internal rectal exam is necessary, it may be performed with the child in the side-lying position or the lithotomy position. Be sure to reassure the patient throughout the examination. Start the exam with a thorough inspection of the anus, noting any lesions, abrasions or fissures. Gently insert a gloved, lubricated index finger into the anus to perform the rectal examination.

Abnormal Findings of the Rectal Examination

ANAL TENDERNESS: May indicate infection or inflammation such as appendicitis or abscess.

ANAL SKIN TAGS: May indicate inflammatory bowel disease or condylomata acuminatum associated with human papilloma virus infection (HPV).

FISSURE: Commonly seen in children with constipation or rectal bleeding.

ANAL ABRASIONS OR TEARS: May be a sign of physical or sexual abuse.

Common Abnormalities of Male Genitalia

Conditions occurring in the infant include:

HYPOSPADIAS is one of the most common congenital abnormalities. It presents with abnormal opening of the urethral orifice on the ventral (under) side of the glans or shaft of the penis. The severity of hypospadias is graded upon the position of the urinary meatus and the extent of ventral penile angulation, or chordee. Circumcision should be avoided in all degrees of hypospadias so as to preserve the foreskin to optimize later surgical choices (Baskin, 2010).

CYPTORCHIDISM or undescended testes, occurs when there is failure of one or both or the testes to descend through the inguinal canal into the scrotum. The scrotum appears underdeveloped and the testes cannot be manipulated into the scrotum. (A retractile testes is out of the scrotum but can be milked down into the scrotum and eventually remain there.) Undescended testes is the most common genitourinary disorder in boys. Many descend spontaneously by six months to one year of age.

HYDROCELES is a collection of serous fluid in the scrotal sac, and is a nontender mass that overlie the testes and spermatic cord. It presents as a bulge or lump in the scrotum that often increases with activity and decreases with rest. The mass transilluminates with a pink or red glow. This fluid generally is reabsorbed spontaneously and no treatment is indicated.

INGUINAL HERNIA is a soft nontender mass or swelling in the inguinal area, scrotum or both. It increases and decreases in size with crying or straining. It does not transilluminate, as it includes abdominal contents rather then fluid. It does not resolve spontaneously but requires surgical repair.

PHIMOSIS presents with a tight pinpoint opening of the foreskin with inability to retract the foreskin to expose the glands penis. This is due to adhesions of the glands and inner layer of the foreskin. In young children, phimosis is a normal or physiologic finding and generally is retractable by four or five years of age. See **Figure 14-5**.

Conditions occurring in early to late childhood include:

PRECOCIOUS PUBERTY presents with an earlier than normal progression of sexual development including pubic hair growth, axillary hair and odor, and penis and testes enlargement with obvious pubertal changes. A multiplicity of conditions linked with excess androgens can cause this, including adrenal or pituitary tumors.

Common causes of painful testicle:

EPIDIDYMITIS refers to the inflammation of the epididymis, a densely coiled tube in which sperm mature and are transported from the testes to the vas deferens. The pain is often relieved with elevation (positive Phren's sign).

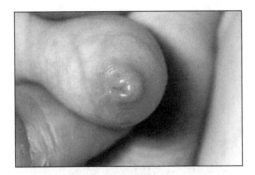

Figure 14-5 Phimosis

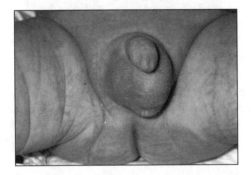

Figure 14-6 Undescended Testis

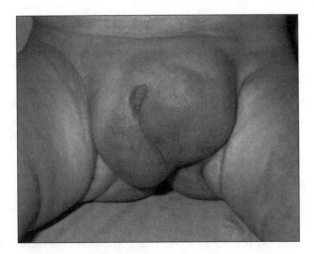

Figure 14-7 Bilateral Inguinal Hernia

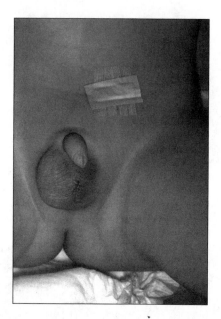

Figure 14-8 The bandage is the result of an operation that involved moving an undescended testis (testicle) from the groin to its correct position in the scrotum, which corrected this boy's cryptorchidism.

Urethral discharge may be present secondary to an STD such as gonorrhea or chlamydial infection. This is best treated with ice pack, elevation of the scrotum, and antibiotics.

ORCHITIS: Acute inflammation of the testis. Clinical presentation includes scrotal swelling, pain, and tenderness with erythema and shininess of the overlying skin. Treatment includes ice pack, nonsteroidal anti-inflammatories, and bed rest (Brenner & Ojo, 2010).

TESTICULAR TORSION: Presents with acute onset due to sudden twisting of the spermatic cord causing interruption of blood supply to the testis. This causes severe pain, and ischemia of the testes requiring emergency surgical intervention.

Conditions occurring in adolescence include:

GENITAL HERPES HSV-2 presents as a cluster of small vesicles with surrounding erythema. These vesicles are painful and erupt on the glands or foreskin and form superficial ulcers. The initial infection lasts seven to ten days and then remains dormant indefinitely. It will present with recurrent infection, although with milder symptoms.

GENITAL WARTS is the most common clinical manifestation of HPV. They present as soft, fleshy painless papules, some may be single or multiple or in a cauliflower like appearance. They occur on the shaft of the penis, behind the corona, or around the genital area. They can also present around the anus where they can grow into large grapelike clusters. They are transmitted through sexual activity.

GONORRHEA presents with a thick white, yellow, or green discharge from the tip of the penis, as well as pain or a burning sensation upon urination. This is transmitted through unprotected sexual intercourse and is treated with antibiotics.

CHLAMYDIA symptoms may be unnoticeable in men, although when they do present they include a whitish or watery discharge from the penis and dysuria when urinating. This STD is transmitted through unprotected intercourse and treated with antibiotics.

SYPHILIS presents as a painless red oval lesion, or chancre, that appears at the site where the bacteria entered the body, such as the penis or vagina. The chancre usually resolves within a few weeks without treatment. Secondary syphilis presents several weeks or months later and is characterized by a macularopapular rash that appears over the body, including the palms of the hands and soles of the feet. This disorder is treated with antibiotics. If untreated, it can eventually cause blindness and dementia.

Sample Charting for Male Genitalia Exam

INFANT: + pulses, without lymphadenopathy, uncircumcised prepuce, testes descended bilaterally, skin without erythema or lesions.

SCHOOL-AGE: + pulses, without lymphadenopathy, foreskin retracts easily, glans without lesions, testes descended bilaterally symmetric without masses or tenderness. Document Tanner stage.

ADOLESCENT: + pulses without lymphadenopathy, penis without lesions, inflammation or discharge. Scrotum: testes descended bilaterally, symmetric without masses or tenderness. Without sign of inguinal hernia (chart Tanner stage). Anus: no fissures, tears, or skin lesions in perianal area. (If internal exam: sphincter tone good, no prolapse, rectal walls smooth, no masses or tenderness).

The Female Reproductive System

Anatomy

External Genitalia

The external genitalia are the female reproductive structures that lie external to the vagina. They include the vulva or covering, the mons pubis, labia, and clitoris. The mons pubis is a fatty rounded area overlying the pubic symphysis. This area is covered with pubic hair after puberty. Two elongated hair-covered fatty skin folds running posterior from the mons pubis are the labia majora or 'larger lips.' The labia majora are the female counterpart to the male scrotum, which means they are derived from the same embryonic tissue. The labia majora encloses the labia minor or 'smaller lips.' These are two thin hair-free skin folds that are counterpart to the ventral penis. The labia minora encloses a recess called the vestibule. This area contains the external opening of the urethra. On both sides of the vaginal opening are two pea-size glands that are counterpart to the bulbourethral glands of the male. When a child reaches puberty, the Bartholin's gland and the Skene's gland release mucus into the vestibule that helps to keep it moist and lubricated during intercourse. Anterior to the vestibule is the clitoris or hill. It is a small protruding structure composed of erectile tissue that is counterpart to the penis of the male. It is hooded by a skin fold called the prepuce of the clitoris. This area is innervated with many sensory nerve endings sensitive to touch and becomes erect with blood during tactile stimulation, which contributes to female sexual arousal. Located between the pubic arch anteriorly is the perineum, which overlies the muscles of the pelvic outlet and posterior portion of the labia majora.

The vagina or sheath is a thin-walled tube approximately 8–10 cm in length in the adult female. It lies between the bladder and the rectum and serves as the birth canal during delivery of an infant as well as for menstrual flow. The wall of the vagina is highly distensible and is marked by transverse ridges or rugae. The pH of the vagina is normally acidic, which helps to keep the vagina infection free. At the distal end of the vaginal orifice is the hymen, which is mucosa that forms an incomplete partition in the vagina. This area tends to be very vascular and bleeds when it is ruptured during the first coitus. It may also rupture during sports activity.

Assessment Considerations: Subjective Information

Newborns and Infants
- Is the child experiencing any burning or pain with urination?
- Does the child cry or hold her genital area? Does she have any history of urinary tract infections?

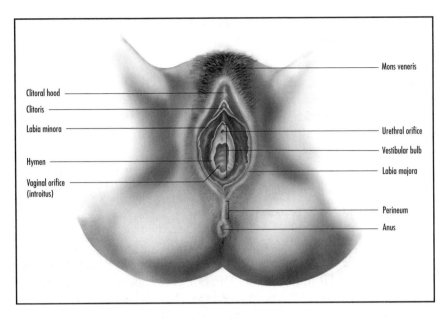

Mons veneris

Clitoral hood

Clitoris

Labia minora

Urethral orifice

Vestibular bulb

Hymen

Labia majora

Vaginal orifice
(introitus)

Perineum

Anus

Figure 14-9 Female External Reproductive Organs

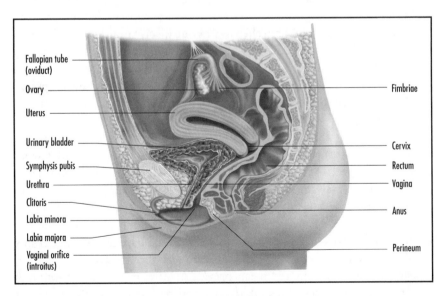

Fallopian tube
(oviduct)

Ovary

Fimbriae

Uterus

Urinary bladder

Cervix

Symphysis pubis

Rectum

Urethra

Vagina

Clitoris

Labia minora

Anus

Labia majora

Vaginal orifice
(introitus)

Perineum

Figure 14-10 Organs of the Female Reproductive System

- Are there any problems with the child's genital area, including redness, swelling, lesions, vaginal discharge, or itching?

Patients Older Than 2 Years of Age

- Has the child started toilet training? Where is she in the process? What steps is the parent taking to facilitate the process?
- Does the child take bubble baths? Bubble bath, foams, and gels cause changes in the vaginal pH level, which can lead to vaginal irritation and infections.
- Has the child had any issues with bed-wetting? How often is this happening? How is the parent handling this?

Preschoolers and Young School-Age Children

- Screen for sexual abuse. Ask the child directly if anyone has ever asked to touch her private area or actually touched her private area. Be sure to let the child know that it is okay to talk about this and that she has not been bad and is not to blame. This is a good time to reiterate that it is not okay for anyone to do this and that she should always tell an adult if this happens.
- Ask the parent if the child is touching her genitalia?

Preadolescents and Adolescents

Approach the adolescent patient in a nonjudgmental manner. Ask questions pertaining to sexual growth and development. Also address sexual activity and behavior. It is important to ask questions appropriate for the patient's age. The patient may be apprehensive about discussing these topics with you. Do not be too assertive in your questioning, but offer information on topics such as pubertal development and sexual changes the adolescent may expect. Ask questions pertaining to sexual growth and development by phrasing them in a non-judgmental way, such as, "when did you first?" rather than by asking, "do you?"

The topics for this age include changes in the patient's genitalia. Ask the patient if she has noticed any physical changes or if she knows what changes to expect. At 9 or 10 years of age, girls begin to develop breasts and pubic hair. Has she discussed these changes with her parents? Is there anyone special she can talk to about these issues? Has she had sexual education at school? Also discuss menstruation. Ask the patient if she has started her period yet. Review the process with the patient and answer any questions she may have. Ask her how she feels about getting her period. Ask her if she was prepared or surprised. Ask the patient about tampon use and hygiene. Discuss sexual activity and behavior. Ask the patient if she is dating, if she has a steady boyfriend or girlfriend, or if she has same-sex interest. Ask her if she has ever had intercourse or engaged in oral sex.

Ask her if she is using birth control, and ask what type of protection she is using. Assess her knowledge of sexually transmitted diseases such as chlamydia, genital herpes (HSV-2), HPV, gonorrhea, and HIV. Also screen for sexual abuse at this time. Finish by asking the patient if she has any questions or concerns.

FAMILY HISTORY: Is there a family history of congenital adrenal hyperplasia, which is the most common cause of pseudohermaphroditism or ambiguous genitalia. Also consider a history of maternal virilization in pregnancy, history of females who are childless or have amenorrhea or androgen insensitivity. Is there a history of consanguinity? (Hour, 2001).

Assessment Considerations: Objective Information

The physical assessment, including *inspection* and *palpation*, is discussed next (Bickley, 2003; Jarvis, 2008). All healthcare providers should be well aware of the normal female anatomy before assessing a female patient. Understanding what is normal will help you identify abnormalities. Generally, gynecologic problems are uncommon in young girls, inspection of the external genitalia and palpation of the breasts should be part of the routine physical examination (Emans, Laufer, Goldstein, 2005). For the older child and adolescent patient, the genital exam can be very stressful. Be sensitive to this when approaching the patient.

The Newborn Period and Infancy

During this period, the genitalia may be enlarged due to the effects of the maternal estrogen. This will diminish during the first year of life. The labia majora and minora have a dull pink color in light-skinned infants and may be hyperpigmented in the dark-skinned infants (Brinkley, 2003). In the first few weeks after delivery there may be a milky white blood-tinged discharge secondary to maternal hormones. Inspect the female genitalia with the infant in the supine position. Assess all structures noting color, size, shape, as well as any abnormalities such as lesions, rashes, and bruising. Assess the hymen, which in infancy appears as a thick structure covering the vaginal opening. You should still be able to assess the opening for any vaginal discharge. Use a relaxed approach and include an explanation as you move through the examination. Always use a good light source. Most children can be examined in the supine or frog leg position.

Examples of Abnormal Findings During the Newborn Period and Infancy

AMBIGUOUS GENITALIA: Masculinization of the female external genitalia. This is a rare condition that is caused by disorders of the endocrine system.

SKIN IRRITATIONS: Due to poor hygiene, pest inhabitants, and infections.

Early and Late Childhood

The external genitalia remains unestrogenized with the labia majora and minora flattened out and the hymenal membrane thin, translucent, and vascular until the female reaches puberty. As puberty progresses, the estrogenization of the vaginal mucosa and lengthening and enlargement of the uterus occur with increasing estrogen exposure. As a result of mucus from the estrogenized mucosa of the vagina and desquamantion of epithelaial cells, leukorrhea is observed, which is a whitish mucoid discharge that starts before menarche and may continue for several years.

Normally, a speculum exam is not necessary for this age. Approach the child in a gentle, nonthreatening manner. Have the patient change into an examination gown with undergarments off and the child in the supine, frog-leg position. Assess the genitalia and inspect all structures, noting color, size, and shape, as well as any abnormalities such as lesions, rashes, and bruising. Assess for pubic hair. Next, assess the inner structures by separating the labia majora. Note the appearance of the labia minora, vaginal opening, and the urethral meatus. Also assess the hymen, which after infancy appears as a thin, translucent structure. Examine the vaginal opening for discharge, lesions, labial adhesions, onset of puberty, and hygiene. Be aware of vaginal bleeding that may be an indication of accidental trauma, sexual abuse, or foreign body. In addition purulent or malodorous discharge should be evaluated for infection and/or foreign body. Bruising or abrasions of the external genitalia may be due to benign causes such as accidental trauma during play or may be do to masturbation. Be aware of any signs of sexual abuse, especially if you have concerns with a patient's history. In the majority of cases, the examination will be unremarkable even with a known history of abuse.

Examples of Abnormal Findings During Early and Late Childhood

PRECOCIOUS PUBERTY: This is defined as the appearance of any secondary sexual characteristics (breast development or pubic hair) before 8 years of age in girls and 9 years of age in boys (pubic hair development) (Pineyard & Zipf, 2005).

VAGINAL DISCHARGE: In early childhood, assess for use of scented soaps, bath soaps, foreign body, and sexually transmitted diseases from sexual abuse.

VAGINAL BLEEDING: Assess for infection, abrasions, foreign body, trauma, sexual abuse, and early menses.

Adolescence

The external genital exam for an adolescent patient is usually the same as for the school-age child. For the nonpelvic genital examination, with the

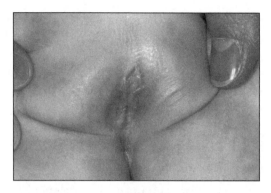

Figure 14-11   Vulval Adhesions in a Child

adolescent in a supine, frog-leg position, inspect all structures, noting color, size, and shape, as well as any abnormalities such as lesions, rashes, and bruising. Note sexual maturity by assessing pubic hair and breast development. Hymenal changes due to estrogen may also be noted. Be mindful that there may be a large difference in the age of patients when they start and finish puberty. Normally, the first signs of puberty are the development of breast buds; however, pubic hair may appear earlier in some patients. These first signs can appear as early as 7 years of age. You may also notice the patient growing taller and her hips widening. Be aware of any signs of sexual abuse, especially if you have any concerns with the patient's history.

If a pelvic exam is necessary, you would follow the same procedure you would use on an adult patient. Be sure to approach the patient in a gentle

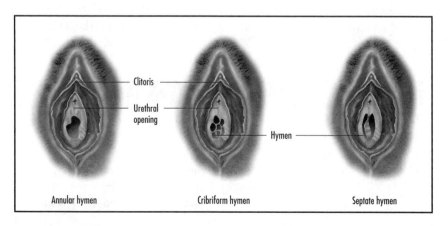

Figure 14-12   Hymens

manner if a pelvic exam needs to be performed. Explaining the steps while reassuring the patient may help to put her at ease. Assure her of privacy and confidentiality. You may want to examine the patient without the parent present. This will allow for an open discussion that may not happen if the parent is in attendance. If this is the adolescent's first pelvic examination, a healthcare provider with experience in performing pelvic examinations is encouraged, according to the American Congress of Obstetricians and Gynecologists.

Examples of Abnormal Findings During Adolescence

AMENORRHEA: Absence of menses in adolescence may be primary or secondary. Primary amenorrhea is defined as absence of menarche by age 14.5 in association with no growth or development of secondary sexual characteristics, or absence of menses by age 16 when secondary sexual characteristics and growth are present. Secondary amenorrhea is defined as cessation of menstrual periods 6 months, or 3 cycles after menstruation has begun (Ball & Bindler, 2008, p. 1243).

DELAYED PUBERTY: A delay should be suspected in girls without pubic hair by 13 years of age.

VAGINAL DISCHARGE: In adolescents, vaginal discharge should be assessed as in the adult patient. The assessment would include testing for sexually transmitted diseases, obtaining wet mounts for yeast and bacterial vaginosis, and foreign body.

Sample Charting for Female Pediatric Genitalia Exam

EXTERNAL: + pulses bilaterally, no lymphadenopathy, labia majoria pink with smooth surface, labia minora light pink in color (color changes to dark pink as tissues becomes estrogenized during puberty), uretheral meatus

TABLE 14–2 TANNER SCALE FOR GIRLS		
Tanner Stage	Pubic Hair	Breasts
1	None	None
2	Sparse	Small breast buds
3	Darker, begins to curl	Breasts and nipples enlarged
4	Coarse, less curly than adult	Continued breast development
5	Adult triangle	Mature; nipple projects

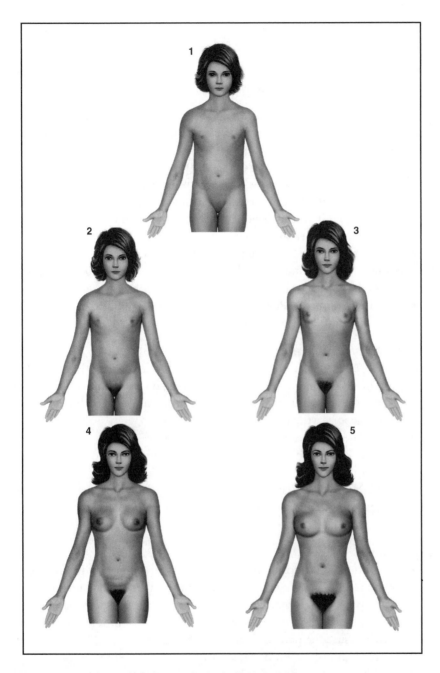

Figure 14-13 Tanner Scale for Female Genitalia Figure 11-17

Source: Adapted from: Marshall, W.A., and Tanner, J.M. Variations in Pattern of Pubertal Changes in Girls. *Archives of Disease in Childhood*. June 1969, 44(235): 291–303. Marshall, W.A., and Tanner, J.M. Variations in the Pattern of Pubertal Changes in Boys. *Archives of Disease in Childhood*. February 1970, 45(239): 13–23.

midline, vaginal introitus tissue moist, color pink. No lesions, no discharge, no erythema or swelling noted. No pubic hair (chart Tanner staging).

Pelvic Exam

The following exam is adapted from Jarvis (2008).

- Inspect the external genitalia thoroughly, noting skin color and hair distribution. Assess for delayed puberty, hygiene, excoriations, swelling, lesions, nodules, or rash.
- Palpate the nodes and pulses. Separate the labia majora and inspect the clitoris, labia minora, urethral opening, vaginal opening, perineum area, and anus. Assess for excoriations, swelling, lesions, nodules, rash, and vaginal discharge. Palpate the Skene and Bartholin glands for tenderness or enlargement.
- Using a properly sized vaginal speculum, inspect the vagina and cervix, noting the vaginal mucosa and the color, size, and position of the cervix. Assess the cervix for inflammation, redness, discharge, and lesions.
- Obtain specimens: Pap, gonorrhea culture/chlamydia, potassium hydroxide test, and saline wet mounts (if necessary).

Sample Charting for Pelvic Exam

- *EXTERNAL*: + pulses bilaterally, no lymphadenopathy, labia majora prominent and hair covered, labia minora, dark pink in color, clitoris nl., uretheral meatus midline, vaginal introitus, pink without lesions, discharge, or erythema or odor.
- *INTERNAL*: + rugae, no discharge, no lesions
- *CERVIX*: Pink, scant discharge (clear/white at cervical os, no odor, no lesions)
- *ANUS*: No fissure, skin lesions in perianal area (If internal exam performed: sphincter tone good, no rectal prolapse, rectal walls smooth, no masses or tenderness)

Rectal Exam

The rectal exam is not normally performed as part of the traditional pediatric examination. If a patient or parent of the patient complains of rectal bleeding or pain, an internal rectal exam may be necessary. It may be performed with the child in the side-lying position or the lithotomy position. Be sure to reassure the patient throughout the examination. Start the exam with a thorough inspection of the anus, noting any lesions, abrasions, or fissures. Gently insert a gloved, lubricated index finger into the anus to perform the rectal examination.

Examples of Abnormal Findings During the Rectal Exam

ANAL TENDERNESS: May indicate infection or inflammation such as appendicitis or abscess

ANAL SKIN TAGS: May indicate inflammatory bowel disease or condylomata acuminatum associated with HPV infection

FISSURE: Commonly seen in children with constipation or rectal bleeding

ANAL ABRASIONS OR TEARS: May be a sign of physical or sexual abuse

Sample Charting for a Normal Rectal Exam

ANUS: No fissure, tears, or skin lesions in perianal area; sphincter tone good; no rectal prolapse; rectal walls smooth; no masses or tenderness.

Case Study: Girl Presenting with Vaginal Symptoms

Amanda is an 11-year-old female who comes into your office with the complaint of vaginal discharge, redness, and pruritus for the past 2 weeks. Her mother describes the discharge as thick and white in color. She tells you that Amanda has been well, has not taken any antibiotics, and is very active with gymnastics. She denies any concerns regarding sexual abuse.

On examination, you observe that Amanda is at Tanner stage 2 for breast development. On vaginal examination, you observe scant mucoid discharge and erythema around the introitus. The hymen is intact, and the rectal exam is normal.

Questions

1. What additional history do you need to obtain?
2. What would you include in your differential diagnosis for prepubescent vulvovaginitis?
3. What pubertal changes would you expect to see in a girl Amanda's age?

Answers

1. Additional history regarding recent streptococcal respiratory infection of a family member is relevant, as it can lead to vaginitis. Questions regarding hygiene are important as well. Due to the anatomic location of the vagina and the anus, the lack of protective pubic hair, the lack of labial fat pads, and the lack of estrogenization, the vulvar

skin is more susceptible to irritation and easily irritated by tight clothing. The use of bubble baths may contribute to vulvovaginitis. The presence of sexual abuse and sexually transmitted disease should be explored as well, even though the concern was previously denied.

2. Differential diagnosis includes leukorrhea, which is physiologic and should not be confused with vulvovaginitis. Leukorrhea is due to the effect of estrogen on the vaginal mucosa, particularly in prepubescent females. Foreign body may produce increased discharge, as well as a foul-smelling discharge. Vulvar and rectal pruritus occur secondary to the itching associated with pinworms. Increased vaginal discharge is associated with sexually transmitted disease if the child has been sexually abused.

3. Pubertal changes you would expect to observe include breast budding (thelarche), which occurs on average between 9 and 13 years of age. This is followed by the appearance of pubic hair (adrenarche), which is related to adrenal development. Menarche occurs next, generally 1.5 to 2.5 years after thelarche. Girls experience a continuous increase in proportion of fat to total body mass during puberty. Females also experience rapid linear growth after the onset of thelarche, and height reaches its peak approximately 1 year later. Final height is determined when hormonal factors close the epiphyseal plates in the long bones (Burns, Dunn, Brady, Starr, & Blosser, 2004).

References

Ball, J. Binder, R. (2008). *Pediatric nursing*. Upper Saddle River, NJ: Pearson.

Ball, J., Binder, R., Cowen, K (2010). *Child health nursing*. Upper Saddle River, NJ: Pearson.

Barkauskas, V., Stoltenberg-Allen, K., Baumann, L., & Darling-Fisher, D. (1998). *Health and physical assessment* (2nd ed.). St. Louis, MO: Mosby-Year Book.

Baskin, L. (2010). Hypospadias. Retrieved from http://www.uptodate.com

Bickley, L. (2003). *Bates' guide to physical examination and history taking* (8th ed.). New York: Lippincott Williams & Wilkins.

Brenner, J. & Ojo, A. (2010). Causes of scrotal pain in children and adolescents. Retrieved from http://www.uptodate.com

Burns, C., Dunn, A., Brady, M., Starr, N., & Blosser, C. (2004). *Pediatric primary care: A handbook for nurse practitioners* (3rd ed.). St. Louis, MO: Saunders.

Emans, S.J, Laufer, M.R., Goldstein, D.P., (2005). Pediatric and Adolescent Gynecology, (5th ed.). Philadelphia: Lippincott Williams & Wilkins,

Hour, C.P., Levitsky, S.L. (2010). Evaluation of infant with ambiguous genitalia. Retrieved from http://www.uptodate.com

Jarvis, C. (2008). *Physical examination and health assessment* (5th ed.). St. Louis, MO: Elsevier.

Shoemaker, C. (2010). Circumcision: Benefits and risks. Retrieved from http://www.uptodate.com

Pineyerd, B. & Zipf, W. B. (2005). Puberty- timing is everything. *Journal of Pediatric Nursing, 20*(2), 75–82.

Resources

Marieb, E. (1998). *Human anatomy and physiology* (3rd ed.). California: The Benjamin Cummings Publishing Co.

National Cervical Cancer and HPV Coalition. (2010). New ACOG guidelines for 2010. Retrieved January, 21, 2010, from http://www.inspire.com/groups/national-cervical-cancer-coalition/discussion/new-acgo-guidelines-for-2010/

Examination of the Breasts and Axillae

Rosemarie A. Fuller

Breast Anatomy

The breast consists of three types of tissue: glands containing the lobes, alveoli, and ducts, which are involved in lactation; supporting structures, including connective and lymphatic tissue, blood vessels, and nerves; and fat tissue, which helps give the breast its form. Each breast is divided into 15–20 lobules with branching ducts and alveoli. Myoepithelial cells surround the glands and eject milk into the ducts.

The breasts, supported by Cooper's ligaments, are located between the second and sixth ribs on either side of the sternum at the midaxillary line. The inframammary crease, beneath the breasts, marks the area where the breasts meet the torso. The upper, outer corner of the breast is called the tail of Spence and extends into the axilla. Breast size is determined by age, amount of fat tissue, history of pregnancy and lactation, elasticity, and heredity.

Anatomic components and functions of the breasts include the following:

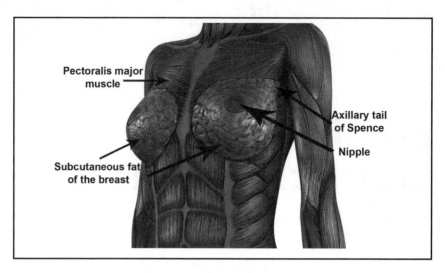

Figure 15-1(a) Anatomy of the Breast (See Color Plate)
Source: ©Sebastian Kaulitzki/Shutterstock, Inc.

AREOLA: Slightly raised, pigmented area behind the nipple containing small protuberances called Montgomery glands, which provide lubrication for the nipple.

NIPPLE: Consists of erectile tissue, which protrudes at the tip of the breast and is surrounded by the areola. Collecting sacs called ampullae are located behind the areola and, when contracted by the smooth muscle surrounding them, eject milk during lactation. The nipple may be flat, protuberant, or inverted. Inverted nipples are fairly common, occurring in about 20% of the population, including men; they are either a hereditary condition or due to scar tissue as a result of trauma to the nipple.

NERVES: The breasts are innervated by the fourth through sixth intercostal nerves and sensory fibers predominantly from the autonomic nervous system. Somatic nerves arise from the supraclavicular and thoracic inter-costal branches and run toward the nipple.

MUSCLES: Underlying the breasts are two muscles—the pectoralis major, which extends to the upper arm, and the pectoralis minor, which extends to the axilla.

LYMPHATIC SYSTEM: Lymphatic drainage is extensive in the breast and is directed toward the axillae. The central lymph nodes are the most fre-quently palpable, are located in the axillae, and receive lymphatic flow

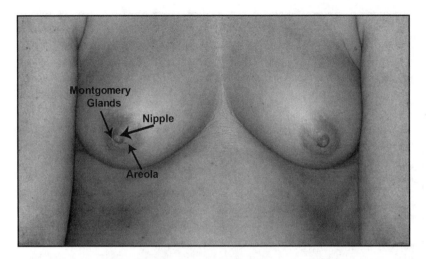

Figure 15-1(b) Anatomy of the Nipple (See Color Plate)

from three other chains: the anterior chain, which drains the anterior chest wall and the breast; the posterior chain, which drains the posterior chest wall; and the lateral chain, which drains the arm. From the central nodes, lymphatic fluid drains toward the infra- and supraclavicular nodes.

BLOOD SUPPLY: Comes from the interior mammary artery to the subscapular, central, and deep axillary arteries.

MALE BREAST: Flat, with a slightly protuberant nipple. Underlying the nipple is a disc of tissue. If this disc enlarges, it produces gynecomastia, or enlargement of the male breast, under the influence of estrogen and testosterone. This is referred to as pubertal gynecomastia and has an onset between ages 10 and 12 years of age, and peaks between 13 and 14 years of age and Tanner stage 3. It generally regresses within 18 months and is uncommon after 17 years of age (Braunstein, 2010).

Assessment Considerations: Subjective Information

Infants

- Did the mother report whitish discharge from either of the infant's breasts in the newborn period, or note that the infant's breasts were enlarged? This is referred to as "witch's milk."

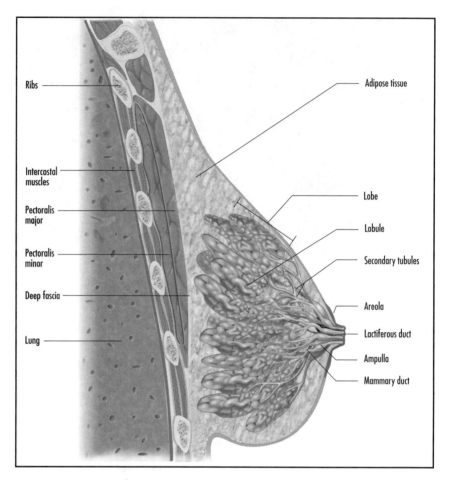

Figure 15-2(a) Anatomy of the Female Breast

School-Age Children and Adolescents

- Has the child noted any changes in the breast, asymmetry in breast development, or breast tenderness? Developing breasts may appear asymmetric and be sensitive to touch. The child may also report a unilateral firm disc-like area of tissue under the areola. This is a breast bud and typically heralds the onset of puberty or the larche.

Family History

- Is there a family history of breast cancer, particularly in the mother or sister?

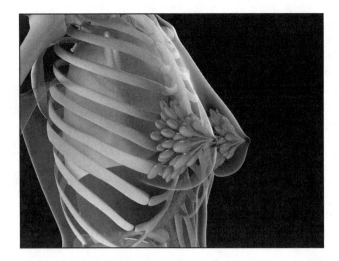

Figure 15-2(b)   Anatomy of the Female Breast

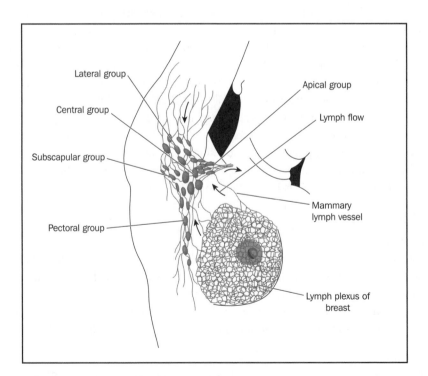

Figure 15-3   Axillary Lymph Nodes (See Color Plate)

Source: © Blamb/ShutterStock, Inc.

- Is there a history of nipple discharge or retraction?
- Is there a history of fibrocystic disease or history of breast surgery?
- Is there a history of congenital adrenal hyperpasia, which is the most common cause of pseudohermaphroditism?
- Is there a history of maternal virilization, or females who are childless, or have amenorrhea, or adrogen insensitivity?
- Is there a history of consanguinity? (Hour, 2010)

Review of Systems

Review any physical changes in a young girl 9 to 10 years of age, which are the signs of puberty. They can include a growth spurt, breast development, axillary hair growth, as well as the onset of menstruation. In addition, review problems such as endocrine disorders.

Breast Development

Breast development begins at about 5 weeks of gestation with formation of the mammary ridges, which are bands of tissue that extend on both sides of the embryo from the upper to lower extremities. At 16 weeks of gestation, lines of secretory alveoli begin to form. By 28 weeks of gestation, maternal hormones enter the fetal circulation, and differentiation of lobules and alveoli occurs. Most of this line disintegrates, but the section that persists forms about 20 pairs of buds, which become the lactiferous sinuses, ducts, and alveoli of the lobes of the breast. Areas of the mammary line that do not disintegrate may persist as accessory nipples after birth. These nipples may be seen anywhere along the site of the mammary line, vary in appearance, and excrete a small amount of milk, called witch's milk, which may be noted in female as well as male babies. Persistence of tissue along this line may also form accessory breasts.

Changes with Age

Newborns

By the time a female infant is born, a nipple and the beginnings of the ductal system have formed. Breast changes continue throughout the lifespan, with lobes (small subdivisions of breast tissue) developing first. During pregnancy, maternal hormones cross the placenta and may cause slight breast enlargement and excretion of milk in both the male and female newborn.

Adolescents

During puberty, mammary glands begin to proliferate under the influence of estrogen. Female sexual development, including breast maturation, begins at about 8 years of age and continues until about 13 years. The growth spurt seen in adolescence begins at about 9 to 10 years of age and corresponds to the appearance of the prepubertal breast. In this stage, the breast is flat with slight elevation of the nipple. As development of secondary sexual characteristics begins, breast buds arise and the areola begins to enlarge. Differentiation of the breast tissue and the areola is then noted as the areola forms a secondary mound above the level of the breast. As the breast matures, the areola becomes absorbed into the breast itself and the nipple projects outward. Along with breast development pubic hair begins to appear and spread. Axillary hair appears about 2 years after pubic hair. Menarche usually occurs at the peak of the growth spurt, around 13 years of age. This progression varies between adolescents and populations; African American women may move more quickly through the stages compared to Caucasian women. Breast asymmetry may be noted during puberty and is generally temporary.

The mature breast is soft, but may feel nodular to palpation, particularly around the time of menstruation in response to hormonal changes. The breasts may enlarge and become painful at this time.

During pregnancy, the thyroid gland and breasts enlarge; the nipples darken and become more erectile. Montgomery glands become more prominent, as do veins in the breasts. A yellowish discharge, colostrum, may be expressed from the nipple.

Hormonal Influence

Secondary sexual characteristics are under the influence of the hypothalamic-pituitary-gonadal axis. This axis regulates production of gonadal steroids and maintains a negative feedback mechanism in response to steroid levels. The hypothalamus is a small hollow structure deep in the brain that releases vasopressin during stress and gonadotropin-releasing hormone (GnRH) during puberty. GnRH is released to the pituitary gland, a small pea-shaped structure just under the hypothalamus. Release of luteinizing hormone (LH) from the pituitary stimulates release of estrogen and testosterone from the ovaries. Follicle-stimulating hormone (FSH) released from the pituitary inhibits the production of these gonadal steroids.

Assessment of the Breasts and Axillae

Observation

The techniques used in assessing the breasts apply to the female as well as the male child. The young child's breasts should be observed for symmetry, dimpling, puckering, or masses. In an adolescent with mature breast development, examine with the young woman in the following additional positions: arms down at sides, hands on hips, hands clasped above the

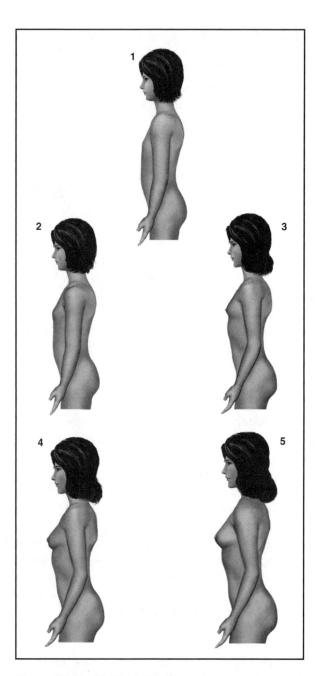

Figure 15-4 Tanner Staging for Female Breast

Source: Adapted from: Marshall, W.A., and Tanner, J.M. Variations in Pattern of Pubertal Changes in Girls. *Archives of Disease in Childhood*. June 1969, 44(235): 291–303. Marshall, W.A., and Tanner, J.M. Variations in the Pattern of Pubertal Changes in Boys. *Archives of Disease in Childhood*. February 1970, 45(239): 13–23.

head, and hands on the knees while leaning forward. Inspect the breasts for symmetry; note any swelling, edema, redness, or warmth, which indicates inflammation. Note lymphatic draining and swelling at the sites of the lymph nodes. Inspect the nipples for symmetry and drainage. As the adolescent lifts her arms and then pushes her hands together, note symmetry of movement, dimpling, and puckering.

The development of breast tissue in the adolescent should be assessed by using the Tanner maturity rating:

- *STAGE 1*: In this prepubertal stage, small elevated nipples are observed.
- *STAGE 2*: Breast budding starts at around 10–11 years of age. Initially, breast buds may be noted only on one side. Pubic hair begins to grow at this stage, and axillary hair follows in about 2 years.
- *STAGE 3*: The breast and nipple enlarge with no demarcation between them at around 12 years of age. This corresponds with the peak of the growth spurt, and menarche often occurs at this point at around 10–12 years of age.
- *STAGE 4*: The breast mound is distinct from the nipple and areola at around 13–14 years of age.
- *STAGE 5*: The mature breast is seen, with projection of the nipple by around 18 years of age (Tanner, 1962).

Palpation

To facilitate palpation, the child should lie in a supine position with the arm raised and a flat towel under the side to be examined. Palpate each breast in either a "spokes of a wheel" pattern or in concentric circles until the entire breast has been palpated. The breasts may have a lumpy texture due to the presence of the lobes underneath the skin, or they may have a nodular texture. Palpate the entire breast as well as the axillae for nodes or masses. If appreciated, they should be described in terms of location, size, shape, consistency, contours, and mobility. Small, well-circumscribed, moveable nodes are normal; however, hard, irregularly shaped nodules fixed to the underlying tissue, and dimpling or flattening of the breast contour are associated with malignancy.

Milk production in a woman unrelated to pregnancy or lactation is termed nonpuerperal galactorrhea. It may result from medications or hormonal influences, particularly of the pituitary gland.

The male breast should also be observed for lumps, swelling, intactness of skin, rashes, signs of infection, or discoloration such as acanthosis nigricans. Acanthosis nigricans is a skin disorder characterized by brownish-black discoloration in the neck, groin, or under the breasts; it is associated with diabetes or malignancy. The nipple should also be gently compressed to assess for discharge.

Breast Self-Examination

Adolescents approximately 20 years of age should be instructed in breast self-examination (American Cancer Society, 2010). This should be performed just after menses or at a consistent time each month. The child should become familiar with the feel of her own breasts. The American Cancer Society endorses the following method for breast self-examination. It is different from previous recommendations in hopes of increasing the chances of a woman identifying an abnormal mass.

While standing in front of a mirror, the woman should press her hands firmly on her hips and look at her breasts for any changes of size, shape, contour, or dimpling, or changes in the skin of the nipple or breast. She should then lie down with the arm of the breast to be examined placed behind her head. In this position, the breast is easier to feel. She should feel for lumps in the breast using the pads of her fingers and applying three intensities of touch: She should first palpate lightly to feel the tissue closest to the skin, then a little more deeply, and finally more deeply still to feel tissue next to the ribs and chest wall. The woman should feel the breast in an up and down pattern, moving from the underarm down the chest wall, inward toward the sternum, upward to the collarbone. The axillae should be felt with the arm only slightly raised to avoid tightening the tissue (American Cancer Society, 2010).

Suggested Write-up of the Breast Exam

INFANT: Breasts are slightly enlarged, nipples flat, small areola, no discharge noted.

SCHOOL-AGE TO PREADOLESCENT: Tanner 2 with bilateral breast buds. No palpable breast masses or nodules. No discharge or tenderness. Document Tanner stage.

ADOLESCENT: Tanner 4, breasts without skin dimpling or retractions. No palpable breast masses or nodules. No discharge or tenderness. Document Tanner stage.

 Red Flags

- Firm, unmovable masses in the breasts, especially accompanied by dimpling.
- Palpable lymph nodes, particularly in the supraclavicular area, may be a sign of lymphoma.

■ Polycystic ovary syndrome is a condition characterized by amenorrhea, infertility, ovarian cysts, alopecia, hirsutism, obesity, and skin tags. The underlying pathophysiology is the production of large amounts of testosterone, preventing release of ova from the ovaries. The condition is associated with a health risk of diabetes and heart disease if untreated.

Case Study: Girl Presenting with Asymmetric Breast Development

A mother brings her 13-year-old daughter to your office. The presenting complaint is that one of the girl's breasts, which are still developing, seems bigger than the other. The mother states that the daughter sustained a mild injury in soccer practice in which the soccer ball struck her in the left breast (the smaller breast). The child's developmental history is otherwise noncontributory.

As you perform an examination, you find no signs of trauma or injury to the breast. The child is at Tanner stage 2 and has completed her growth spurt; she has not yet begun to menstruate.

Question

What would you discuss with this mother and daughter regarding pubertal development?

Answer

The first visible sign of sexual maturation in the female is breast buds. During this stage, asymmetric breast development is common. This stage is followed by the growth of pubic hair. Menarche occurs approximately 2 years after breast development starts and after the adolescent growth spurt. During the growth spurt, acceleration in height and weight is not uniform. Generally, weight begins to increase first, followed in several months by an increase in height. In females, the adolescent growth spurt accompanies the first signs of puberty (pubic hair and breast development).

References

American Cancer Society. (2010). *Detailed guide: Breast cancer*. Retrieved from http://www.cancer.org/Cancer/BreastCancer/DetailedGuide/index.

Braunstein, G. (2010). Epidemiology and pathogenesis of gynecomastia. Retrieved from http://www.uptodate.com

Hour, C. P. & Levitsky, S. L. (2010). Evaluation of infant with ambiguous genitalia. Retrieved from http://www.uptodate.com

Tanner, J. M. (1962). *Growth at adolescence*. Oxford, UK: Blackwell Scientific taken from *Jarvis Physical Examination & Health Assessment* (5th ed.). Saunders.

Resources

Hale, T., & Hartmann, P. (2007). *Textbook of human lactation.* Amarillo, TX: Hale Publishers.

Jarvis, C. (2000). *Physical examination and health assessment* (3rd ed.). Philadelphia: Saunders.

Lawrence, R., & Lawrence, R. (2005). *Breastfeeding: A guide for the medical profession* (6th ed.). Philadelphia: Elsevier.

Sadler, T. W. (2009). *Langman's medical embryology: North American edition* (11th ed.). Philadelphia: Lippincott Williams & Wilkins.

Integration of the Examination: Putting It All Together

An Integrated Examination of the Infant

The previous chapters have discussed the examination of each system individually, addressing the assessment techniques of inspection, palpation, percussion, and auscultation. Integration of the physical examination incorporates these four assessment techniques in coordination with the sequencing of the exam.

When performing a physical examination on an infant, the baby should be wearing only a diaper. There is no specific order that should be followed; instead, *seize the opportunity* and examine the part of the body that is most accessible and that will cause the least amount of disruption. For example, if the baby is lying quietly over the mother's shoulder, take this opportunity to listen to lung sounds and heart sounds while observing for respiratory excursion, as well as inspecting the skin and the back. Auscultating the heart and lung sounds in a quiet baby allows for clearer interpretation of any abnormal heart sounds or adventitious lung sounds. Throughout the exam, observe the infant's alertness, response to handling, and

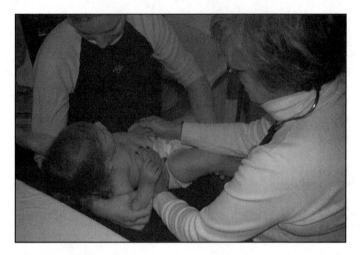

Figure 16-1   Palpating the Abdomen

ability to be quieted and/or consoled. Note the quality of the cry and the parent's responsiveness and ability to quiet and comfort the baby. It is important to have the parent nearby, not only to reassure the infant, but also so you can observe the nature of their interaction.

After listening to heart and lung sounds, it may be more advantageous to continue the exam with the child on the table, as a young infant is generally not fearful when placed on the examination table. Before placing your hands on the baby's skin, be sure they are warmed. Be gentle and use a soft touch. Avoid abrupt movements, as they may startle the infant.

The integrated exam of the infant incorporates assessment of the skin into each system. This assessment of the skin includes inspection for color, degree of uniformity, cyanosis or pallor, hydration, rash or inflammation, pigmentation, nevi, jaundice, texture, turgor, lanugo, temperature, and edema. The following exam is described in an approachable order that causes the least amount of crying and/or discomfort for the infant

Chest and Lungs

- Inspect the thorax for size, symmetry, and respiratory excursion, noting retractions, tugging, or stridor.
- Inspect the thorax for distance between nipples, extranumerary nipples, and a prominent or depressed sternum.
- Inspect the posterior thorax for musculoskeletal development and spinal abnormalities.
- Palpate the anterior chest for masses, tenderness, and temperature.

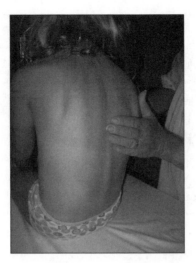

Figure 16-2   Palpation and Assessment of the Skin

- Palpate the nipples for breast tissue.
- Palpate the posterior chest, including spinous processes, for masses, tenderness, and temperature.
- Palpate the chest for tactile fremitus in the crying infant.
- Auscultate the anterior chest for adventitious sounds.
- Auscultate the posterior chest for adventitious sounds.

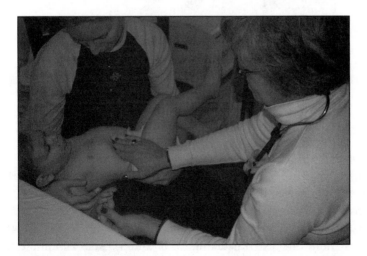

Figure 16-3   Palpation of the Liver

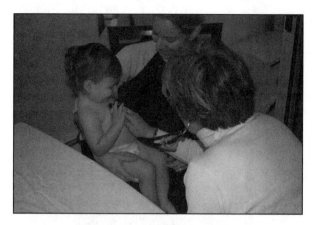

Figure 16-4 Introducing the Stethoscope

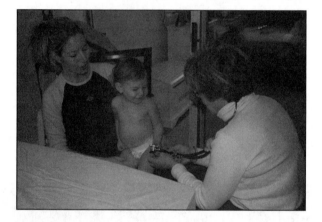

Figure 16-5 Introducing the Stethoscope

Heart

- Inspect for general observation of cyanosis and clubbing of the nail beds of fingers and toes.
- Inspect the chest for pulsations, heaves, and lifts.
- Palpate the precordium for the point of maximum impulse (PMI).
- Auscultate the heart, listening for S_1 and S_2. Also auscultate for any splitting, murmurs, rubs, or possibly S_3 or S_4.

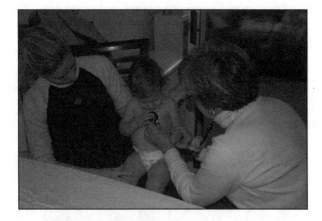

Figure 16-6   Introducing the Stethoscope

Abdomen

- Inspect for size and contour, noting scaphoid or distended appearance, and also noting pulsations.
- Inspect the umbilicus, noting the presence of vessels—one vein and two arteries (if a neonate).
- Auscultate all four quadrants for bowel sounds.
- Lightly palpate all four quadrants for muscle tone and distention.
- Palpate more deeply, noting the size of the liver, spleen, and possible masses.
- Percuss the abdomen, assessing for the size of the liver and spleen, noting areas of tympany versus dullness.
- Palpate the inguinal area for lymphadenopathy.
- Palpate for femoral pulses, checking for symmetry in pulse pressure.

Lower Extremities

- Inspect the legs for movement, size, shape, alignment, lesions, and color, noting any color change or swelling at joint areas.
- Inspect the feet, noting the number of toes, how toenails are cut, alignment, longitudinal arch, lesions, and cleanliness. Inspect between the toes for skin breakdown or rash.
- Inspect muscles for bulk, contour, symmetry, and strength.
- Palpate the dorsalis pedis pulse if possible. Also palpate the feet and legs for tenderness and temperature, and put the joints through passive range of motion.

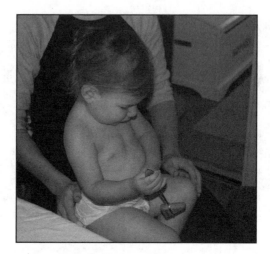

Figure 16-7 Introducing the Reflex Hammer

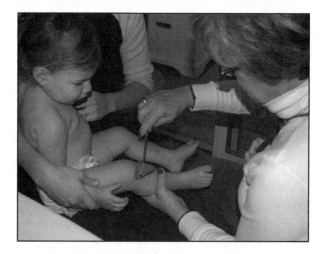

Figure 16-8 Patella Reflex

- Using your reflex hammer, elicit the plantar reflex and the Achilles and patellar reflexes bilaterally.
- Assess the hips using the Barlow and Ortolani maneuvers to detect hip dislocation.

Upper Extremities

- Inspect the hands, noting the number and configuration of the fingers. Also note how the fingernails are cut and their cleanliness.

- Inspect the palms for palmar creases.
- Inspect the arms for size, shape, movement, color, and lesions, noting any color change or swelling at joint areas.
- Inspect muscles for bulk, contour, symmetry, and strength.
- Palpate brachial and/or radial pulses.
- Palpate the arms and hands for tenderness and temperature. Put the joints through passive range of motion.
- Using your reflex hammer, elicit the triceps, biceps, and brachioradialis reflexes.
- Place your fingers in the infant's palms to assess palmar grasp reflex.
- Place your fingers in the infant's palms and gently pull the infant to a sitting position, assessing grasp, strength, and head control.

Genitals and Rectum

Males

- Inspect the external genitalia, noting placement of the urinary meatus, whether the child is circumcised, and whether diaper rash or other lesions are present.
- Inspect the scrotum for rugae, and note any ambiguity of structures.
- Palpate the scrotum for testes, presence of hernia, or hydrocele.
- Palpate the penis, noting if the foreskin is retractable.
- Transilluminate the scrotum when concerned about masses other than testes.
- Inspect the rectum for skin tags, warts, and erythema. Assess sphincter tone.

Females

- Inspect the labia and vulvar vestibule, noting any edema, lesions, erythema, or ambiguity of structures.
- Inspect the urethral and vaginal orifices, noting any discharge, odor, or erythema.
- Inspect the rectum for skin tags, warts, and erythema. Assess sphincter tone

Central Nervous System

- Assess for tone through vertical suspension by holding the infant in an upright position with your hands under the axillae, assessing for slip through.
- Assess for tone through horizontal suspension by holding the infant horizontally, assessing for flexion at the elbow, hip, knee, and ankle.
- Assess infant reflexes based on the age of the infant:
    - *PALMAR GRASP*: Present at birth, integrated by 3 months
    - *ROOTING*: Present at birth, integrated at 3–4 months

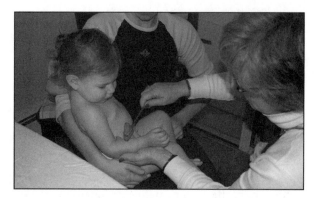

Figure 16-9 Brachioradialis Reflex

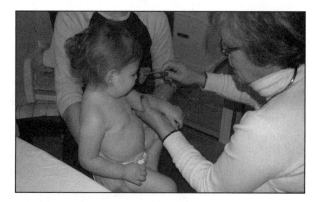

Figure 16-10 Bicep Reflex

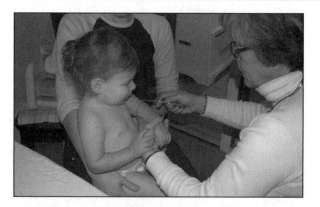

Figure 16-11 Tricep Reflex

> - *SUCKING*: Present at birth, integrated at 3–4 months
> - *PALMAR GRASP*: Present at birth, integrated at 3–6 months
> - *PLANTAR GRASP*: Present at birth, integrated at 10 months
> - *MORO*: Present at birth, integrated by 6 months
> - *PLACING*: Present at birth integrated at 6–8 weeks
> - *STEPPING*: Present at birth, integrated at 6–8 weeks
> - *ASYMMETRIC TONIC NECK (FENCING)*: Present at birth, integrated at 4–6 months
> - *GALANT*: Present at birth, integrated at 2 months
- Assess later reflexes:
  > - *LANDAU*: Appears at 3 months, integrated 15 months to 2 years
  > - *PARACHUTE*: Appears at 6–8 months, never becomes integrated

Back

With the patient in a prone position on the examination table:

- Inspect the spine for alignment and for symmetry of muscular development. Note any tufts of hair, dimples, or lesions.
- Palpate each spinal process for any defects.
- Holding the legs together, inspect the symmetry of the gluteal folds, checking for hip dislocation.

Head

- Inspect the head, noting any abnormal shape and head circumference.
- Inspect the scalp for lesions such as cradle cap.
- Palpate the fontanelles, both anterior and posterior; palpate for overriding sutures.

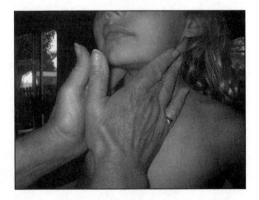

Figure 16-12 Palpation of Posterior Cervical Nodes

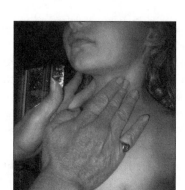

Figure 16-13 Palpation of Anterior Cervical Nodes

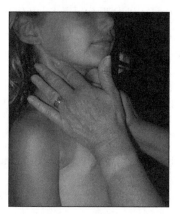

Figure 16-14 Palpation of Tonsillar Nodes

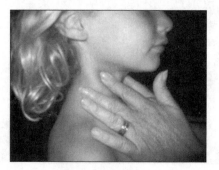

Figure 16-15 Palpation of Anterior Cervical Nodes

Neck

- Holding the infant and allowing his or her head to gently fall back to hyperextension, inspect the neck for webbing and/or excess skin folds. Inspect for alignment of the head with the neck.
- Palpate the neck for masses, thyroid gland, and muscle tone.
- Palpate for lymphadenopathy.
- Palpate the clavicles for crepitus and integrity.
- With the infant in a supine position, rotate the head through passive range of motion.
- Assess for the tonic neck reflex.
- Observe for the neck-righting reflex in the older infant.

Eyes

- Inspect the eyes, noting placement, configuration, eyebrows, eyelashes, drainage, lacrimal apparatus, and palpebral fissures.
- Inspect the sclera and conjunctiva, cornea, iris, pupils, and lens.
- Assess for the direct and consensual light reflexes.
- Assess for the corneal light reflex.
- With your ophthalmoscope, inspect for the bilateral red reflex.
- Inspect eye movements, noting nystagmus and ability to track a ball or face.

Nose

- Inspect the nose for placement and configuration.
- Determine patency of each nostril.
- Inspect the mucosa, septum, and turbinates.
- Palpate for tenderness.

Mouth

- Inspect the lips, gums, oral cavity, hard and soft palate, and posterior pharynx.
- Inspect the tongue for color and characteristics.
- Inspect for presence of teeth, noting color, number, surface characteristics, and alignment.
- With a gloved hand, palpate the hard and soft palates, assessing for a cleft. Evaluate the sucking reflex.
- Stroke each side of the mouth to stimulate the rooting reflex.
- Assess the gag reflex (cranial nerve [CN] X).
- Assess the frenulum for tongue thrust ability.

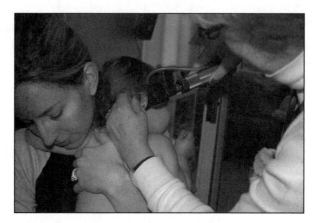

Figure 16-16   Use of Ososcope to Assess the Ear

Ears

- Inspect the ears for placement, configuration, and alignment, noting pits, sinuses, or skin tags.
- Palpate the auricles for tenderness.
- Assess the ear canal and tympanic membrane using the otoscope and insufflator.
- Assess gross hearing by eliciting a response to loud noise, such as by clapping out of the infant's view.

If abnormalities are found or parts of the examination could not be performed, try to reassess those areas that you are concerned about in a different position, in different lighting, or when the room is quiet and the child is more relaxed. You may find that at the end of the exam both parent and child are more comfortable, yielding a more compliant child.

An Integrated Exam of the Child

When performing a physical examination on a child, just as with the infant, there is no specific order that should be followed, especially when examining a toddler. If you are examining an older school-age child or adolescent, the established sequence of the head-to-toe exam may be followed. Otherwise, be flexible, without rigid guidelines, and *seize the opportunity* to evaluate those parts of the exam that are easily accessible and that will cause the least disruption or discomfort. Always save the mouth and ear exam for last, as they are the most intrusive and require the child's cooperation.

In most cases, when entering the exam room, you will find the young child sitting on the parent's lap. Start by pulling up a chair so you are eye level with the child, but keep a reasonable distance, approximately 2 feet away, so you are not too close. Start by talking to the parent and reviewing the history, allowing the child to examine and/or play with your instruments such as a stethoscope or reflex hammer. While obtaining (or updating) the history, maintain eye contact with the parent when asking questions; this demonstrates interest and concern in what the parent is saying. Ask questions if background information needs clarification, often rewording what the parent has said. Establish a relaxed, comfortable, and trusting environment for both the parent and the child by speaking in a soft tone. Remember, if the parent displays a level of comfort and relaxation, the child will pick up on the parent's body language, becoming more relaxed and, ultimately, more cooperative. The child who is calm, comfortable, and trusting will allow you the opportunity to perform a more thorough exam.

Before placing your hands on the child or using any equipment, sharpen your observation skills. Much can be gleaned by just observing the undressed child sitting on the parent's lap or playing with toys in the examination room, or even exploring the room and "checking things out." Observations to look for include physical characteristics of the child, as well as play behaviors. Note fine and gross motor skills, perceptual and cognitive skills, language skills, and self-care skills, as well as parent–child interactions.

Physical characteristics of the child should be observed starting at the top and gradually scanning downward. Be observant when watching the child at play. You will have more time to comprehensively assess each system during the actual examination. Areas to concentrate on are the following:

- Does the child's head appear normal in size and shape? Is it tilted toward one side?
- Does the child's hairline appear low? Are facies within normal? If not, what specifically stands out to you, such as placement or shape of the eyes, shape of the nose, or asymmetry of facial features?
- Is skin tone even? Smooth? Are there obvious birth marks or rashes? Unusual lesions?
- Does the child's neck appear normal? Is it webbed? Does the child easily move his or her head from side to side?
- If the child is undressed, does his or her chest appear normal, without specific disfiguration such as depression of the sternum?
- Do respirations appear regular without tugging or retractions or evidence of difficulty breathing?
- Is the child's abdomen protuberant or flat?

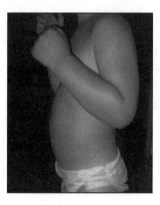

Figure 16-17   Protuberant Abdomen

- When walking, does the child show any marked inversion or eversion of the feet? Are the child's legs markedly bowed? Do the knees touch when walking (knock-kneed)?
- Do the child's feet turn in? Does the child frequently trip? Does the child walk on his or her toes?
- Do you notice any involuntary movements or tremors?

Observation of behavioral characteristics that underline developmental milestones is supported by Dworkin (1989) in the concept of developmental surveillance:

> Surveillance encompasses all primary care activities related to the monitoring of the development of the child. It includes obtaining a relevant developmental history, making accurate and informative observations of the child, and eliciting and attending to parental concerns. Emphasis is placed on monitoring development within the context of the child's overall well-being, rather than viewing development in isolation during a testing session.

Behavioral observations of the child should help you answer the following questions:

- Does the child leave the parent's side to explore toys in the room?
- How does the child manipulate toys when playing? Does the child use a pincer grasp, play with one toy only, examine the toy(s) closely, or randomly go from toy to toy?
- Does the child appear coordinated during play, such as while stacking blocks?

- Does the child imitate behavior, perhaps while playing with your instruments or pretending to feed a doll?
- Does the child appear coordinated when walking? Is the child steady on his or her feet? Does the child frequently fall? Does the child go from sitting to standing easily?
- Does the child appropriately use expressive language? Note difficulties in verbal expression, stuttering, and difficulties with word retrieval.
- Does the parent–child interaction appear normal? Does the child look to the parent for approval? Note the tone of the parent's voice. Is it comforting? Demanding? Punitive?
- Does the parent direct or encourage the child?
- Who appears to be in control, the parent or the child?
- Does the child's level of awareness and interaction with the parent appear appropriate?
- Does the child smile? Is the child playful?
- Do you note fearfulness in the child? If the child is crying, is the parent soothing and comforting?
- Does the child respond appropriately to questions? Ask the child to bring you a certain color crayon, for example.
- Is the child quiet? Does the child respond to your questions? Does the child ask you questions?
- Does the child make eye contact when answering you?

The actual examination is often confirmatory, particularly after obtaining a detailed history and interpreting careful observation of the child. When you are ready to perform the physical exam, note that if the child is comfortably sitting on the parent's lap, it may prove beneficial to do the exam with the child on the parent's lap. Ask the parent if putting the child on the table will cause too much disruption, informing the parent that you can also perform the exam with the child on his or her lap. The child's comfort and participation are key factors in obtaining a comprehensive examination.

In integrating the physical exam, it is helpful to examine the child in several different positions: sitting up, supine, and standing. Start by assessing the child in a sitting position, whether on the parent's lap or on the exam table. If the child is apprehensive, it is helpful to start from a distal point and gradually move closer. With the child in a sitting position, the provider can start the exam by first inspecting the feet and legs and then checking the hands and arms.

Integrating the exam implies that when examining the hands and arms, you are also assessing the skin, the musculoskeletal system, and the central nervous system. Integration of the physical exam in an organized sequence makes it easier for the patient, so the patient is not going from a sitting to a standing to a supine position several times. It also allows the provider to execute the exam in a logical and organized pattern. It is important to remember that when examining a child, you should *seize the opportunity* and examine those areas most accessible without causing fearfulness or discomfort in the child.

The following is an example of an integrated examination in a child.

Skin

Inspect the skin throughout the exam, noting skin characteristics for each system. Assessment includes color, degree of uniformity, cyanosis or pallor, hydration, rash or inflammation, pigmentation, nevi, jaundice, texture, turgor, temperature, edema, and lanugo (associated with eating disorders in the older child).

Lower Extremities

- Inspect the legs for movement, size, shape, alignment, lesions, and color, noting any color change or swelling at joint areas.
- Inspect the feet, noting the number of toes, how toenails are cut, alignment, longitudinal arch, lesions, and cleanliness. Inspect between the toes for skin breakdown or rash.
- Inspect muscles for bulk, contour, symmetry, and strength.
- Palpate the dorsalis pedis pulse bilaterally if possible. Also palpate the feet and legs for tenderness and temperature, and the joints for range of motion.
- Using your reflex hammer, elicit the plantar reflex and the Achilles and patellar reflexes bilaterally.

Upper Extremities

- Inspect the arms for size, shape, movement, color, and lesions, noting any color change or swelling at joint areas.
- Inspect the hands, noting the number and configuration of the fingers. Inspect the fingernails for biting. Inspect for palmar creases and cleanliness.
- Inspect muscles for bulk, contour, symmetry, and strength.
- Palpate radial and/or brachial pulses.
- Palpate the arms and hands for tenderness and temperature, and the joints for range of motion.
- Elicit biceps, triceps, and brachioradialis reflexes bilaterally.

Head

- Inspect the head, noting size and shape, hairline, position of auricles, and alignment with the neck. Inspect the face for symmetry, noting any abnormal or unusual facies. Inspect for skin characteristics. Inspect the scalp for lesions and infestations.
- Palpate the head for depressions and tenderness. Check the hair for texture, distribution, and quantity.
- Palpate the temporomandibular joint for crepitation. Palpate the frontal and maxillary sinuses.
- Test the temporal and masseter muscles for strength (CN V).
- Test the patient's ability to clench teeth, squeeze eyes shut, wrinkle forehead, smile, stick out tongue, and puff out cheeks (CN V and VII).
- Test for light sensation of forehead, cheeks, and chin (CN V).

Eyes

- Inspect the eyes, noting placement, configuration, eyebrows, eyelashes, drainage, lacrimal apparatus, and palpebral fissures.
- Inspect the sclera and conjunctiva, cornea, iris, pupils, and lens.
- Assess the direct and consensual light reflexes and accommodation (CN III).
- If age appropriate, assess visual acuity (CN II).
- Assess for color vision, if age appropriate.
- If cooperative, assess the extraocular muscles, cover/uncover test, and corneal light reflex (CN III, IV, and VI).

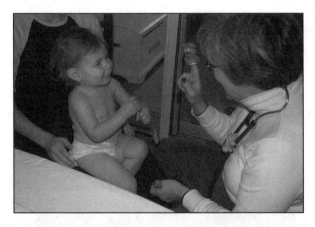

Figure 16-18   Following an Object Assessment of Extraocular Muscles

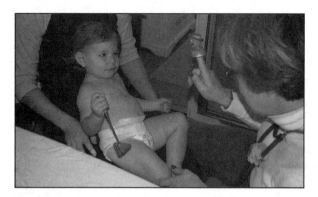

Figure 16-19 Example of Following an Object to Assess Extraocular Muscles

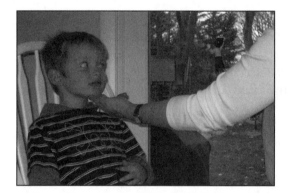

Figure 16-20 Example of Following an Object to Assess Extraocular Muscles

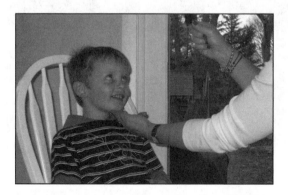

Figure 16-21 Example of Following an Object to Assess Extraocular Muscles

- Assess for the red reflex; if cooperative, assess the fundus (CN II).
- Evaluate visual fields by confrontation (CN II).

Ears

- Inspect the ears for placement, configuration, and alignment, noting skin tone, lesions, pits, or skin tags.
- Palpate the auricles for tenderness.
- Assess the ear canal and tympanic membrane using the otoscope and insufflator.
- Assess for hearing by audiometry (CN VIII).

Nose

- Inspect the nose for placement and configuration.
- Determine patency of each nostril.
- Inspect the mucosa, septum, and turbinates.
- Palpate for tenderness.
- Assess sense of smell—i.e., olfactory function (CN I).

Neck

- Inspect the neck for webbing, range of motion, strength, and resistance (CN XI).
- Palpate the neck for lymphadenopathy, including the pre-auricular, postauricular, occipital, tonsillar, submaxillary, submental, superficial cervical, posterior cervical, deep cervical, and supraclavicular areas.
- Palpate for the position of the trachea and size of the thyroid.

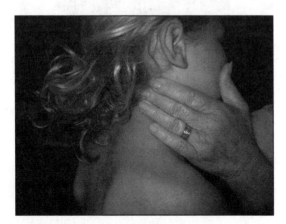

Figure 16-22 Palpating Posterior Cervical Nodes

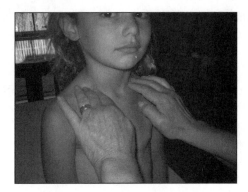

Figure 16-23   Palpating Superclavicular Nodes

Mouth

- Inspect the lips, oral cavity, and posterior pharynx, noting the tonsils and their size.
- Inspect the tongue for color, characteristics, and movement (CN XIII).
- Inspect the teeth, noting the color, number, surface characteristics, and alignment.
- Assess the gag reflex (CN X)
- Assess the frenulum for tongue thrust ability.

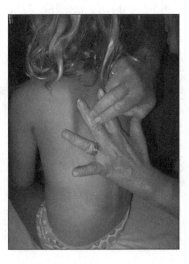

Figure 16-24   Percussion of Lungs

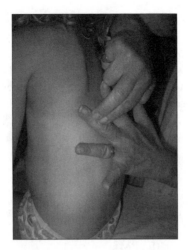

Figure 16-25   Percussion of Lungs

Chest and Lungs

- Inspect the thorax for configuration, respiratory movements, size, shape, and deformity.
- Inspect the breasts and nipples, noting placement and/or asymmetry.
- In females, assess the breasts for Tanner stage.
- Inspect respirations for excursion, depth, rhythm, and pattern.
- Inspect the posterior chest for symmetry and musculoskeletal development.

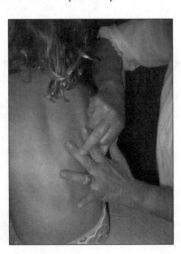

Figure 16-26   Percussion of Lungs

- Palpate the posterior chest for temperature, tenderness, and masses.
- Palpate the scapulae and spinous processes for tenderness.
- Percuss the costovertebral angle for tenderness.
- Inspect the anterior chest for symmetry and musculoskeletal development.
- Palpate the anterior chest for temperature, tenderness, and/or masses.
- Auscultate the posterior chest for breath sounds, noting any adventitious sounds.
- Auscultate the anterior chest for breath sounds, noting any adventitious sounds.

Heart

- Inspect the anterior chest for any precordial movement.
- Palpate the chest wall for thrills, heaves, and pulsations.
- Palpate the heart for the PMI.
- Auscultate the heart, listening for cardiac sounds, S_1 and S_2, noting any murmurs, splitting, rubs, and S_3 or S_4.

After performing the portion of the exam in which the child is in the sitting position, complete the exam with the child in a supine position, either on the examination table or lying on the parent's lap.

Abdomen

- Inspect the abdomen for lesions, striae, pulsations, and contour.
- Auscultate the abdomen in all four quadrants for bowel sounds.
- Palpate the abdomen lightly, noting any tenderness, distention, or masses.

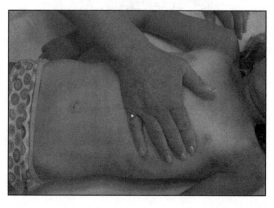

Figure 16-27   Palpating for the PMI (Point of Maximum Impulse)

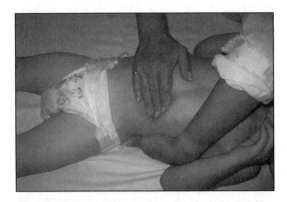

Figure 16-28   Palpation of the Spleen

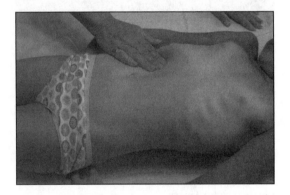

Figure 16-29   Palpating the Liver

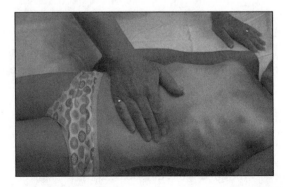

Figure 16-30   Palpating the Spleen

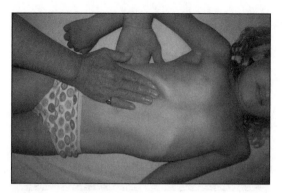

Figure 16-31 Palpation of the Liver

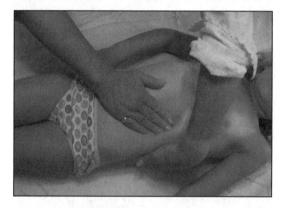

Figure 16-32 Palpation of the Spleen

- Palpate more deeply, noting the size of the liver, spleen, and any other palpable masses.
- Palpate the inguinal area for lymphadenopathy.
- Palpate the femoral pulses, and compare them to the radial pulses.
- Percuss the abdomen, assessing for the size of the liver and spleen, noting areas of tympany versus dullness.

Genitals

Males

- Inspect the external genitalia, noting placement of the urinary meatus. Note whether the child is circumcised. Assess the skin tone and lesions.
- Inspect the scrotum for fullness, rugae, and symmetry.

- Palpate the testes bilaterally. If the testes are difficult to assess, ask the child to sit in the tailor position with legs crossed or to sit on a chair with heels on the chair and hands on his knees. This position places pressure on the abdominal wall, which helps push the testicles into the scrotum.
- Palpate the testes for tenderness or masses.
- Palpate for retraction of the foreskin.
- Assess the Tanner stage.

Female
- Inspect the external genitalia with the child's legs in the frog position. Inspect the labia and vulvar vestibule and the urethral and vaginal orifices.
- Inspect for skin tone, lesions, discharge, erythema, and odor.
- Assess the Tanner stage.

Rectum

- Inspect the rectal area for lesions, skin tone, and erythema.
- Inspect the rectal area for sphincter tone and for lesions such as warts, skin tags, and erythema.

Back

- Inspect the child's back, noting spinal alignment from the anterior, posterior, and lateral views, as well as when the child bends over to touch his or her toes.
- Observe the child's gait for any in-toeing, limping, or other abnormality.

Central Nervous System

- When assessing the CNS, ask the child to perform tasks that will elicit age-appropriate responses, as they may differ from the young child to the adolescent.
- Assess for mental status, including attention span, memory, reading, writing, and math skills, all of which need to be assessed in conjunction with the child's age. It is beneficial in determining mental status to talk to the child about school, what he or she is learning, school activities, friends, play activities, and favorite things to do.
- Assess the cranial nerves (see Chapter 13).
- Assess for proprioception.
- Assess for sensory response.
- Assess motor strength.
- Elicit deep tendon reflexes.

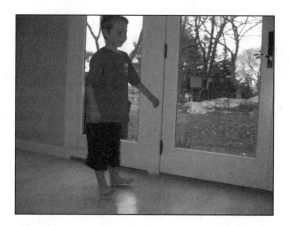

Figure 16-33   Walking on Heels

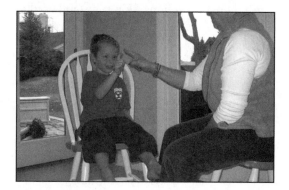

Figure 16-34   Finger to Nose Test

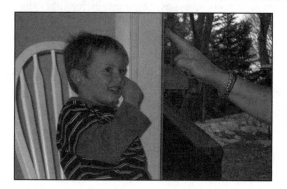

Figure 16-35   Finger to Nose Test

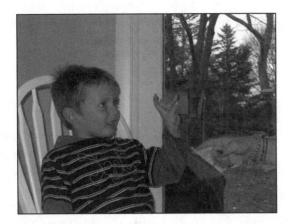

Figure 16-36   Finger to Finger Test

Physiologic Differences Between the Child and the Adult

It is important to keep in mind that children are not just little adults; they differ not only in size and shape, but in physiology as well. As the child develops and approaches adulthood, such as during late adolescence, there is less of a physiologic difference.

The following is a summary of the differences between the child and the adult.

EYES: In the infant, the lens is more spherical and cannot accommodate for both near and far objects. This means that the infant sees best at a distance of approximately 20 cm (8 inches). Also, in the young infant, the optic nerve is not fully myelinated, which decreases the infant's ability to distinguish between colors. As the child grows, the eye matures and vision improves, reaching normal adult size at approximately 14 years of age. A child attains normal vision of 20/20 by 6 or 7 years of age. Development of the eye occurs in conjunction with increasing cognitive development; as acuity improves, the brain is able to interpret the messages received through the visual input.

EARS: As the child matures, the eustachian tube changes in size. It is initially horizontal and narrow, which results in decreased drainage during upper respiratory infections. As the child matures, the eustachian tube broadens and angles in a more downward position, allowing for better drainage. In infants, the end of the eustachian tube opens during sucking, which increases the likelihood of increased incidence of otitis media when the infant takes the bottle, particularly in a supine position. The eustachian tube also equalizes air pressure between the middle ear and the outside, which allows for better drainage of secretions from the middle ear.

SKIN: In the infant, the skin is thin with little subcutaneous fat and provides less protection against burns and bruises and less protection against hypothermia. The epidermis is loosely bound to the dermis, which causes blistering due to separation of the layers. The apocrine sweat glands are nonfunctional and mature during puberty. The eccrine sweat glands produce sweat in response to heat in the infant and achieve full function during puberty. There is less melanin in the skin of infants, which means they need additional protection against ultraviolet light. Melanin reaches adult levels during puberty.

UPPER AIRWAY: In the infant, the nasal passages are relatively small and more easily obstructed and/or occluded with discharge or foreign bodies. Because newborns and young children are obligate nose breathers, they are particularly vulnerable. The oral cavity is small with a relatively large tongue, which increases the risk of obstruction. Lymph tissue such as tonsils and adenoids grow rapidly during childhood until approximately 12 years of age, potentially leading to sleep apnea problems in the child. The trachea is much narrower and its cartilage more elastic and collapsible, which makes it more vulnerable to edema and inflammation. Hyperextension or flexion of the neck can easily crimp or obstruct the airway. In the child, the larynx and glottis are higher and more anterior in the neck, which increases the risk of aspiration.

LUNGS: The intercostal muscles are immature in the young child, making the rib cage more elastic and flexible. As a result, during respiratory distress, the negative pressure causes retractions. Due to the higher oxygen consumption in children than in adults, there is a greater metabolic rate. This higher metabolic rate and higher oxygen requirement eventually leads to muscle fatigue when muscles tire more easily with prolonged effort. Ultimately, this change in the metabolic rate, particularly during periods of respiratory distress, leads to hypoxemia.

CARDIOVASCULAR SYSTEM: In an infant and very young child, the muscle fibers of the heart are immature and less well developed. Subsequently, the heart is more sensitive to pressure overload, meaning there is less compliance of the ventricles to achieve adequate stroke volume (the amount of blood ejected with each contraction). This ultimately places the young child at risk for bradycardia, which is an initial response to hypoxemia and may herald cardiac arrest.

ABDOMEN: Due to the small capacity of the infant's stomach, the infant requires small frequent meals and has an increased frequency of stool. Also, because of the relaxed cardiac sphincter in infants, reflux is common until 1 year of age. Digestive enzymes are not present in sufficient quantities until 4–6 months of age. By 2 years of life, stomach capacity has increased to accommodate three meals per day, and the digestive processes are matured. In addition, the liver and spleen, due to their relatively large size and increased vascularity, are more susceptible to injury and less protected by the ribs.

MUSCULOSKELETAL SYSTEM: The majority of skull growth occurs by 2 years of age, with the skull reaching adult size by 16 years. The fontanelles in the skull, anterior and posterior, contain a fibrous membrane that allows for growth of the brain and skull. The anterior fontanelle closes at approximately 18 months, and the posterior fontanelle closes between 2 and 3 months of age. In children, the long bones are porous and less dense than those of the adults, resulting in more fractures. As the child grows, the cartilage cells at the epiphyses remain cartilaginous, which allows for continued growth until approximately 20 years of age. At this time, skeletal maturation is complete, the epiphyseal plate closes, and the cartilage cells are replaced by bone cells, eventually leading to the deposition of calcium and increased strength. As the child grows, the muscles do not increase in number, but instead increase in length and circumference. During this period, there is rapid bone growth, which facilitates healing of fractures but also often leads to growing pains as muscles are pulled during periods of rapid bone growth. Until puberty, the ligaments and tendons are stronger than bone, but as the cartilage is gradually replaced by bone, it is stronger than the ligaments and tendons. This change explains the decrease in fractures and the increase in injuries to ligaments and tendons in late adolescence. Muscle strength continues to increase until approximately the mid-20s.

CENTRAL NERVOUS SYSTEM: In infants, the head is large in proportion to the body, the neck muscles are poorly developed, and the bones of the skull are not fused—all of which make the infant prone to brain injury and skull fractures. The dura, which is firmly attached to the skull in children, is more apt to tear and bleed with injury. In infants and children, the vertebral bodies are wedge shaped, which allows for increased spinal mobility. Also there are cartilaginous vertebral bodies and incomplete ossification of the vertebral bodies, factors that lead to an increased risk of cervical spine injuries. The child's spinal cord attains adult characteristics around 8 to 9 years of age when the vertebral bodies lose their wedge shape and are completely formed and ossified. This all leads to increased spinal stability.

Appreciating the various stages in child development is helpful when approaching a child and gaining his or her cooperation in order to conduct a comprehensive assessment. Sensitivity to the underlying assumptions that guide development is key in your approach and actual implementation of the physical examination. Stein and Dixon (1992) researched developmentally supportive care based on the following assumptions:

- Development is a self-fueling, ongoing process that requires physical and emotional energy.
- Development occurs in stages, is dynamic, and is interactional.
- Development is influenced by the child and his or her environment.
- Development occurs in "spurts and lulls." Periods of disorganization, disharmony, and turbulence are usually followed by periods of harmony, balance, and organization as new skills are integrated.
- All areas of development are interrelated.

The following is a developmental approach to the pediatric examination. It incorporates a review of developmental principles based on Piaget's Stages of Cognitive Development (1972), Erikson's Stages of Psychosocial Development (1963), and Freud's Stages of Psychosexual Development (Craig & Dunn, 2007). (This text does not intend to portray an in-depth analysis of developmental theorists. For more detailed analysis of theorists, refer to a text on developmental theory.)

Infants

AGES: Birth to 1 year

DEVELOPMENT:
> *PIAGET*: Sensorimotor
> *ERIKSON*: Trust vs. mistrust
> *FREUD*: Oral stage

DEVELOPMENTAL OVERVIEW: During the first year, sensorimotor development is experienced as the infant explores and learns about the environment through his or her senses, through reaching out, and through oral exploration of objects. This is a period when trust is established through touch, comfort, and feeding. Stranger anxiety begins to be displayed around 7–9 months of age. A child responds to his or her own name and begins to understand a few words, such as "no-no" and "bye-bye." Gross motor skills develop during the first year, from sitting up, rolling over, crawling, pulling to stand, and walking. An infant begins to finger-feed near the end of the first year and starts to use a sippy cup.

POSITION FOR THE EXAM: For the younger infant, the exam can be performed on an exam table with the parent in full view. With an older infant who is very apprehensive, you may need to perform most of the exam with the infant on the parent's lap.

PREPARATION: Undress the child, leaving only the diaper on. Be sure the temperature in the room permits undressing, speak in a soft gentle tone, use bright-colored toys and rattles to gain the infant's attention, and use a pacifier if necessary.

SEQUENCE OF EXAM: When the child is quiet, start with auscultation of the heart and lungs, then progress to palpation of the abdomen. Proceed with the exam, always performing more traumatic procedures such as examination of the ears and throat last.

Toddlers

AGES: 1–3 years

DEVELOPMENT:
- ➤ *PIAGET*: Preoperational
- ➤ *ERIKSON*: Autonomy vs. shame/doubt
- ➤ *FREUD*: Anal stage

DEVELOPMENTAL OVERVIEW: During this period, the toddler shows increasing curiosity and explorative behavior. The child begins to point to body parts, follows simple directions, and stacks blocks. The child is striving for independence. Negativism and temper tantrums are common. This period is the beginning of magical thinking. By 2 years of age, a toddler can go up and down stairs one step at a time, kick a ball, and imitate behavior. By 3 years of age, the child can ride a tricycle; knows his or her name, age, and sex; copies a circle; has some self-care skills such as feeding and dressing; and derives gratification from control over bodily excretions.

POSITION FOR THE EXAM: The exam can be performed with the child sitting on the parent's lap.

PREPARATION: Remove outer clothing, but leave diaper or underpants on. Allow the toddler to inspect and hold your equipment, and speak in soft tones, using simple, short sentences. Demonstrate parts of the exam on a doll or parent before conducting them on the child. Tell the child what you are going to do rather than asking the child whether you can. For example, say, "I am going to check your tummy now." Perform as much of the exam on the parent's lap as possible, if the child is cooperative there.

Preschoolers

AGES: 3–6 years

DEVELOPMENT:
- ➤ *PIAGET*: Preoperational stage
- ➤ *ERIKSON*: Industry vs. guilt
- ➤ *FREUD*: Phallic stage

DEVELOPMENTAL OVERVIEW: During this period, magical thinking and egocentrism play a central role. The child becomes increasingly verbal and can sing a song, draw a person with three parts, distinguish fantasy from reality, and give his or her first and last name. The child likes to initiate play activities such as throwing a ball overhand. During this period, the child identifies with the parent of the opposite sex; by the end, however, the child has identified with the same-sex parent.

POSITION FOR THE EXAM: The exam can be conducted on the table, although if the child is fearful, initiate the exam with the child sitting on the parent's lap.

PREPARATION: Ask the child to undress down to the underwear. Inform the child what you are going to do and what the child can do to help you, and praise the child for helping you and being cooperative. Allow the child to look at and touch your equipment, and role-play by listening to the doll's heart. Ask if the child wants to help you by placing his or her hand on the diaphragm of the stethoscope as you listen to the heart and lungs.

The exam can generally be performed in a head-to-toe sequence, although if the child is fearful, start distally by looking at the extremities and gradually move in closer, saving the ears and mouth for last.

School-Age Children

AGES: 6–12 years

DEVELOPMENT:
- ➤ *PIAGET*: Concrete operational stage
- ➤ *ERIKSON*: Industry vs. inferiority
- ➤ *FREUD*: Latent stage

DEVELOPMENTAL OVERVIEW: This is a period of concrete thinking, and an interest in learning and the ability to understand cause and effect are primary features. Academic achievements in the classroom—the child's ability to attend school, stay focused, and succeed—are important. School activities and sports contribute to a sense of accomplishment and self-worth. Modesty emerges with the older school-age child, particularly as his or her body starts to change, so respect for privacy is important.

POSITION FOR THE EXAM: The exam can be performed on the examination table in a head-to-toe sequence.

PREPARATION: Ask the child to undress to the underwear. Offer the child a hospital gown to put on. Draw the curtain to allow the child privacy or step out of the room while the child is changing. Use age-appropriate vocabulary when explaining use of the equipment, and explain what you are going to do. Asking children what they are studying in school or what their favorite subject is, is a good way to encourage conversation and alleviate concern or fear.

Adolescents

AGES: 13–18 years

DEVELOPMENT:
- ➤ *PIAGET*: Formal operational stage
- ➤ *ERIKSON*: Identity vs. identity diffusion
- ➤ *FREUD*: Genital stage

DEVELOPMENTAL OVERVIEW: The period of adolescence includes early, middle, and late stages. This is overall a period when the adolescent is striving for independence and control. In early adolescence, puberty defines the characteristic behaviors, which include mood swings, preoccupation with body image and physical changes, and intense friendships with the same sex. In middle adolescence, characteristic behaviors include strong peer group influence, family conflicts and ambivalence about emerging independence, excessive physical activity, emergence of sexual drives and dating, and experimentation with sex, drugs, and risk-taking behaviors. Late adolescence is characterized by the transition to adulthood and assuming adult roles such as college, work, or vocational training. The adolescent relates to family as an adult, establishes ethical and moral value systems, pursues realistic career goals, and establishes a sexual identity.

POSITION FOR THE EXAM: The exam can be performed in a head-to-toe sequence.

PREPARATION: Ask the adolescent to undress in private, always assuring privacy by drawing a curtain or by stepping out of the room. Conduct the exam without the parent in the room, unless the adolescent prefers the parent to be present. Inform the adolescent about each part of the exam, covering body parts not being examined to ensure privacy. Provide reassurance of normalcy during the course of the exam. Acknowledge and discuss concerns about the breast, pelvic, and testicular examination.

References

Craig, G. J. & Dunn, W.L. (2007). *Understanding human development.* Upper Saddle River, NJ: Pearson.

Dworkin, P. H. (1989). British and American recommendations for developmental monitoring: The role of surveillance. *Pediatrics, 83,* 619–622.

Erikson, E. (1963). *Childhood and society.* New York: Norton.

Piaget, J. (1972). *The child's conception of the world.* Totowa, NJ: Littlefield Adams.

Stein, M. T., & Dixon, S. D. (1992). *Encounters with children.* St. Louis, MO: Mosby.

Resources

Ball, J., Bindler, R., & Cowen, K. (2010). *Child health nursing* (2nd ed.). Upper Saddle River, NJ: Pearson.

Barkauskas, V., Stoltenberg-Allen, K., Baumann, L., & Darling-Fisher, D. (1998). *Health and physical assessment* (2nd ed.). St. Louis, MO: Mosby-Year Book.

Burns, C., Dunn, A., Brady, M., Starr, N., & Blosser, C. (2004). *Pediatric primary care: A handbook for nurse practitioners* (3rd ed.). St. Louis, MO: Saunders.

Jarvis, C. (2008). *Physical examination and health assessment* (5th ed.). St. Louis, MO: Elsevier.

Potts, N., & Mandleco, B. (2007). *Pediatraic nursing* (2nd ed.). Victoria, Australia: Thomson, Delmar Learning.

Photo Credits

Chapter 2

2.1b 1 © Fashon Studio/ShutterStock, Inc.; **2.1b 2** © Martin Allinger/ShutterStock, Inc.; **2.1b 3** © Feverpitch/ShutterStock, Inc.; **21b 4** © Monkey Business Images/ShutterStock, Inc.; **2.1b 5** © Monkey Business Images/ShutterStock, Inc.; **2.1b 6** © Anton Albert/ShutterStock, Inc.

Chapter 3

3.1 © Raia/ShutterStock, Inc.; **3.2** © Catchlight Visual Services/Alamy Images; **3.11** © Martin Kubát/ShutterStock, Inc.; **3.12a** © Joanna Zielinska/Fotolia.com; **3.12b** © greenland/ShutterStock, Inc.; **3.12c** © Paul Moore/Dreamstime.com; **3.12d** © Jason Stitt/ShutterStock, Inc.; **3.21a** © AVAVA/ShutterStock, Inc.; **3.21b** © Francois Etienne du Plessis/ShutterStock, Inc.; **3.21c** © Antonia Reeve/Photo Researchers, Inc.; **3.21d** Courtesy of Invicta Education; **3.22** © Darren Brode/ShutterStock, Inc.; **3.23** © Ilya Andriyanov/ShutterStock, Inc.; **3.24** © Ia64/Dreamstime.com; **3.25** © CHASSENET/age fotostock; **3.26** © Thomas M Perkins/ShutterStock, Inc.; **3.27** © Fred Goldstein/Dreamstime.com

Chapter 5

5.3a © Simon Krzic/ShutterStock, Inc.; **5.3b** Courtesy of CDC; **5.3c** © Joy Brown/ShutterStock, Inc.; **5.3d** Courtesy of CDC; **5.3e** Courtesy of CDC; **5.3f** Courtesy of Joe Miller/CDC; **5.4** © Tracy Dominey/Photo Researchers, Inc.; **5.5** © Jeffrey Williams/Dreamstime.com; **5.6** Courtesy Dr. Charlie Goldberg; **5.7** Courtesy of Dr. Kenneth Greer; **5.8** © Dr. P. Marazzi/Photo Researchers,

Inc.; **5.9** © Wellcome Images/Custom Medical Stock Photo; **5.10** Courtesy of Dr. Kenneth Greer; **5.11** Courtesy of CDC; **5.12** © Dr P. Marazzi/Photo Researchers, Inc.; **5.13** Courtesy of Dr. Heinz F. Eichenwald/CDC; **5.14** © Dr. P. Marazzi/ Photo Researchers, Inc.; **5.15** © Dr. Chris Hale/Photo Researchers, Inc.; **5.16** © Dr P. Marazzi/Photo Researchers, Inc.; **5.17** Courtesy of CDC; **5.18** Courtesy of CDC; **5.19** © Tom Myers/Photo Researchers, Inc.; **5.20** © Dr P. Marazzi/Photo Researchers, Inc.; **5.21** Courtesy of Dr. Lucille K. Georg/CDC; **5.22** © leschnyhan/ Fotolia.com; **5.23** © Dr P. Marazzi/Photo Researchers, Inc.; **5.24** © Dr P. Marazzi/ Photo Researchers, Inc.; **5.25** Courtesy of Dr. Hermann/CDC; **5.26** Courtesy of Leonard V. Crowley, MD, Century College; **5.27** © Mark Clarke/Photo Researchers, Inc.; **5.28** © Radist/Dreamstime.com; **5.29** Courtesy of Dr. Gavin Hart/CDC; **5.30** Courtesy of CDC; **5.31** Courtesy of Dr. Kenneth Greer; **5.34** © John Watney/Photo Researchers, Inc.; **5.35** Courtesy of Dr. John Noble, Jr./CDC; **5.36** © Science Photo Library/Photo Researchers, Inc.; **5.37** Courtesy of CDC; **5.38** Courtesy of CDC; **5.39** © Rob Byron/ShutterStock, Inc.; **5.40** Courtesy of CDC; **5.41** Courtesy of CDC; **5.42** © SPL/Photo Researchers, Inc.

Chapter 6

6.5 © Lucian Coman/Dreamstime.com; **6.9** © Dr. P. Marazzi/Photo Researchers, Inc.; **6.10** © Dr P. Marazzi/Photo Researchers, Inc.; **6.11** © Custom Medical Stock Photo; **6.13** © bsites/ShutterStock, Inc.; **6.15** © Terence Mendoza/ShutterStock, Inc.; **6.16** © Terence Mendoza/ShutterStock, Inc.; **6.17** © LightScribe/Fotolia.com; **6.18** © Pascal Goetgheluck/Photo Researchers, Inc.; **6.19** © Phanie/Photo Researchers, Inc.; **6.22** © StockLite/ShutterStock, Inc.; **6.23** Courtesy of Vision Assessment Corporation; **6.25** © Dr. P. Marazzi/Science Photo Library/Photo Researchers, Inc.; **6.26** © Medical-on-Line/Alamy Images; **6.27** © Dr P. Marazzi/Photo Researchers, Inc.; **6.28** © Dr. P. Marazzi/Science Photo Library/Photo Researchers, Inc.; **6.29** © Dr P. Marazzi/Photo Researchers, Inc.; **6.30** © Dr. M.A. Ansary/Photo Researchers, Inc.; **6.31** © Science Source/Photo Researchers, Inc.; **6.32** © Dr P. Marazzi/Photo Researchers, Inc.

Chapter 7

7.13 Courtesy of CDC; **7.14** © Dr. P. Marazzi/Science Photo Library/Photo Researchers, Inc.; **7.22** © Dr. P. Marazzi/Science Photo Library/Photo Researchers, Inc.; **7.23** Printed with permission of Catherine Watson Genna, BS, IBCLC.

Chapter 8

8.12a © ASK_H/Fotolia.com; **8.12b** © Zzvet/ShutterStock, Inc.; **8.13** © Biophoto Associates/Photo Researchers, Inc.; **8.14** © Dr P. Marazzi/Photo Researchers, Inc.; **8.15** © Annabella Bluesky/Photo Researchers, Inc.; **8.16** © Dr P. Marazzi/Photo Researchers, Inc.; **8.18** © Dr P. Marazzi/Photo Researchers, Inc.; **8.19** © Guniita/ Dreamstime.com; **8.20** © Dr P. Marazzi/Photo Researchers, Inc.; **8.21** © Dr P. Marazzi/Photo Researchers, Inc.; **8.22** Courtesy of Dr. Hisham Yehia El Batawi; **8.23** © SPL/Photo Researchers, Inc.; **8.24** © SPL/Photo Researchers, Inc.; **8.25** © Scott Camazine/Photo Researchers, Inc.; **8.26** © Wellcome Images/Custom Medical Stock Photo; **8.27** © Wellcome Images/Custom Medical Stock Photo; **8.28** ©

Dr. M.A. Ansary/Photo Researchers, Inc.; **8.29** Courtesy of CDC; **8.30** © Dr. P. Marazzi/Photo Researchers, Inc.; **8.31** © Prof. Tony Wright/Inst. of Laryngology & Otology/Photo Researchers, Inc.

Chapter 9

9.10a © Dr. P. Marazzi/Photo Researchers, Inc.; **9.10b** © Living Art Enterprises, LLC/Photo Researchers, Inc.; **9.16a** © mmm/ShutterStock, Inc.; **9.16b** © Daniel W. Slocum/ShutterStock, Inc.

Chapter 10

10.10 Courtesy of Jane Needham

Chapter 11

11.16 © Dr. P. Marazzi/Science Photo Library/Photo Researchers, Inc.; **11.17** © SPL/Photo Researchers, Inc.; **11.19** Courtesy of Leonard V. Crowley, MD, Century College; **11.21** © Sebastian Kaulitzki/Dreamstime.com

Chapter 12

12.4 © Steve Gschmeissner/Photo Researchers, Inc.; **12.37a** © James Steidl/ShutterStock, Inc.; **12.37b** © Sebastian Kaulitzki/ShutterStock, Inc.; **12.48** © Wellcome Images/Custom Medical Stock Photo; **12.49** © Dr. P. Marazzi/Photo Researchers, Inc.; **12.50** © Dr. P. Marazzi/Photo Researchers, Inc.; **12.51** © CNRI/Photo Researchers, Inc.; **12.55** © medicalpicture/Alamy Images; **12.57a** © aniad/ShutterStock, Inc.; **12.57b** © Biophoto Associates/Photo Researchers, Inc.

Chapter 14

14.3 © KEENE/age fotostock; **14.5** © Dr. P. Marazzi/Photo Researchers, Inc.; **14.6** © Dr. P. Marazzi/Photo Researchers, Inc.; **14.7** © Dr. P. Marazzi/Photo Researchers, Inc.; **14.8** © Dr. P. Marazzi/Photo Researchers, Inc.; **14.11** © Dr. P. Marazzi/SPL/Photo Researchers, Inc.

Chapter 15

15.1a © Sebastian Kaulitzki/ShutterStock, Inc.; **15.1b** © Image Source Limited/Phototake; **15.2b** © Sebastian Kaulitzki/ShutterStock, Inc.

Color Plate Inserts

CP5.3a © Simon Krzic/ShutterStock, Inc.; **CP5.3b** Courtesy of CDC; **CP5.3c** © Joy Brown/ShutterStock, Inc.; **CP5.3d** Courtesy of CDC; **CP5.3e** Courtesy of CDC; **CP5.3f** Courtesy of Joe Miller/CDC; **CP5.7** Courtesy of Dr. Kenneth Greer; **CP5.10** Courtesy of Dr. Kenneth Greer; **CP5.11** Courtesy of CDC; **CP5.14** © Dr. P. Marazzi/Photo Researchers, Inc.; **CP5.20** © Dr P. Marazzi/Photo Researchers, Inc.; **CP5.34** © John Watney/Photo Researchers, Inc.; **CP5.36** © Science Photo

Index

Pages numbers followed by *t* and *f* denote tables and figures, respectively.